Acute Leukemia

Guest Editor

MARTIN S. TALLMAN, MD

HEMATOLOGY/ONCOLOGY CLINICS OF NORTH AMERICA

www.hemonc.theclinics.com

Consulting Editors
GEORGE P. CANELLOS, MD
NANCY BERLINER, MD

December 2011 • Volume 25 • Number 6

SAUNDERS an imprint of ELSEVIER, Inc.

W.B. SAUNDERS COMPANY
A Division of Elsevier Inc.

1600 John F. Kennedy Blvd. • Suite 1800 • Philadelphia, PA 19103-2899

http://www.theclinics.com

HEMATOLOGY/ONCOLOGY CLINICS OF NORTH AMERICA Volume 25, Number 6
December 2011 ISSN 0889-8588, ISBN 13: 978-1-4557-1197-0

Editor: Patrick Manley

Hematology/Oncology Clinics (ISSN 0889-8588) is published bimonthly by Elsevier Inc., 360 Park Avenue South, New York, NY 10010-1710. Months of issue are February, April, June, August, October, and December. Business and Editorial Offices: 1600 John F. Kennedy Blvd., Ste. 1800, Philadelphia, PA 19103–2899. Customer Service Office: 3251 Riverport Lane, Maryland Heights, MO 63043. Periodicals postage paid at New York, NY and at additional mailing offices. Subscription prices are $353.00 per year (domestic individuals), $576.00 per year (domestic institutions), $173.00 per year (domestic students/residents), $401.00 per year (Canadian individuals), $705.00 per year (Canadian institutions) $477.00 per year (international individuals), $705.00 per year (international institutions), and $233.00 per year (international and Canadian students/residents). International air speed delivery is included in all *Clinics* subscription prices. All prices are subject to change without notice. **POSTMASTER:** Send address changes to *Hematology/Oncology Clinics of North America*, Elsevier Health Sciences Division, Subscription Customer Service, 3251 Riverport Lane, Maryland Heights, MO 63043. Customer Service (orders, claims, online, change of address): Elsevier Health Sciences Division, Subscription Customer Service, 3251 Riverport Lane, Maryland Heights, MO 63043. Tel: 1-800-654-2452 (U.S. and Canada); 314-447-8871 (outside U.S. and Canada). Fax: 314-447-8029. E-mail: journalscustomerservice-usa@elsevier.com (for print support); journalsonlinesupport-usa@elsevier.com (for online support).

Reprints. For copies of 100 or more, of articles in this publication, please contact the Commercial Reprints Department, Elsevier Inc., 360 Park Avenue South, New York, New York 10010-1710; Tel.: 212-633-3813, Fax: 212-462-1935, E-mail: reprints@elsevier.com.

Hematology/Oncology Clinics of North America is covered in *MEDLINE/PubMed (Index Medicus), EMBASE/ Excerpta Medica, and BIOSIS.*

Printed in the United States of America.

Contributors

CONSULTING EDITORS

GEORGE P. CANELLOS, MD
William Rosenberg Professor of Medicine, Department of Medical Oncology, Dana-Farber Cancer Institute, Boston, Massachusetts

NANCY BERLINER, MD
Chief, Division of Hematology, Brigham and Women's Hospital; Professor of Medicine, Harvard Medical School, Boston, Massachusetts

GUEST EDITOR

MARTIN S. TALLMAN, MD
Chief, Leukemia Service; Professor of Medicine, Department of Medicine, Memorial Sloan-Kettering Cancer Center, Weill Cornell Medical College, New York, New York

AUTHORS

OMAR ABDEL-WAHAB, MD
Instructor, Leukemia Service and Human Oncology and Pathogenesis Program, Memorial Sloan-Kettering Cancer Center, New York, New York

JESSICA K. ALTMAN, MD
Assistant Professor of Medicine, Department of Medicine, Robert H. Lurie Comprehensive Cancer Center, Northwestern University Feinberg School of Medicine, Chicago, Illinois

MUHAMED BALJEVIC, MD
Resident in Internal Medicine, Department of Medicine, Weill Cornell Medical Center, New York and Presbyterian Hospital, New York, New York

RENIER BRENTJENS, MD, PhD
Associate Attendent, Leukemia Service, Department of Medicine, Memorial Sloan-Kettering Cancer Center; Department of Medicine, Weill Cornell Medical College, New York, New York

DAN DOUER, MD
Professor of Medicine and Leader, Acute Lymphoblastic Leukemia Program, Department of Medicine, Memorial Sloan-Kettering Cancer Center, Weill Cornell Medical College, New York, New York

ADELE K. FIELDING, MB BS, PhD, FRCP, FRCPath
Senior Lecturer in Haematology, UCL; Chair, UK National Cancer Research Institute (NCRI) Adult ALL Subgroup, University College London, London, United Kingdom

CHEZI GANZEL, MD
Department of Hematology, Shaare Zedek Medical Center, Jerusalem, Israel

DAVID GRIMWADE, PhD, FRCPath
Professor of Molecular Haematology, Cancer Genetics Laboratory, Department of Medical and Molecular Genetics, Guy's Hospital, King's College London School of Medicine, London, United Kingdom

JOSEPH G. JURCIC, MD
Associate Member, Leukemia Service, Department of Medicine, Memorial Sloan-Kettering Cancer Center; Associate Professor of Medicine, Weill Cornell Medical College, New York, New York

HILLARD M. LAZARUS, MD, FACP
Department of Medicine, University Hospitals Case Medical Center, Case Comprehensive Cancer Center, Cleveland, Ohio

ROSS L. LEVINE, MD
Associate Member, Leukemia Service and Human Oncology and Pathogenesis Program, Memorial Sloan-Kettering Cancer Center, New York, New York

MARK R. LITZOW, MD
Professor of Medicine and Director, Myeloid Disease-Oriented Group, Division of Hematology, Mayo Clinic, Rochester, Minnesota

KRZYSZTOF MRÓZEK, MD, PhD
Research Scientist, Comprehensive Cancer Center, James Cancer Hospital and Solove Research Institute, The Ohio State University, Columbus, Ohio

JAE H. PARK, MD
Assistant Attending, Leukemia Service, Department of Medicine, Memorial Sloan-Kettering Cancer Center; Department of Medicine, Weill Cornell Medical College, New York, New York

JAY PATEL, BSc
Human Oncology and Pathogenesis Program, Memorial Sloan-Kettering Cancer Center, New York, New York

OANA PAUN, MD
Department of Medicine, University Hospitals Case Medical Center, Case Comprehensive Cancer Center, Cleveland, Ohio

TODD L. ROSENBLAT, MD
Assistant Member, Leukemia Service, Department of Medicine, Memorial Sloan-Kettering Cancer Center; Instructor in Medicine, Weill Cornell Medical College, New York, New York

JACOB M. ROWE, MD, FACP
Director, Department of Hematology, Shaare Zedek Medical Center, Jerusalem; Department of Hematology and Bone Marrow Transplant, Rambam Medical Center; Emeritus Professor, Technion, Israel Institute of Technology, Haifa, Israel

CRAIG SAUTER, MD
Assistant Attending, Adult Bone Marrow Transplant Service, Department of Medicine, Memorial Sloan-Kettering Cancer Center; Department of Medicine, Weill Cornell Medical College, New York, New York

DAVID P. STEENSMA, MD, FACP
Associate Professor of Medicine, Harvard Medical School; Adult Leukemia Group, Department of Hematological Malignancies, Dana-Farber Cancer Institute; Attending Physician, Brigham and Women's Hospital, Boston, Massachusetts

EYTAN STEIN, MD
Fellow in Medical Oncology/Hematology, Department of Medicine, Memorial
Sloan-Kettering Cancer Center, Weill Cornell Medical College, New York, New York

MARTIN S. TALLMAN, MD
Chief, Leukemia Service; Professor of Medicine, Department of Medicine, Memorial
Sloan-Kettering Cancer Center, Weill Cornell Medical College, New York, New York

Contents

Preface: Acute Leukemias   xi

Martin S. Tallman

Clinical Implications of Novel Mutations in Epigenetic Modifiers in AML   1119

Omar Abdel-Wahab, Jay Patel, and Ross L. Levine

> Increased understanding of the molecular genetics of acute myeloid leuke-
> mia (AML) has uncovered several mutations in genes with a role in the epi-
> genetic regulation of gene transcription, including mutations in *TET2*,
> *IDH1*, *IDH2*, and *DNMT3a*. This article reviews recent studies investigating
> the clinical importance of these mutations in AML, and specifically dis-
> cusses the efficacy of molecular analysis for these mutations in refining
> prognosis in AML and informing therapeutic management of patients
> with AML.

Diagnostic and Prognostic Value of Cytogenetics in Acute Myeloid Leukemia   1135

David Grimwade and Krzysztof Mrózek

> The last 4 decades have seen major advances in understanding the ge-
> netic basis of acute myeloid leukemia (AML), and substantial improve-
> ments in survival of children and young adults with the disease. A key
> step forward was the discovery that AML cells harbor recurring cytoge-
> netic abnormalities. The identification of the genes involved in chromo-
> somal rearrangements has provided insights into the regulation of
> normal hematopoiesis and how disruption of key transcription factors
> and epigenetic modulators promote leukemic transformation. Cytogenet-
> ics has been widely adopted to provide the framework for development of
> risk-stratified treatment approaches to patient management.

Prognostic Factors in Adult Acute Leukemia   1163

Chezi Ganzel and Jacob M. Rowe

> The prognostic factors in adult acute leukemia have undergone a major
> change over the past decade and are likely to be further refined in the com-
> ing years. Age is the single most important prognostic factor in both acute
> myeloid leukemias and in acute lymphoblastic leukemias. Recurring cyto-
> genetic abnormalities and molecular markers have become crucial for the
> prognosis of patients and for new directions in the development of tar-
> geted therapies. No less important is the development of a personalized
> approach to therapy as determined by the response to therapy using in-
> creasingly sensitive technologies.

**Induction and Postremission Strategies in Acute Myeloid Leukemia: State of the
Art and Future Directions**   1189

Todd L. Rosenblat and Joseph G. Jurcic

> Advances in the understanding of the molecular pathogenesis of acute
> myeloid leukemia have led to the identification of diagnostic and prognostic

markers, resulting in further refinement of karyotype-based risk classification. This article presents strategies for induction therapy of younger adults and approaches to postremission therapy based on prognostic features. Although some older adults may benefit from intensive chemotherapy and reduced-intensity hematopoietic stem cell transplantation, development of less intensive therapies for older patients who are not candidates for these modalities is an area of active investigation. Novel molecularly targeted agents and other investigational chemotherapeutic drugs now entering late-stage development are also discussed.

Curing All Patients with Acute Promyelocytic Leukemia: Are We There Yet?   1215

Muhamed Baljevic, Jae H. Park, Eytan Stein, Dan Douer, Jessica K. Altman, and Martin S. Tallman

The introduction of *all*-trans retinoic acid to anthracycline-based chemotherapy has revolutionized the prognosis of patients with acute promyelocytic leukemia (APL). The introduction of arsenic trioxide enabled the therapeutic approach of rationally targeted frontline protocols with minimal or no traditional cytotoxic chemotherapy and without compromise of previously established outstanding outcomes with anthracycline-based regimens. Although most of the current investigative efforts in APL are focused on developing potentially curative therapy without the exposure to toxicities and risks of DNA-disrupting agents, the cure rate can further be increased by implementing meticulous supportive care strategies that counter early coagulopathy-related deaths.

Oddballs: Acute Leukemias of Mixed Phenotype and Ambiguous Origin   1235

David P. Steensma

Historically, acute leukemias that do not fit neatly into the broad categories of "acute myeloid leukemia" or "acute lymphoblastic leukemia" have caused considerable confusion and frustration for clinicians and pathologists. These misfit cases include bilineage and biphenotypic leukemias (collectively termed "mixed phenotype acute leukemias" in the 2008 World Health Organization Classification of Tumors of Hematopoietic and Lymphoid Tissues), as well as acute undifferentiated leukemias and other miscellaneous atypical cases. In this review, the author discusses the definitions, history, clinical behavior, and current treatment approaches to acute leukemias of Sambiguous lineage.

Current Therapeutic Strategies in Adult Acute Lymphoblastic Leukemia   1255

Adele K. Fielding

Approximately half of all adults with acute lymphoblastic leukemia now survive long term. This article summarizes the current approaches to treating acute lymphoblastic leukemia in adults, with a focus on a pragmatic approach to decision making. Coupled with a particularly punishing and often complex combination chemotherapy treatment regimen, treatment-related morbidity and mortality are frequent, and this article focuses on these situations. The field will change significantly over the next few years with many ongoing clinical studies and molecular insights which will be translated into providing prognostic information and novel therapeutic targets.

Cellular Therapies in Acute Lymphoblastic Leukemia   1281

Jae H. Park, Craig Sauter, and Renier Brentjens

Most adult patients with acute lymphoblastic leukemia (ALL) will die of the disease. The prognosis in all patients with relapsed or refractory disease is uniformly poor. Although allogeneic hematopoietic stem cell transplantation (allo-HSCT) from a related donor offers significant benefit for some patients, most lack a suitable related donor. Therefore, alternative approaches, including unrelated, umbilical cord blood, and haploidentical allo-HSCT, are being studied. Reduced-intensity conditioning further extends access to allo-HSCT for older more-comorbid patients. Modified adoptive T-cell regimens, including infusion of enriched tumor-targeted donor and genetically targeted autologous T cells, and natural killer cells genetically modified to target ALL are under investigation.

Novel Therapeutic Approaches for Acute Lymphoblastic Leukemia   1303

Mark R. Litzow

Success in therapy for adults with acute lymphoblastic leukemia (ALL) has lagged behind that of children with ALL. However, the application of pediatric-intensive regimens to young and middle-aged adults suggests improved outcomes without excessive toxicity. A promising area in the treatment of adult ALL is the addition of monoclonal antibodies in various forms to chemotherapy in adults with ALL. New chemotherapeutic approaches show promise, and early-phase clinical trials with these drugs are under way.

Novel Transplant Strategies in Adults with Acute Leukemia   1319

Oana Paun and Hillard M. Lazarus

Autologous and allogeneic hematopoietic cell transplantation (HCT) is regularly used as a curative treatment option for patients with various disorders, including acute leukemia in adults. The past decade has witnessed dramatic improvements in the reduction of treatment-related mortality (TRM), in part attributable to improved supportive care but also due to better graft selection and donor-to-recipient matching regimens, and the emergence of reduced-intensity conditioning in place of myeloablative conditioning. Despite these advances, HCT remains plagued by the risk of relapse or failure due to graft-versus-host disease, infectious complications, and TRM. This article reviews new approaches that may improve overall patient outcome.

Index   1341

FORTHCOMING ISSUES

February 2012
Gynecologic Cancer
Ross Berkowitz, MD,
Guest Editor

April 2012
Consultative Hematology
Fred Schiffman, MD, and
Anthony Mega, MD, *Guest Editors*

June 2012
New Drugs for Malignancy
Franco Muggia, MD,
Guest Editor

RECENT ISSUES

October 2011
Chronic Myelogenous Leukemia
Daniel J. DeAngelo, MD, PhD,
Guest Editor

August 2011
Renal Cell Cancer
Toni K. Choueiri, MD,
Guest Editor

June 2011
Testis Cancer
Timothy Gilligan, MD,
Guest Editor

THE CLINICS ARE NOW AVAILABLE ONLINE!
Access your subscription at:
www.theclinics.com

Preface

Acute Leukemias

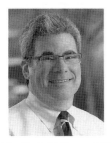

Martin S. Tallman, MD
Guest Editor

The acute leukemias represent a heterogeneous group of malignant hematopoietic stem cell disorders with myeloid characteristics. Remarkable insights have occurred in our understanding of the molecular genetics involved in the development of these diseases. Advances have been made in identifying prognostic factors, both molecular and clinical, that can help guide therapy. The ability to carry out hematopoietic cell transplantation (HCT), in older patients or those not otherwise suitable candidates for intensive transplant strategies using reduced-intensity conditioning regimens and the availability of alternative donors as the stem cell source for those who lack a satisfactory donor, can now provide a graft-versus-leukemia effect to more patients who may benefit. Finally, drug development with new agents with novel mechanisms of action, many of which are directed at specific leukemia-cell-related molecular targets, has proceeded rapidly. All of these exciting areas are authoritatively addressed in this volume.

In the first article, Drs Abdel-Wahab, Patel, and Levine inform us of new genetic mutations in acute myeloid leukemia (AML) that impact on prognosis and help guide therapeutic decisions. This may be particularly important for patients with a normal karyotype, which is a very heterogenous group of AMLs, in which discovery of recurrent genetic mutation can now define specific subtypes for whom different post-remission approaches are now better defined. More clinical prognostic factors in both AML and acute lymphoblastic leukemia (ALL) are discussed by Drs Ganzel and Rowe. They make the important point that many of the more clinical prognostic factors used in the past may be supplanted by cytogenetics and molecular genetics. Precious few advances in induction and post-remission strategies in AML during the last 2 decades have been reported. However, recent studies suggest dose intensification of anthracyclines among younger patients and dose reduction in consolidation intensity may be changing routine practice. Although the immunoconjugate gemtuzumab ozogamicin has been withdrawn from the commercial market, several studies discussed by Drs Rosenblat and Jurcic suggest this agent may have a role in the core binding factor

Hematol Oncol Clin N Am 25 (2011) xi–xii
doi:10.1016/j.hoc.2011.10.003
0889-8588/11/$ – see front matter © 2011 Elsevier Inc. All rights reserved.

hemonc.theclinics.com

AML. They also identify matched unrelated donor transplantation as a promising treatment for patients with high-risk AML.

In a very comprehensive way, Dr David Steensma describes acute leukemias of mixed phenotype and ambiguous lineage in the context of the World Health Organization 2008 classification. Dr David Grimwade provides important data on specific cytogenetic subtypes of AML. Three articles are devoted to ALL. The first by Dr Adele Fielding addresses current therapeutic strategies for both Philadelphia-negative and -positive ALL. Major advances have occurred among patients with Philadelphia-positive disease with the addition of tyrosine kinase inhibitors (TKI) to chemotherapy. The role of transplantation in the TKI era and the role of TKI as maintenance after transplantation both remain to be studied. In the second, Dr Mark Litzow outlines novel strategies including the addition of monoclonal antibodies to conventional chemotherapy as well as the very exciting agent Blinatumomab, a bispecific T-cell engager that combines an anti-CD19 antibody targeted to B cells and an anti-CD3 antibody targeted to T-cell recruiting T cells and therefore the immune system. This agent appears in preliminary studies to have remarkable activity in ALL. Another promising new therapeutic approach involves a cellular immunologic strategy of adoptively transferred autologous CD19-targeted T cells, discussed by Drs Park, Sauter, and Brentjens after a thorough presentation of the role of allogeneic HCT in ALL. Acute promyelocytic leukemia (APL) is an uncommon subtype of AML that has unique biologic and clinical characteristics. It has emerged as highly curable, whereas it once was the most lethal at diagnosis and during induction because of often catastrophic bleeding. Drs Baljevic, Park, Stein, Douer, Altman, and Tallman discuss recent developments in induction and post-remission therapy for patients with APL tailored in a risk-adapted manner that leads to a very high cure rate and, for the first time, using approaches without or, at most, only minimal, chemotherapy when both all-trans-retinoic acid and arsenic trioxide are given.

Finally, the role of HCT is addressed in the article by Dr Lazarus with a focus on new transplant strategies. The heterogeneity of the acute leukemias is amply demonstrated by the fact that we can cure most patients with one subtype (APL) with novel targeted agents with less chemotherapy and others (patients with AML and primary induction failure) can only be cured with intensive transplant approaches that rely on the innate immune system. We hope the student of the acute leukemias, at any level of sophistication, will find this issue both helpful and, in fact, inspirational. As Henry David Thoreau wrote, "How many a man has dated a new era in his life from the reading of a book."

Martin S. Tallman, MD
Leukemia Service, Department of Medicine
Memorial Sloan-Kettering Cancer Center
Weill Cornell Medical College
1275 York Avenue
New York, NY 10065, USA

E-mail address:
TallmanM@mskcc.org

Clinical Implications of Novel Mutations in Epigenetic Modifiers in AML

Omar Abdel-Wahab, MD[a],*, Jay Patel, BSc[b], Ross L. Levine, MD[a]

KEYWORDS

• TET2 • IDH1 • IDH2 • DNMT3a • Epigenetics • AML

EPIGENETIC MODIFIERS MUTATED IN AML

Conventional and molecular cytogenetics are essential components of risk stratification and therapeutic decision making in the clinical management of patients with acute myeloid leukemia (AML). In addition to structural chromosomal alterations, molecular analysis of mutations have been incorporated into the World Health Organization (WHO) and European Leukemia Net (ELN) AML classification; specifically, mutations in *FLT3*, *NPM1*, and *CEBPA* are now broadly accepted in routine clinical practice.[1] In particular, mutations in these three genes allow the stratification of patients with cytogenetically normal AML (CN-AML) into prognostic risk categories, and can be used to guide the use of postremission therapy, including allogeneic stem cell transplantation. Currently, patients with CN-AML with either a *CEBPA* or a *NPM1* mutation without a concurrent *FLT3-ITD* are classified as having favorable-risk AML in the ELN Classification along with patients with core-binding factor leukemias (t(8;21)(q22;q22), inv(16)(p13.1q22), or t(16;16)(p13.1;q22)).[1] Similarly, adult AML with mutations in *NPM1* or *CEBPA* has been classified as a provisional disease entity in the current WHO classification of AML.[2]

In addition to these three clinically used molecular abnormalities, an increasing number of additional mutations are being identified in patients with myeloid malignancies, including AML. Mutations in a large proportion of these newly discovered genetic

This work was supported in part by grants from the National Institutes of Health (U54CA143798-01, Physical Sciences Oncology Center) and the Starr Cancer Consortium and Howard Hughes Medical Institute to Dr Levine. Dr Abdel-Wahab is a Basic Research Fellow of the American Society of Hematology.
The authors have nothing to disclose.
[a] Leukemia Service and Human Oncology and Pathogenesis Program, Memorial Sloan-Kettering Cancer Center, 1275 York Avenue, Box 20, New York, NY 10065, USA
[b] Human Oncology and Pathogenesis Program, Memorial Sloan-Kettering Cancer Center, 1275 York Avenue, Box 20, New York, NY 10065, USA
* Corresponding author.
E-mail address: abdelwao@mskcc.org

Hematol Oncol Clin N Am 25 (2011) 1119–1133
doi:10.1016/j.hoc.2011.09.013
0889-8588/11/$ – see front matter © 2011 Elsevier Inc. All rights reserved.

hemonc.theclinics.com

abnormalities are in genes that impact the epigenetic regulation of gene expression, including mutations in *TET2*, *IDH1*, *IDH2*, and *DNMT3a*. A precedence for the clinical importance of mutations in epigenetic modifiers in acute leukemia is already well established with the characterization of chromosomal translocations and partial tandem duplications in *MLL1* (*MLL*-PTD), the main human histone lysine methyltransferase. The *MLL*-PTD mutation was the first adverse prognostic molecular marker identified in CN-AML. Two initial correlative studies identified that patients with CN-AML with the *MLL*-PTD mutation experienced significantly shorter remission compared with wild-type counterparts.[3,4] Subsequent studies have reported variable effects of the *MLL*-PTD on outcome, possibly related to the more-intensive consolidation therapy administered to patients in recent studies.[5]

This article reviews the progression of clinical understanding of the clinical importance of mutations in *TET2*, *IDH1*, *IDH2*, *DNMT3a* in AML and discusses the potential use of analyzing these mutations in refining prognostication and affecting choice of induction or postremission therapy in AML.

MUTATIONS AND DELETIONS IN *TET2*: A POTENTIALLY IMPORTANT PROGNOSTICATOR IN CN-AML

TET2 is member of the Tet family of enzymes, Fe(Ii)-, α-ketoglutarate–dependent enzymes with a previously unknown function, specially the ability to convert 5-methylcytosine to 5-hydroxymethylcytosine,[6] an enzymatic activity that is now believed to be critical in mediating DNA demethylation.[7] Somatic mutations in *TET2* were first identified in 2009 and occur throughout the coding region of *TET2* as deletion mutations, missense, nonsense, and frameshift mutations in patients with myeloproliferative neoplasms (MPN) and myelodysplastic syndromes (MDS). The presence of deletions, nonsense, and frameshift mutations in *TET2* provided genetic data suggesting that TET2 functions as a tumor suppressor in myeloid malignancies.

Shortly after the initial description of *TET2* mutations, the authors reported that *TET2* was mutated in 10.1% of patients with AML and that *TET2* mutations were associated with significantly decreased overall survival in a single-institution cohort of 119 patients with AML (including de novo and secondary AML).[8] Since then, a series of studies have been performed to identify the clinical correlates and potential prognostic importance of *TET2* mutations in AML in more detail (**Table 1**). The first study to focus exclusively on the clinical effect of *TET2* mutations on prognosis in de novo AML was performed by Nibourel and colleagues.[9] This study found a trend toward a higher frequency of *TET2* mutations among patients with AML who did not experience a complete remission compared with those who did (27% vs 17%, respectively; *P* = not significant). However, the authors found that *TET2* mutations had no effect on disease-free or overall survival. Unfortunately, the survival analyses were restricted to only 54 patients, all of whom experienced a complete remission, likely masking any effect of *TET2* mutations on outcome.

Four larger subsequent studies evaluating the clinical correlates of *TET2* mutations in de novo AML have been reported.[10–12] The first, presented in abstract form at the 2010 American Society of Hematology Annual Meeting, evaluated the effect of *TET2* mutations in 783 patients who were prospectively treated in the AML HD98A Study of the German AML Study Group.[10] Although *TET2* mutations were found in 7.6% of patients (60 patients), the investigators did not observe a significant impact of *TET2* mutations on clinical outcome in the entire cohort or the subset of patients with CN-AML (this included analysis of overall, event-free, and relapse-free survival). When interpreting the results of this study, one must consider that all patients

Table 1
Prognostic studies of *TET2* mutations in AML

Reference	Number of Patients	Mutational Frequency	Clinical Implications Investigated	Patient Population/Comments
Abdel-Wahab et al[8]	119	10.1%	*TET2* mutations found to be associated with OS	Patients with de novo and secondary AML included
Nibourel et al[9]	147	19.7%	*TET2* mutations not found to affect OS or DFS although enriched in patients who did not experience CR (*P* = not significant)	Survival analysis limited to 54 patients with de novo AML who experienced CR
Gaidzik et al[10]	783	7.6%	No effect of *TET2* mutations on clinical outcome (EFS, RFS, OS) or response to therapy in any subgroup	Limited to young adult patients with AML (aged 16–60 years) treated on AML HD98A study
Metzeler et al[11]	427	23%	Shorter EFS and DFS and lower CR among patients with *TET2*-mutant genotype with *NPM1* or *CEBPA* mutations without *FLT3-ITD*	Analysis limited to de novo CN-AML
Kosmider et al[52]	247	19.8%	No effect on CR or OS	Limited to secondary AML secondary from MDS and therapy-related AML Very diverse therapies (included best supportive care in 20%)
Chou et al[12]	486	13.2%	*TET2* mutations associated with adverse risk in intermediate-risk AML (n = 171)	Analysis limited to de novo AML
Patel et al[13]	398	10%	*TET2* mutations associated with adverse risk in intermediate-risk AML regardless of *FLT3-ITD* status	Analyzed patients from phase III trial of patients with de novo AML aged 16- to 60 years on standard- or high-dose daunorubicin induction

Abbreviations: CN-AML, cytogenetically normal acute myeloid leukemia; CR, complete remission; DFS, disease-free survival; EFS, event-free survival; MDS, myelodysplastic syndromes; OS, overall survival; RFS, relapse-free survival; TTF, time-to-treatment failure.

analyzed were treated using an intense response-adapted double-induction and first consolidation therapy, which is distinct from the commonly used standard induction chemotherapy regimens consisting of an anthracycline plus cytarabine, which are standard of care in the United States, United Kingdom, and elsewhere.

Very recently, Chou and colleagues[12] studied the effect of *TET2* mutations on a cohort of 486 patients with de novo AML treated with standard induction chemotherapy. In this study, *TET2* mutations were not associated with differences in overall survival, complete remission, or disease-free survival in the entire cohort. However, *TET2* mutations were clearly associated with shorter overall survival in 171 patients with intermediate-risk cytogenetics (median not reached in patients with the *TET2*–wild-type genotype vs 22.1 months in those with the *TET2*-mutant genotype; $P = .0076$). This study also found that patients with CN-AML with *FLT3-ITD*$^+$/*TET2*-mutant and *NPM1*–wild-type/*TET2*-mutant genotypes also had worsened outcome compared with their *TET2*–wild-type counterparts.

Metzeler and colleagues[11] specifically investigated the prognostic impact of *TET2* mutations in CN-AML. In an analysis of 427 patients with CN-AML who received cytarabine/daunorubicin-based first-line therapy, the authors found that *TET2* mutations adversely affected survival in patients within the ELN favorable-risk category of CN-AML (patients who have mutated *NPM1* and/or *CEBPA* without *FLT3-ITD* mutations). *TET2*-mutated patients in this subset had significantly shorter event-free and disease-free survival because of a lower complete remission rate only among patients with favorable-risk CN-AML.

The authors recently completed an analysis of the effect *TET2* mutations on 398 patients enrolled on the ECOG E1900 trial.[13] This phase III prospective trial randomized adults younger than 60 years with AML to standard-dose (45 mg/m^2) or dose-intensified (90 mg/m^2) daunorubicin as part of induction therapy.[14] Although 10% of the patients analyzed had a *TET2* mutation, the adverse effect of *TET2* mutations was not seen in the overall cohort. However, a clear association was seen between *TET2* mutations and adverse overall survival in the subset of patients with intermediate-risk AML. Moreover, *TET2* mutations were found to be associated with worsened overall survival in patients with intermediate-risk AML, regardless of the presence of the *FLT3-ITD* mutation, suggesting that mutations in *TET2* may be an important prognosticator in patients with intermediate-risk AML.

In addition to these studies, which focused mostly on patients with de novo AML (many of whom were genotyped pretreatment), a set of smaller studies focused on the effect of *TET2* mutations in patients with secondary AML. The authors noted that *TET2* mutations are a frequent event at leukemic transformation of MPNs, occurring in 43% patients for whom paired MPN/secondary AML (sAML) samples were available, suggesting that *TET2* mutations are a common event in transformation from MPN to AML.[15] Recently, Kosmider and colleagues[16] performed a retrospective study of the effect of *TET2* mutation on clinical outcome in 247 patients with AML from an antecedent MDS (n = 201) or therapy-related AML (n = 46). They found no clear effect of *TET2* mutations (19.8% of cohort) on survival in this cohort; however, the different therapies administered were very heterogeneous, ranging from supportive care to induction chemotherapy or allogeneic stem cell transplantation. Future studies of large, clinical trial cohorts of homogenously treated secondary AML are needed to assess the prognostic significance of *TET2* mutations in this context.

Despite all of these studies, no clearly consistent clinical or molecular features specific to AML patients with *TET2* mutations have been shown, except that *TET2* mutations are exclusive of *IDH1/2* mutations in AML.[17] This robust finding clearly indicates epistasis between *TET2* and *IDH1/2* mutations, and led to functional studies showing that 2-hydroxyglutarate, the metabolite produced by neomorphic *IDH1/2* mutations, inhibits the function of the TET family of enzymes.[17,18] At least two studies have also noted a positive correlation between *TET2* and *NPM1* mutations, but this has not been a consistent finding among all studies.[12,19] Moreover, Chou and colleagues[12] reported a correlation between *TET2* and *ASXL1* mutations in AML. However, this finding may be confounded by the inclusion in their analysis of a frequent nucleotide variant in *ASXL1*, which does not seem to represent a bona fide somatic mutation.[20]

Given the finding that patients with AML with *TET2* mutations are characterized by a DNA hypermethylation,[17] nascent efforts have been made to investigate whether patients with a *TET2*-mutated genotype may have differential rates of response to DNA methyltransferase inhibitors (DNMTIs) compared with their wild-type counterparts. A French study of 86 patients with MDS and secondary AML reported that patients with *TET2* mutations had a high response rate to 5-azacitidine compared with the *TET2*–wild-type group (82% vs 45%, respectively). However, no effect on survival was seen based on mutational status, and the study group was heterogeneous with few additional genetic parameters studied.[21] In contrast, other groups have found that *TET2* alterations in a similar cohort of patients may actually predict for decreased responsiveness to demethylating therapies.[22] The small number of patients included in these studies and the limited genetic characterization of the patients in these cohorts must be considered. Larger studies with more comprehensive genetic evaluation will be critical in determining whether mutations in genetic factors suspected to be important in regulating DNA methylation (*TET2*, *IDH1/2*, and *DNMT3a* mutations, among others) affect response to DNMTIs or other epigenetic therapies. Moreover, the questions remain whether *TET2* mutations actually result in global hypermethylation of DNA in all diseases in which *TET2* mutations exist and, if so, what is the proper methodology to detect this altered methylation. Ko and colleagues[23] found that patients with *TET2* mutations with different chronic myeloid malignancies actually had a relative hypomethylation of DNA compared with their wild-type counterparts using Infinium 27K methylation arrays (Illumina, San Diego, CA). These findings will need to be clarified in future studies with more-comprehensive genotyping and multiple methodologies to assay DNA methylation and hydroxymethylation.

GAIN-OF-FUNCTION MUTATIONS IN *IDH1* AND *IDH2* IN AML

Somatic mutations in human cytosolic isocitrate dehydrogenase 1 (*IDH1*) and mitochondrial isocitrate dehydrogenase 2 (*IDH2*) are now well-recognized recurrent genetic alterations in AML.[24] The mutations in *IDH1* occur at R132 and were initially reported to cause loss of the enzyme's normal ability to catalyze the conversion of isocitrate to α-ketoglutarate. Subsequently, investigators discovered that these mutations also conferred a neomorphic gain-of-function: the novel nicotinamide adenine dinucleotide phosphate (NADPH)–dependent reduction of α-ketoglutarate to the metabolite $R(-)$-2-hydroxyglutarate (2HG), which is normally only found in trace amounts in normal cells.[25] Similarly, mutations have been described in *IDH2* at arginine 172, the residue analogous to *IDH1-R132*, in addition to mutations at a different arginine in IDH2's active site, R140. Currently, no mutations at *IDH1* or *IDH2* in residues outside of these sites have been shown to result in altered enzymatic activity (nor are nucleotide variants at the IDH1 single nucleotide polymorphism rs11554137 known to have functional importance).[26]

Because of the relative ease of genotyping *IDH1* and *IDH2* mutations and ability to multiplex testing for both *IDH1* and *IDH2* mutations simultaneously using a variety of modalities,[27,28] several large studies have been quickly performed in patients with AML to determine the clinical and prognostic relevance of *IDH1/2* mutations in AML (**Table 2**). Although no unifying result common to all of these studies has been found, multiple studies have reported a statistically significant co-occurrence of *NPM1* mutations and *IDH1* or *IDH2* mutations.[17,29–32] In terms of effects on clinical outcome,

Table 2
Prognostic studies of *IDH1/2* mutations in AML

Reference	Number of Patients	Mutational Frequency	Clinical Implications Investigated	Patient Population/ Comments
IDH1-R132, IDH2-R140, and *IDH2-R172* codons sequenced				
Abbas et al[29]	893	17% (*IDH1* 6% and *IDH2* 11%)	No effect on overall cohort or CN-AML overall; Adverse effect of *IDH1* mutations on OS and EFS in subset of patients with *FLT3*–wild-type/*NPM1*–wild-type genotype	Patients were culled from multiple different HOVON AML protocols (HO04, HO04A, HO029, HO029, HO42, HO42A, HO43).
Paschka et al[34]	805	16% (*IDH1* 7.6%, *IDH2* 8.7%)	No effect on overall cohort or patients with CN-AML overall; Adverse effect of *IDH1* or *IDH2* mutants on patients with CN-AML with *NPM1*-mutant/*FLT3*–wild-type genotype	All patients were on AMLSG HD98A or HD95 studies and younger than 60 years
Marcucci et al[53]	358	33% (14% *IDH1*, 19% *IDH2*)	*IDH1* mutations associated with worsened DFS and *IDH2-R172* mutation associated with lower CR	All patients with de novo CN-AML from multiple CALGB trials (9621, 19808, 8525, 8923, 9420, 9720, or 10201)
Rockova et al[54]	439	15.4% (7.2% *IDH1*, 8.2% *IDH2*)	No effect of *IDH* mutations on overall cohort but combined with gene expression analysis, *IDH2* associated with a distinctive improved survival	De novo AML and MDS RAEBt patients, all younger than 60 years, treated on HOVON protocols between 1987 and 2006
Only *IDH1-R132* and *IDH2-R172* codons sequenced				
Boissel et al[19]	520	12.6% (*IDH1* 9.6%, *IDH2-R172* 3.0%)	*IDH1* mutations found to be associated with higher RR and shorter OS in patients with CN-AML with *NPM1* or *CEBPA* mutations but no *FLT3* mutations; *IDH2-R172* mutations were associated with higher RR and shorter OS in patients with CN-AML overall	Adult patients with AML of all ages and assigned to French Acute Leukemia French Association -9801 and -9802 trials

Only IDH1 or IDH2 sequenced

Study	n	Frequency	Clinical finding	Patient description
Schnittger et al[55]	1414	6.6% IDH1	IDH1-R132 mutations associated with decreased EFS	Adult patients with AML of all ages and assigned to AMLSG to receive induction either with a standard-dose (cytarabine, daunorubicin, and 6-thioguanine) and a high-dose (cytarabine and mitoxantrone) combination, or with two courses of the high-dose combination
Green et al[32]	1333	8% IDH1	No effect on overall cohort or CN-AML overall. Adverse effect on relapse in patients with FLT3–wild-type genotype but favorable effect in FLT3/ITD mutant patients.	All patients were on UK MRC AML10 or AML12 trials
Green et al[31]	1473	10% IDH2	IDH2-R140Q mutation found to be have favorable effect for RFS and OS in overall cohort and FLT3–wild-type/NPM1-mutant subset	All patients were on UK MRC AML10 or AML12 trials
Chou et al[30]	493	5.5% IDH1	No effect of IDH1-R132H on clinical outcome	Patients with IDH1-mutant genotype followed serially, and 61.1% of patients who experienced relapse had reemergence of the IDH1 mutation at relapse
Thol et al[56]	272	12.1% IDH2	No impact of IDH2 mutations on response to therapy, OS, and RFS in patients with CN-AML	All patients with CN-AML, younger than 60 years
Wagner et al[57]	275	10.9% IDH1	No effect of IDH1R132H on clinical outcome	All patients with CN-AML, younger than 60 years, and treated on AML Suddeutsche Hamoblastose Gruppe trials 0295 or 0199

Abbreviations: AMLSG, German–Austrian AML Study Group; CALGB, Cancer and Leukemia Group B; CN-AML, cytogenetically normal acute myeloid leukemia; CR, complete remission rate; DFS, disease-free survival; EFS, event-free survival; HOVON, Dutch-Belgian Cooperative Group on Hemato-Oncology in Adults; OS, overall survival; RAEBt, refractory anemia with excess blasts in transformation; RFS, relapse-free survival; TTF, time-to-treatment failure; UK MRC, United Kingdom Medical Research Council.

differing effects on clinical outcome seem to be associated with the different *IDH1/2* alleles (*IDH1-R132, IDH2-R140, IDH2-R172*).[31] This finding has been hypothesized to be related to the biologic finding of differing 2HG production with the different *IDH1/2* mutant alleles in vitro,[26,33] a possibility to be tested in future trials correlating metabolite measurement with clinical outcome in AML.

The two largest studies correlating *IDH1/2* mutations with outcome in AML analyzed more than 1000 patients treated on two United Kingdom Medical Research Council Trials (see **Table 2**), who were also tested for *FLT3-ITD/TKD*, *NPM1*, and *CEBPa* mutations.[31,32] In both studies, patients with either *IDH1* or *IDH2* mutations were significantly enriched with *NPM1* mutations. Among the entire cohort of patients, the investigators found that patients with an *IDH2-R140Q* mutation had an improved overall survival and decreased response rate. This finding was even more striking among the subset of patients with the *FLT3–wild-type/NPM1*-mutant genotype who had similar survival to the most favorable subsets of patients. In contrast, *IDH2-R172* mutations had a neutral effect on outcome and response to therapy, whereas *IDH1-R132* mutations seemed to impart worsened outcome on patients with the *FLT3–wild-type* genotype. The latter finding of an adverse effect of *IDH1-R132* mutations on subsets of patients with AML with the *FLT3–wild-type* genotype were also reported by and Abbas and colleagues[29] and Paschka and colleagues.[34] However the prognostic impact of *IDH1/2* mutations and the relevance of other co-occurring disease alleles on outcome require further investigation.

Currently, the large number of individual studies of *IDH1* and *IDH2* mutation effects on clinical outcome in AML make this subject ripe for meta-analysis, because subset analysis based on combinations of *FLT3/NPM1/CEBPA* genotypes have resulted in a multitude of varying results, likely related to limits in sample size. In addition, because the different *IDH* mutant alleles result in a novel gain-of-function, small molecule inhibitors of these mutations may emerge as a novel therapeutic option for patients with *IDH*-mutant AML.

MUTATIONS IN *DNMT3A* IN AML

From June 2010 to April 2011, three groups independently reported mutations in the DNA methyltransferase 3A gene (*DNMT3a*) in patients with AML (**Table 3**).[35–37] Since that time, *DNMT3a* mutations have been further described in additional AML cohorts and in patients with MDS[38] and MPN.[39] Somatic mutations in the other DNMTs (*DNMT1, DNMT3A, DNMT3L*) have not been described in AML or other malignancies.

The aggregate of data from the clinical studies performed thus far suggest that *DNMT3a* mutations are correlated with adverse overall survival in adult patients with AML.[35,36,40] The initial report describing *DNMT3a* mutations in AML identified the recurrent *R882* mutation but included too few patients to identify associations between mutations and clinical parameters.[37] However, two subsequent discovery studies identified mutations throughout the coding region of *DNMT3a* and included sufficiently large retrospective analyses to conclude that patients with *DNMT3a* mutations had significantly worsened overall survival, regardless of age, cytogenetic status, or *FLT3-ITD* mutational status.[35,36]

Ley and colleagues[35] performed whole genome sequencing in AML to identify *DNMT3a* mutations, and found that patients with these mutations had a median survival of 12.3 months compared with 41.1 months in their *DNMT3a–wild-type* counterparts (*P*<.0001). Similar findings were seen regardless of whether the analysis was restricted to *DNTM3A-R882* mutations only or non-*R882* mutations only, suggesting that the prognostic importance of *DNMT3a* mutations did not differ based on the

	Number of	Mutational	Clinical Implications	Patient Population/
Reference	Patients	Frequency	Investigated	Comments
Yamashita et al[37]	75	4.1%	None	Also identified mutations in *JAK3* in 3.1% of patients with AML
Ley et al[35]	282	22.1% (overall); 33.7% of intermediate-risk subset	Shorter OS in patients with mutations overall and in intermediate-risk patients regardless of *FLT3* status	
Yan et al[36]	112	20.5%	Shorter OS and TTF in patients with mutations	Outcome analysis was restricted to patients with FAB M5 AML only (n = 91)
Thol et al[40]	489	17.8%	*DNMT3A* mutations associated with shorter OS but not associated with RFS or CR in the entire cohort In CN-AML, *DNMT3A* mutations independently predicted shorter OS and lower CR rate but not RFS Furthermore, *DNMT3A* mutations had an unfavorable effect on OS, RFS, and CR rate in patients with *NPM1*–wild-type/ *FLT3-ITD* CN-AML, but not in low-risk patients	This study limited *DNMT3a* mutational analysis to last exon in most patients, which may have affected mutational frequency and altered correlative studies

Table 3
Prognostic studies of *DNMT3a* mutations in AML

Abbreviations: CN-AML, cytogenetically normal acute myeloid leukemia; CR, complete remission rate; FAB M5 AML = Myelo-monocytic acute myeloid leukemia (M5 subtype of French American British AML classification). OS, overall survival; RFS, relapse-free survival; TTF, time-to-treatment failure.

specific mutation. Yan and colleagues[36] identified *DNMT3a* mutations in patients with M5 AML through exome sequencing. Specifically examining the effect of *DNMT3a* mutations on the outcome of 91 patients with M5 AML, they found an abysmal effect of *DNMT3a* mutations on overall survival and time-to-treatment failure, such that patients with the *DNMT3a*-mutant genotype had a median survival of 7 months compared with 19.5 months in patients with the *DNMT3a*–wild-type genotype ($P = .004$). In addition to the effects of *DNMT3a* mutation in adult patients with AML overall, two studies have indicated an adverse effect of *DNMT3a* mutations on patients with intermediate-risk AML and CN-AML, specifically.[35,40] Ley and colleagues[35] also found that *DNMT3a* mutations imparted an adverse effect on overall survival regardless of *FLT3-ITD* mutational status.

DNMT3a mutational studies in patients with myeloid malignancies have clearly indicated that mutations can occur throughout the coding region of *DNMT3a* as nonsense, frameshift, and missense mutations. A recurrent heterozygous mutation at residue Arginine 882 accounts for 40% to 60% of *DNMT3a* mutations. Although the finding of mutations throughout the open reading frame suggests that *DNMT3a* mutations result in a loss-of-function, the finding of a recurrent heterozygous point mutation suggests that missense *DNMT3a* mutations may, in fact, result in gain-of-function or acquisition of a novel function. The only functional data to date has shown that *R882* mutations result in a loss of methyltransferase in in vitro assays.[37] However, in AML cells, *R882* mutations always occur with retention of the wild-type allele, requiring reevaluation of the methyltransferase activity of the *R882* mutant in the context of coexpression of wild-type *DNMT3a*. Ley and colleagues[35] investigated the effect of *DNMT3a* mutations on global DNA methylation in AML blast samples using liquid chromatography–tandem mass spectrometry but did not identify a clear effect of *DNMT3a* mutations on overall levels of DNA methylation using this methodology.

The largest *DNMT3a* mutational analysis performed thus far limited mutational analysis to the last exon.[40] Despite this limited approach to mutational profiling, this study also noted a significantly worsened overall survival among all patients with AML and CN-AML with *DNMT3a* mutations. Future studies to validate this more-limited sequencing approach in AML will be necessary to confirm whether a more focused approach can be used to genotype for the most common disease alleles until full-length resequencing becomes feasible in the clinical setting.

NOVEL EPIGENETIC GENE MUTATIONS IN PEDIATRIC AML

Compared with studies among adults with AML, fewer studies of the frequencies and effects of mutations in *TET2*, *IDH1/2*, and *DNMT3a* have been performed in pediatric patients with AML (**Table 4**). These studies, however, show that mutations in all of these genes are rare among pediatric patients with AML, occurring in fewer than 5%.[41–44] These findings highlight potentially important biologic differences between pediatric and adult AML regarding the role of somatic alterations in epigenetic modifiers.

POTENTIAL USE OF *TET2*, *IDH1/2*, AND *DNMT3A* ALTERATIONS FOR MINIMAL RESIDUAL DISEASE DETECTION

Increased identification of cytogenetic and molecular abnormalities in patients with AML has led to an interest in identifying the presence of these genetic alterations in patient samples at diagnosis, remission, and relapse. These studies inform about not only the biologic contributions of these mutations to myelopoiesis but also their potential use in minimal residual disease detection (not yet a well-studied or standardized practice in AML management). It has recently been shown that *FLT3-ITD* mutations and mutations in *RUNX1*, when present at diagnosis, often are not present in blasts of the same individuals at relapse.[45,46] Since the discovery of mutations in *TET2*, *IDH1/2*, and *DNMT3a* in AML, increasing data have shown the durability of these mutations after treatment in serial samples from patients with AML. Most of these data have come from the AML investigators at the National Taiwan University. These studies have shown that *TET2* mutations, when present at diagnosis, are frequently not present at AML relapse, whereas mutations in *IDH1* are most commonly retained at AML relapse.[12,30] In a recent large study of 486 patients sequenced for *TET2*, 23 patients were found to have *TET2* mutations, 13 of whom eventually

Table 4
Prognostic studies of *TET2*, *IDH1/2*, and *DNMT3a* mutations in pediatric patients with AML

Reference	Number of Patients	Gene	Mutational Frequency	Clinical Implications Investigated
Andersson et al[41]	515	*IDH1* and *IDH2*	3.5%	No effect on clinical parameters One *IDH* mutation found in a patient with ALL (N = 288)
Damm et al[42]	460	*IDH1* and *IDH2*	4%	Patients with *IDH* mutations had improved OS in univariate analysis only
Ho et al[43]	180	*DNMT3a*	0%	N/A
Ho et al[43]	180	*IDH1* and *IDH2*	2.2%	N/A
Langemeijer et al[44]	151	*TET2*	3.8%	N/A; no *TET2* mutations seen in 47 patients with ALL

Abbreviations: ALL, acute lymphoblastic leukemia; CR, complete remission rate; OS, overall survival; RFS, relapse-free survival; TTF, time-to-treatment failure.

developed AML relapse and 6 (46%) of whom were wild-type for their documented *TET2* mutation at disease relapse. In contrast, every patient who harbored an *IDH1* mutation at diagnosis and had a sample taken at relapse had the same *IDH1* mutation at relapse. Further retrospective and prospective serial molecular studies to evaluate the durability of these molecular alterations at diagnosis and relapse will be very informative and necessary for future studies aiming to understand the potential efficacy of minimal residual disease monitoring in AML.

SUMMARY

The studies highlighted in this article suggest that mutations in *TET2* mutations may impart adverse outcome in patients with CN-AML, whereas mutations in *DNMT3a* may have adverse implications in a broader set of patients with AML. The data with *IDH* enzyme mutations are less clear, in that individual *IDH1* and *IDH2* mutations may have different clinical effects and the data so far have not suggested a uniform effect on outcome.

Despite the exciting data indicating that mutational testing for these alterations may be clinically useful, several challenges to understanding their clinical relevance remain. First, patients may simultaneously have mutations in multiple genes described in this article (*FLT3, NPM1, CEBPa, DNMT3a, IDH1/2*, or *TET2*), and in additional genes not mentioned earlier (*Ras*,[47] *PTEN*,[48] *PHF6*,[49] *ASXL1*,[15] and *RUNX1*[45]). Furthermore, comprehensive sequencing studies of well-annotated, homogeneously treated patient cohorts are needed to understand the clinical implications of integrated mutational profiling in AML.

An additional challenge to using mutational analysis for *TET2* and *DNMT3a* in clinical use is identifying a means for rapid molecular testing of these mutations. This challenge may be met by the use of non–polymerase chain reaction–based methods of target enrichment, such as hybrid capture, followed by next-generation sequencing technologies. Moreover, clinical studies evaluating the biochemical consequences of mutations in some of these genes (eg, production of 2-HG in bodily fluids from patients with *IDH*-mutant AML or increased hydroxymethylcytosine levels in pretreatment blast DNA in patients with *TET2/IDH* mutant AML) may also prove to be useful in identifying biomarkers. Alternatively, protein-based technologies such as immunohistochemistry or mass spectrometry may be used in the clinical setting to detect the mutant proteins or loss of expression of specific proteins in patients with mutations.

An additional area of importance highlighted by these discoveries is the increasing realization that several of these genes encode enzymes or result in alterations in enzymatic activities, which may represent novel, tractable therapeutic targets for patients with AML. This finding may hopefully lead to the development of novel targeted therapeutics for patients with specific genetic alterations in AML. This development may be occurring now with the advent of *DOT1L*-targeted therapy for leukemic cells with translocations involving *MLL1*.[50,51] Studies to identify whether the neomorphic enzymatic activity of *IDH1/2* mutations may be targetable or if the downstream effects of *TET2* mutations can be targeted are ongoing and may lead to the development of rational epigenetic therapies that improve outcomes for patients with AML.

REFERENCES

1. Dohner H, Estey EH, Amadori S, et al. Diagnosis and management of acute myeloid leukemia in adults: recommendations from an international expert panel, on behalf of the European LeukemiaNet. Blood 2010;115(3):453–74.
2. Swerdlow S, Campo E, Harris NL, et al. WHO classification of tumours of haematopoietic and lymphoid tissues. Lyon (France): IARC Press; 2008.
3. Caligiuri MA, Strout MP, Lawrence D, et al. Rearrangement of ALL1 (MLL) in acute myeloid leukemia with normal cytogenetics. Cancer Res 1998;58(1):55–9.
4. Dohner K, Tobis K, Ulrich R, et al. Prognostic significance of partial tandem duplications of the MLL gene in adult patients 16 to 60 years old with acute myeloid leukemia and normal cytogenetics: a study of the Acute Myeloid Leukemia Study Group Ulm. J Clin Oncol 2002;20(15):3254–61.
5. Whitman SP, Ruppert AS, Marcucci G, et al. Long-term disease-free survivors with cytogenetically normal acute myeloid leukemia and MLL partial tandem duplication: a Cancer and Leukemia Group B study. Blood 2007;109(12):5164–7.
6. Tahiliani M, Koh KP, Shen Y, et al. Conversion of 5-methylcytosine to 5-hydroxymethylcytosine in mammalian DNA by MLL partner TET1. Science 2009; 324(5929):930–5.
7. Guo JU, Su Y, Zhong C, et al. Hydroxylation of 5-methylcytosine by TET1 promotes active DNA demethylation in the adult brain. Cell 2011;145(3): 423–34.
8. Abdel-Wahab O, Mullally A, Hedvat C, et al. Genetic characterization of TET1, TET2, and TET3 alterations in myeloid malignancies. Blood 2009;114(1): 144–7.
9. Nibourel O, Kosminder O, Cheok M, et al. Association of TET2 alterations with NPM1 mutations and prognostic value in de novo acute myeloid leukemia (AML) [abstract 163]. Blood 2009;114(22).
10. Gaidzik V, Schlenk RF, Paschka P, et al. TET2 mutations in acute myeloid leukemia (AML): results on 783 patients treated within the AML HD98A study of the AML Study Group (AMLSG) [abstract 97]. Blood 2010;116(21).
11. Metzeler KH, Maharry K, Radmacher MD, et al. TET2 mutations improve the New European LeukemiaNet Risk Classification of Acute Myeloid Leukemia: a Cancer and Leukemia Group B Study. J Clin Oncol 2011;29(10):1373–81.
12. Chou WC, Chou SC, Liu CY, et al. TET2 mutation is an unfavorable prognostic factor in acute myeloid leukemia patients with intermediate-risk cytogenetics. Oncogene 2011;118(14):3803–10.

13. Patel J, Abdel-Wahab O, Gonen M, et al. High-throughput mutational profiling in AML: mutational analysis of the ECOG E1900 Trial [abstract 851]. Blood 2010; 116(21):851.
14. Fernandez HF, Sun Z, Yao X, et al. Anthracycline dose intensification in acute myeloid leukemia. N Engl J Med 2009;361(13):1249–59.
15. Abdel-Wahab O, Manshouri T, Patel J, et al. Genetic analysis of transforming events that convert chronic myeloproliferative neoplasms to leukemias. Cancer Res 2010;70(2):447–52.
16. Kosmider O, Delabesse E, de Mas VM, et al. TET2 mutations in secondary acute myeloid leukemias: a French retrospective study. Haematologica 2011;96(7): 1059–63.
17. Figueroa ME, Abdel-Wahab O, Lu C, et al. Leukemic IDH1 and IDH2 mutations result in a hypermethylation phenotype, disrupt TET2 function, and impair hematopoietic differentiation. Cancer Cell 2010;18(6):553–67.
18. Xu W, Yang H, Liu Y, et al. Oncometabolite 2-hydroxyglutarate is a competitive inhibitor of alpha-ketoglutarate-dependent dioxygenases. Cancer Cell 2011; 19(1):17–30.
19. Boissel N, Nibourel O, Renneville A, et al. Prognostic impact of isocitrate dehydrogenase enzyme isoforms 1 and 2 mutations in acute myeloid leukemia: a study by the Acute Leukemia French Association Group. J Clin Oncol 2010;28(23): 3717–23.
20. Abdel-Wahab O, Kilpivaara O, Patel J, et al. The most commonly reported variant in ASXL1 (c.1934dupG;p.Gly646TrpfsX12) is not a somatic alteration. Leukemia 2010;24(9):1656–7.
21. Itzykson R, Kosmider O, Cluzeau T, et al. Impact of TET2 mutations on response rate to azacitidine in myelodysplastic syndromes and low blast count acute myeloid leukemias. Leukemia 2011;25(7):1147–52.
22. Pollyea DA, Raval A, Kusler B, et al. Impact of TET2 mutations on mRNA expression and clinical outcomes in MDS patients treated with DNA methyltransferase inhibitors. Hematol Oncol 2011;29(3):157–60.
23. Ko M, Huang Y, Jankowska AM, et al. Impaired hydroxylation of 5-methylcytosine in myeloid cancers with mutant TET2. Nature 2010;468(7325):839–43.
24. Mardis ER, Ding L, Dooling DJ, et al. Recurring mutations found by sequencing an acute myeloid leukemia genome. N Engl J Med 2009;361(11):1058–66.
25. Dang L, White DW, Gross S, et al. Cancer-associated IDH1 mutations produce 2-hydroxyglutarate. Nature 2009;462(7274):739–44.
26. Ward P, Cross J, Lu C, et al. Identification of additional IDH mutations associated with oncometabolite R(-)-2-hydroxyglutarate production. Oncogene 2011. [Epub ahead of print].
27. Chou WC, Huang YN, Huang CF, et al. A single-tube, sensitive multiplex method for screening of isocitrate dehydrogenase 1 (IDH1) mutations. Blood 2010; 116(3):495–6.
28. Tefferi A, Lasho TL, Abdel-Wahab O, et al. IDH1 and IDH2 mutation studies in 1473 patients with chronic-, fibrotic- or blast-phase essential thrombocythemia, polycythemia vera or myelofibrosis. Leukemia 2010;24(7):1302–9.
29. Abbas S, Lugthart S, Kavelaars FG, et al. Acquired mutations in the genes encoding IDH1 and IDH2 both are recurrent aberrations in acute myeloid leukemia (AML): prevalence and prognostic value. Blood 2010;116(12):2122–6.
30. Chou WC, Hou HA, Chen CY, et al. Distinct clinical and biologic characteristics in adult acute myeloid leukemia bearing the isocitrate dehydrogenase 1 mutation. Blood 2010;115(14):2749–54.

31. Green CL, Evans CM, Zhao L, et al. The prognostic significance of IDH2 mutations in AML depends on the location of the mutation. Blood 2011;118(2):409–12.

32. Green CL, Evans CM, Hills RK, et al. The prognostic significance of IDH1 mutations in younger adult patients with acute myeloid leukemia is dependent on FLT3/ITD status. Blood 2010;116(15):2779–82.

33. Ward PS, Patel J, Wise DR, et al. The common feature of leukemia-associated IDH1 and IDH2 mutations is a neomorphic enzyme activity converting alpha-ketoglutarate to 2-hydroxyglutarate. Cancer Cell 2010;17(3):225–34.

34. Paschka P, Schlenk RF, Gaidzik VI, et al. IDH1 and IDH2 mutations are frequent genetic alterations in acute myeloid leukemia and confer adverse prognosis in cytogenetically normal acute myeloid leukemia with NPM1 mutation without FLT3 internal tandem duplication. J Clin Oncol 2010;28(22):3636–43.

35. Ley TJ, Ding L, Walter MJ, et al. DNMT3A mutations in acute myeloid leukemia. N Engl J Med 2010;363(25):2424–33.

36. Yan XJ, Xu J, Gu ZH, et al. Exome sequencing identifies somatic mutations of DNA methyltransferase gene DNMT3A in acute monocytic leukemia. Nat Genet 2011;43(4):309–15.

37. Yamashita Y, Yuan J, Suetake I, et al. Array-based genomic resequencing of human leukemia. Oncogene 2010;29(25):3723–31.

38. Walter MJ, Ding L, Shen D, et al. Recurrent DNMT3A mutations in patients with myelodysplastic syndromes. Leukemia 2011;25(7):1153–8.

39. Abdel-Wahab O, Pardanani A, Rampal R, et al. DNMT3A mutational analysis in primary myelofibrosis, chronic myelomonocytic leukemia and advanced phases of myeloproliferative neoplasms. Leukemia 2011;25(7):1219–20.

40. Thol F, Damm F, Ludeking A, et al. Incidence and prognostic influence of DNMT3A mutations in acute myeloid leukemia. J Clin Oncol 2011;29(21):2889–96.

41. Andersson AK, Miller DW, Lynch JA, et al. IDH1 and IDH2 mutations in pediatric acute leukemia. Leukemia, in press.

42. Damm F, Thol F, Hollink I, et al. Prevalence and prognostic value of IDH1 and IDH2 mutations in childhood AML: a study of the AML-BFM and DCOG study groups. Leukemia. [Epub ahead of print].

43. Ho PA, Kutny MA, Alonzo TA, et al. Leukemic mutations in the methylation-associated genes DNMT3A and IDH2 are rare events in pediatric AML: a report from the Children's Oncology Group. Pediatr Blood Cancer 2011;57(2):204–9.

44. Langemeijer SM, Jansen JH, Hooijer J, et al. TET2 mutations in childhood leukemia. Leukemia 2011;25(1):189–92.

45. Tang JL, Hou HA, Chen CY, et al. AML1/RUNX1 mutations in 470 adult patients with de novo acute myeloid leukemia: prognostic implication and interaction with other gene alterations. Blood 2009;114(26):5352–61.

46. Shih LY, Huang CF, Wu JH, et al. Internal tandem duplication of FLT3 in relapsed acute myeloid leukemia: a comparative analysis of bone marrow samples from 108 adult patients at diagnosis and relapse. Blood 2002;100(7):2387–92.

47. Schlenk RF, Dohner K, Krauter J, et al. Mutations and treatment outcome in cytogenetically normal acute myeloid leukemia. N Engl J Med 2008;358(18):1909–18.

48. Liu TC, Lin PM, Chang JG, et al. Mutation analysis of PTEN/MMAC1 in acute myeloid leukemia. Am J Hematol 2000;63(4):170–5.

49. Van Vlierberghe P, Patel J, Abdel-Wahab O, et al. PHF6 mutations in adult acute myeloid leukemia. Leukemia 2011;25(1):130–4.

50. Bernt KM, Zhu N, Sinha AU, et al. MLL-rearranged leukemia is dependent on aberrant H3K79 methylation by DOT1L. Cancer Cell 2011;20(1):66–78.

51. Daigle SR, Olhava EJ, Therkelsen CA, et al. Selective killing of mixed lineage leukemia cells by a potent small-molecule DOT1L inhibitor. Cancer Cell 2011; 20(1):53–65.
52. Kosmider O, Gelsi-Boyer V, Ciudad M, et al. TET2 gene mutation is a frequent and adverse event in chronic myelomonocytic leukemia. Haematologica 2009; 94(12):1676–81.
53. Marcucci G, Maharry K, Wu YZ, et al. IDH1 and IDH2 gene mutations identify novel molecular subsets within de novo cytogenetically normal acute myeloid leukemia: a Cancer and Leukemia Group B study. J Clin Oncol 2010;28(14): 2348–55.
54. Rockova V, Abbas S, Wouters BJ, et al. Risk stratification of intermediate-risk acute myeloid leukemia: integrative analysis of a multitude of gene mutation and gene expression markers. Blood 2011;118(4):1069–76.
55. Schnittger S, Haferlach C, Ulke M, et al. IDH1 mutations are detected in 6.6% of 1414 AML patients and are associated with intermediate risk karyotype and unfavorable prognosis in adults younger than 60 years and unmutated NPM1 status. Blood 2010;116(25):5486–96.
56. Thol F, Damm F, Wagner K, et al. Prognostic impact of IDH2 mutations in cytogenetically normal acute myeloid leukemia. Blood 2010;116(4):614–6.
57. Wagner K, Damm F, Gohring G, et al. Impact of IDH1 R132 mutations and an IDH1 single nucleotide polymorphism in cytogenetically normal acute myeloid leukemia: SNP rs11554137 is an adverse prognostic factor. J Clin Oncol 2010; 28(14):2356–64.

Diagnostic and Prognostic Value of Cytogenetics in Acute Myeloid Leukemia

David Grimwade, PhD, FRCPath[a],*, Krzysztof Mrózek, MD, PhD[b]

KEYWORDS

- Cytogenetics • Acute myeloid leukemia • Diagnosis
- Prognosis

The last 4 decades have seen major advances in understanding the genetic basis of acute myeloid leukemia (AML), paralleled by substantial improvements in survival of children and younger adults with the disease. A key step forward was the discovery in the 1970s by pioneers in the field such as Rowley and colleagues[1,2] that AML cells harbor recurring cytogenetic abnormalities, such as t(8;21)(q22;q22) in AML[1] and t(15;17)(q22;q21) in acute promyelocytic leukemia,[2] which was enabled by the introduction of chromosome banding techniques.[3,4] This paved the way for the identification of the genes involved in chromosomal rearrangements, which has provided major insights into the regulation of normal hematopoiesis and how disruption of key transcription factors and epigenetic modulators promote leukemic transformation. To date, more than 100 balanced chromosomal rearrangements (translocations, insertions, and inversions) have been identified and cloned,[5] with evidence suggesting that these are critical initiating events in the pathogenesis of AML. It has become apparent that karyotype analysis identifies biologically distinct subsets of AML that differ in their response to therapy and treatment outcome (reviewed in Refs.[6–9]). This information has been taken into account in the latest revision of the World Health Organization (WHO) classification,[10,11] and cytogenetics has been widely adopted to provide the framework for development of risk-stratified treatment approaches to patient management.

[a] Cancer Genetics Laboratory, Department of Medical & Molecular Genetics, Guy's Hospital, King's College London School of Medicine, 8th Floor, Guy's Tower, London SE1 9RT, UK
[b] Comprehensive Cancer Center, James Cancer Hospital & Solove Research Institute, Room 1232 A, The Ohio State University, 300 West Tenth Avenue, Columbus, OH 43210-1228, USA
* Corresponding author.
E-mail address: david.grimwade@genetics.kcl.ac.uk

Hematol Oncol Clin N Am 25 (2011) 1135–1161
doi:10.1016/j.hoc.2011.09.018
0889-8588/11/$ – see front matter © 2011 Elsevier Inc. All rights reserved.

hemonc.theclinics.com

CYTOGENETIC ENTITIES RECOGNIZED IN THE WHO CLASSIFICATION OF AML

The latest (2008) revision of the WHO classification[10,11] is organized in a hierarchical fashion, with the first group to be distinguished being AML with particular balanced translocations or inversions (and their molecular counterparts), defined as "AML with recurrent genetic abnormalities" (**Box 1**), which includes the t(15;17)(q22;q21), the diagnostic hallmark of acute promyelocytic leukemia (APL), which is one of the common molecular subtypes of AML, accounting for ~12% of cases. Cloning of the translocation breakpoints in the early 1990s[12–14] showed that the t(15;17) leads to fusion of the gene encoding the myeloid transcription factor RARA (Retinoic Acid Receptor Alpha) with a previously unknown gene designated *PML* (ProMyelocytic Leukemia), which has subsequently been found to be involved in growth suppression and regulation of apoptosis (reviewed by Brown and colleagues[15]). Although most APL cases harbor an underlying *PML-RARA* fusion formed as a result of the t(15;17), often cytogenetically cryptic insertion events or more complex rearrangements (discussed later); in approximately 1% to 2% of APL cases, *RARA* is fused to an alternative partner.[16] These latter cases are designated AML with a variant *RARA* translocation in the revised WHO classification, which include those involving *ZBTB16* (*PLZF*), *NPM1*, *NUMA*, *FIP1L1*, and *BCOR*, formed as a result of the t(11;17)(q23;q21), t(5;17)(q35;q21), t(11;17)(q13;q21), t(4;17)(q12;q21), and t(X;17)(p11;q21), respectively, and *PRKAR1A* and *STAT5B* genes following rearrangements involving 17q.[17–23] The nature of the fusion partner has an important bearing on disease biology, particularly the response to molecularly targeted therapies (ie, all-*trans* retinoic acid [ATRA] and arsenic trioxide [ATO].[24] Sensitivity to ATRA, which targets the ligand-binding domain in the RARα moiety in the C-terminal region of the fusion proteins (as well as wild-type RARα), has been documented in APL subtypes involving PML, NPM1, NUMA, and FIP1L1[24]; whereas PLZF-RARα and STAT5B-RARα have both been associated with primary resistance to retinoids and a poorer prognosis.[23,25,26] In the case of t(11;17)(q23;q21)/*PLZF-RARA*–associated APL, the retinoid insensitivity is compounded by expression of the reciprocal RARα-PLZF fusion product, which functions as a transcriptional activator targeting PLZF-binding sites, leading to upregulation of cellular retinoic acid binding protein I (CRABP1), which sequesters retinoic acid, limiting its access to the nucleus.[27] To date, sensitivity to ATO has only been shown in *PML-RARA*–positive APL, reflecting the capacity of arsenic to bind directly to the PML moiety of the fusion protein inducing its degradation via the proteosome.[28] The importance of deregulation of retinoid signaling pathways in the pathogenesis of APL has been underlined by a recent report of a case with classic morphologic features, but with t(11;12)(p15;q13), leading to fusion of an alternative RAR family member (RARγ) with *NUP98*, which is a recurrent target of chromosomal translocations in AML.[29]

Approximately 10% of AML are classified as having core binding factor (CBF) leukemia with balanced chromosomal rearrangements that disrupt genes encoding components of a heterodimeric transcription factor complex comprising RUNX1 (AML1, CBFα) and CBFβ, which plays a critical role in hematopoiesis.[30] The CBFα subunit is targeted by the t(8;21)(q22;q22), which fuses *RUNX1* (*AML1*, *CBFA2*) to the gene encoding the *RUNX1T1* (formerly *ETO* [Eight Twenty-One]) transcriptional repressor, thereby potentially silencing *RUNX1* target genes.[30,31] The β subunit is targeted by the inv(16)(p13.1q22) or the less common t(16;16)(p13.1;q22), in which it is fused to the gene encoding myosin heavy chain (*MYH11*). Although alternative fusion partners of *CBFB* have not been reported to date, *RUNX1* is a recurrent translocation target in non-CBF acute leukemias, where it can be fused to *ETV6* (*TEL*) as a result of

---

Box 1
Cytogenetic abnormalities used in the WHO (2008) classification of AML

Cytogenetic abnormalities used to define entities within the WHO category of "AML with recurrent genetic abnormalities"

t(8;21)(q22;q22); *RUNX1-RUNX1T1*

inv(16)(p13.1q22) or t(16;16)(p13.1;q22); *CBFB-MYH11*

t(15;17)(q22;q12); *PML-RARA*

t(9;11)(p22;q23); *MLLT3-MLL*

t(6;9)(p23;q34); *DEK-NUP214*

inv(3)(q21q26.2) or t(3;3)(q21;q26.2); *RPN1-EVI1*

t(1;22)(p13;q13); *RBM15-MKL1*

Cytogenetic abnormalities sufficient to diagnose the WHO category of "AML with myelodysplasia-related changes"

Complex karyotype

    (defined as 3 or more unrelated abnormalities, none of which can be a translocation or inversion associated with AML with recurrent genetic abnormalities)

Unbalanced abnormalities

    −7 or del(7q)

    −5 or del(5q)

    i(17q) or t(17p)

    −13 or del(13q)

    del(11q)

    del(12p) or t(12p)

    del(9q)

    idic(X)(q13)

Balanced abnormalities

    t(11;16)(q23;p13.3)[a]

    t(3;21)(q26.2;q22.1)[a]

    t(1;3)(p36.3;q21.1)

    t(2;11)(p21;q23)[a]

    t(5;12)(q33;p12)

    t(5;7)(q33;q11.2)

    t(5;17)(q33;p13)

    t(5;10)(q33;q21)

    t(3;5)(q25;q34)

[a] A translocation commonly occurring in therapy-related AML. Before this translocation can be used as evidence for diagnosis of AML with myelodysplasia-related changes, therapy-related disease should be excluded.
    Data from Vardiman JW, Thiele J, Arber DA, et al. The 2008 revision of the World Health Organization (WHO) classification of myeloid neoplasms and acute leukemia: rationale and important changes. Blood 2009;114(5):937–51.

the cytogenetically cryptic t(12;21)(p13;q22) in pediatric acute lymphoblastic leukemia (ALL), or to a range of partners in AML,[32,33] including *EVI1/MDS1* as a result of t(3;21)(q26;q22) in "AML with myelodysplasia (MDS)-related changes" (see **Box 1**). *RUNX1* has also been implicated in therapy-related leukemias arising following exposure to drugs targeting topoisomerase II.[34,35]

The *MLL* (Myeloid/Lymphoid or Mixed-Lineage Leukemia) gene located at 11q23 is a further recurrent translocation target in acute leukemia, with more than 60 partner genes now characterized.[36] MLL is an epigenetic regulator that plays a critical role in hematopoiesis, modulating *HOX* gene expression.[37] The commonest *MLL* translocation observed in AML is the t(9;11)(p22;q23), which occurs in ~2% of cases and leads to fusion of *MLL* with *MLLT3* (formerly known as *AF9*). The t(9;11)(p22;q23), which has been associated with a relatively favorable outcome in some pediatric[38] and adult[39] AML studies, is distinguished as a separate entity in the latest WHO classification. Apart from the t(9;11), the most frequent other *MLL* translocations observed in AML are t(6;11)(q27;q23) involving *MLLT4* (*AF6*), t(11;19)(q23;p13.3) involving *MLLT1* (*ENL*), t(11;19)(q23;p13.1) involving *ELL*, and complex rearrangements between 10p12 and 11q23 (eg, a reciprocal translocation and an inversion of an 11q segment translocated to 10p12 or inverted insertion of an 11q segment into 10p12 or a 10p segment into 11q23), in which the fusion partner is *MLLT10* (*AF10*).[40,41] Although most translocations involving *MLL* occur in de novo leukemia, the locus is a recurrent translocation target in therapy-related leukemias,[42] particularly those arising following exposure to the epipodophyllotoxin class of topoisomerase II poisons.[43] Such cases are classified within the WHO as "therapy-related AML".

The remaining subtypes of AML distinguished as separate disease entities by cytogenetics are those characterized by the t(6;9)(p23;q34), inv(3)(q21q26.2) or t(3;3)(q21;q26.2) and t(1;22)(p13;q13). The t(6;9)(p23;q34) is found in ~1% of AML and leads to fusion of the *DEK* gene at 6p23 with *NUP214* (*CAN*), which encodes a component of the nuclear pore complex.[44,45] The inv(3) or t(3;3) occurs in a similar proportion of AML cases and is associated with upregulation of the zinc finger transcription factor EVI1, which is involved in normal hematopoiesis. AML with inv(3) or t(3;3) may present de novo, or secondary to prior MDS and is characterized by a normal or increased presenting platelet count and abnormal megakaryopoiesis with micromegakaryocytes in the marrow.[46] *EVI1* has long been implicated in leukemogenesis, having been identified as a recurrent integration target in murine retroviral mutagenesis screens[47,48]; further evidence has recently been provided by characterization of 2 cases of MDS associated with insertional activation of *EVI1* occurring as a complication of gene therapy for chronic granulomatous disease.[49] Analysis of these 2 cases provided important insights into potential mechanisms underlying acquisition of additional cytogenetic abnormalities in AML, with both cases showing loss of chromosome 7 (monosomy 7), which is well recognized as a frequent secondary abnormality in cases with inv(3) or t(3;3). Forced overexpression of *EVI1* was found to disrupt normal centrosome duplication, suggesting that activation of *EVI1* as a result of retroviral insertion or chromosomal translocation leads to genomic instability, giving rise to acquisition of additional changes such as monosomy 7 involved in progression to MDS and AML.

AML with t(1;22)(p13;q13) is extremely rare (to date, only ~40 cases have been reported worldwide[5]) and is associated with acute megakaryoblastic leukemia occurring in infants and young children (<3 years of age), particularly those without Down syndrome. The translocation fuses *RBM15* (for RNA-binding motif protein 15, also known as *OTT*) with *MKL1* (MegaKaryocyte Leukemia 1 or *MAL*),[50,51] which is involved in normal megakaryocyte maturation.[52]

Apart from distinguishing AML with recurrent genetic abnormalities (as described earlier), for cases lacking one of these aberrations (or their molecular counterparts), cytogenetics has also been used in the latest WHO classification as a criterion (in conjunction with ≥20% leukemic blasts in the marrow) to define a subgroup of "AML with MDS-related changes", as detailed in **Box 1**. Some of these cytogenetic entities are common, such as monosomy 5 and 7 (−5 and −7) or deletion of the long arms of these chromosomes [del(5q) and del(7q)], which often occur as part of a complex karyotype. However, although −7 is recurrently observed both as a sole chromosome aberration and as part of a complex karyotype, −5 is rare in patients with noncomplex karyotypes.[53] Moreover, most patients with a complex karyotype with −5 detected using banding techniques (eg, G-banding) also do not harbor true monosomy 5, because segments from a seemingly missing chromosome 5 can be found using spectral karyotyping[54] or fluorescence in situ hybridization (FISH)[55] in marker chromosomes or unbalanced structural aberrations only partially identified by G-banding. Although balanced translocations such as the t(11;16)(q23;p13.3), t(3;21)(q26.2;q22.1) involving *MLL* and *RUNX1*, respectively, and the t(3;5)(q25;q34) that generates the *NPM1-MLF1* fusion[56] may be initiating lesions in the development of leukemia, many of the changes considered as "MDS-related" entail loss of chromosomal segments or whole chromosomes, which are poorly understood at the molecular level and may represent secondary and cooperating lesions in AML pathogenesis (reviewed in Refs.[57,58]). Some of the aberrations designated MDS related, especially balanced translocations and idic(X)(q13), are extremely rare,[59] making it challenging to characterize their biologic features and establish their impact on the clinical outcome.

INFLUENCE OF PATIENT AGE ON CYTOGENETIC PROFILE IN AML

AML is uncommon, with an overall incidence of approximately 4 cases per 100,000 population.[60] Age has a major bearing on disease frequency and biology, with AML being particularly uncommon in children (0.6 cases/100,000), accounting for ~20% of acute leukemias arising in this age group (<16 years). The disease increases in incidence in adults (2 cases/100,000 for ages 16–60 years), and is becoming an increasing health care problem as the population ages (incidence 9.7/100,000 for ages 60–74 years; incidence 20.2/100,000 for ages ≥75 years).

The pattern of cytogenetic abnormalities differs according to age. In infants, translocations involving the *MLL* gene account for a greater proportion of cases than in other age groups. In a series comprising 62 infants with AML (<1 year of age), 11q23 abnormalities were identified in 35%, with t(9;11) accounting for half of the cases.[61] Apart from the t(1;22) associated with acute megakaryoblastic leukemia (described earlier), which is detected in ~5% of infant AML, translocations involving the *ETV6* (*TEL*) locus at 12p13 have also been particularly associated with AML presenting in this age group. The distinct pattern of cytogenetic abnormalities observed in AML presenting in infancy, compared with older children and adults, merits consideration for the potential reasons underlying this phenomenon and raises some interesting issues concerning the biology of these disorders. Many of the leukemias presenting in infancy develop in utero and hence the initiating mutations may arise in embryonic hematopoietic stem/progenitor cell populations, which may be distinct from the cellular origins of AML presenting in older children or in adulthood. The characteristics of the stem/progenitor cells, particularly in terms of nuclear architecture and the nature of the genes that are actively transcribed, may have a critical bearing on the chromosomal regions that are most susceptible to DNA damage and aberrant repair, which may provide an explanation for why rearrangements of *MLL* and *ETV6* are particularly prevalent in both AML and ALL arising in children. Moreover, it is clear that fusion genes created by these translocations are extremely potent, giving rise to overt leukemia within short latency periods from occurrence of the initiating mutation.

In older children and younger adults, recurring balanced translocations/inversions, particularly t(15;17), t(8;21), and inv(16) or t(16;16), between them account for ~30% of AML, whereas cytogenetic entities now defined as "MDS-related" in the WHO classification, particularly −5/del(5q), −7/del(7q), and complex karyotype, occur in ~15% of cases. In older adults, there is a particular expansion of AML cases with chromosomal losses and gains, with an increase in cases with MDS-related changes including complex karyotype. This expansion mirrors the increased prevalence of secondary AML in older adults against the background of an antecedent hematological disorder, particularly MDS or myeloproliferative neoplasm, or occurring as a complication of treatment with chemotherapy and/or radiotherapy (which is an increasing problem as more patients survive their primary tumors).

CYTOGENETICS AS A PROGNOSTIC FACTOR

Cytogenetics is the most powerful independent prognostic factor in AML and provides the framework for risk-stratification schemes that have been generally adopted to guide the treatment approach. Cytogenetic analysis is now considered a mandatory component of the diagnostic work-up of patients with suspected AML.[62] Apart from identifying patients with particular subtypes of AML who may benefit from molecularly targeted therapies [ie, ATRA/ATO in t(15;17)/*PML-RARA*-associated APL and tyrosine kinase inhibitors for patients with t(9;22)/*BCR-ABL1*-associated AML], karyotype analysis has been used to distinguish groups of patients with substantially different probabilities of achieving a complete remission (CR) and risks of relapse, particularly as a tool to guide transplantation in first CR. The major cooperative trial groups have typically distinguished between favorable, intermediate (standard), and adverse cytogenetic risk groups. However, several notable differences between the various classification systems have been described (**Table 1**), which not only carries implications for patient management, but may also be a confounding factor when comparing trial results, particularly when drawing conclusions as to which groups of patients are most (and least) likely to benefit from allogeneic transplant in first CR. The t(15;17), t(8;21), and inv(16) or t(16;16) comprise the favorable risk group in most classification schemes; although some classifications do not include t(15;17), its favorable prognostic significance has been shown in numerous other studies. However, there has been a lack of consensus concerning the prognostic relevance of additional cytogenetic abnormalities in patients with CBF leukemia (see **Table 1**). In particular, the Southwest Oncology Group (SWOG) exclude from the favorable risk group those patients in whom the t(8;21) occurs as part of complex karyotype (defined as 3 or more abnormalities) and/or those in whom there is a deletion of the long arm of chromosome 9 [del(9q)], who account for 16% and 12% of patients with this subtype of CBF leukemia.[53] The exclusion of the patients with del(9q) is based on an early, small study in which patients with this additional change were noted to have a poorer outcome.[63] However, this finding has not been substantiated on analysis of much larger patient numbers[53,64–66]; complex karyotype has also not been found to adversely affect the treatment outcome of patients with t(8;21)[53,64] [or those with inv(16) or t(16;16)[64]]. The SWOG group has also categorized del(16q) as favorable risk alongside the inv(16), although it is now clear that del(16q) cases are

Table 1
Risk-group assignments of patients with particular cytogenetic abnormalities in major collaborative studies of adult AML

Risk-group Assignment	MRC (Grimwade et al,[70] 1998)	SWOG/ECOG[a] (Slovak et al,[170] 2000)	CALGB[b] (Byrd et al,[64] 2002)			GIMEMA/AML10 (Suciu et al,[171] 2003)	GERMAN AMLCG (Schoch et al,[172] 2003)	HOVON/SAKK (Cornelissen et al,[71] 2007)	MRC Refined (Grimwade et al,[53] 2010)
			CR Rate	**CIR**	**OS**				
Favorable	t(15;17), t(8;21), inv(16)/t(16;16)	t(15;17), t(8;21) [lacking del(9q) and complex karyotype], inv(16)/t(16;16)/del(16q)	t(8;21), inv(16)/t(16;16)	t(8;21), t(16;16)	t(8;21), inv(16)/t(16;16), del(9q)[c]	t(8;21), inv(16)/t(16;16)	t(15;17), t(8;21), inv(16)/t(16;16)	t(8;21) with WBC <20×10⁹/L, inv(16)/t(16;16) and lacking adverse abn	t(15;17), t(8;21), inv(16)/t(16;16)
Intermediate	Normal karyotype, +8, +21, +22, del(7q), del(9q), abn(11q23), other structural/numerical abn	Normal karyotype, +6, +8, −Y, del(12p)	Normal karyotype, −Y, del(5q), t(6;9), t(6;11), −7, loss of 7q, +8 sole, +8 with 1 other abn, del(9q), t(9;11), del(11q), +11, t(11;19)(q23;p13.1), +13, del(20q), +21	Normal karyotype, −Y, t(9;11), del(9q), +8 sole, +8 with 1 other abn, +11, +13	Normal karyotype, −Y, del(5q), loss of 7q, t(9;11), +11, del(11q), abn(12p), +13, del(20q), +21	Normal karyotype, −Y	Normal karyotype, abn other than favorable or adverse	Normal karyotype, other noncomplex abn, pts without karyotype	Normal karyotype, abn other than favorable or adverse
Adverse	abn(3q), −5/del(5q), −7, complex karyotype [≥5 abn, excluding pts with favorable changes]	−5/del(5q), −7/del(7q), abn(3q), abn(9q), abn(11q), abn(20q), abn(21q), abn(17p), t(6;9), t(9;22), complex karyotype (≥3 abn)	inv(3) or t(3;3), abn(12p), complex karyotype [≥3 abn, excluding pts with t(8;21), inv(16)/t(16;16) and t(9;11)]	−7, +21, complex karyotype [≥3 abn, excluding pts with t(8;21), inv(16)/t(16;16) and t(9;11)]	inv(3) or t(3;3), t(6;9), t(6;11), −7, +8 sole, +8 with 1 other abn, t(11;19) (q23;p13.1), complex karyotype [≥3 abn, excluding pts with t(8;21), inv(16)/t(16;16) and t(9;11)]	complex karyotype (unspecified), abn(3q), −5/del(5q), −7/del(7q), t(6;9), t(9;22), abn(11q23), absence of favorable abn[d]	inv(3)/t(3;3), −5/del(5q), −7/del(7q), abn(11q23), del(12p), abn(17p), complex karyotype (≥3 abn)	abn(3q), −5/del(5q), −7/del(7q), abn(11q23), t(6;9), t(9;22), complex karyotype (≥3 abn), pts with intermediate cytogenetics with a late CR, reached after cycle II of induction	abn(3q) [excluding t(3;5)], inv(3)/t(3;3), add(5q)/del(5q)/−5, add(7q)/del(7q)/−7 (excluding pts with favorable karyotype), t(6;11), t(10;11), t(11q23) [excluding t(9;11) and t(11;19)], t(9;22), −17/abn(17p), complex karyotype ≥4 abn, excluding pts with favorable or adverse changes)

Abbreviations: CALGB, Cancer and Leukemia Group B; CIR, cumulative incidence of relapse; ECOG, Eastern Cooperative Oncology Group; MRC, Medical Research Council; OS, overall survival; abn, abnormality; pts, patients; SWOG, Southwest Oncology Group.

a All other, unclassified abnormalities were considered to have unknown risk.

b Abnormalities not specified as conferring favorable, intermediate, or adverse risk were not included in the risk assessment model.

c Favorable for a group of 13 patients with del(9q) that included 6 who underwent transplantation off protocol; intermediate for nontransplanted patients treated with chemotherapy only.

d The abnormalities listed were denoted as "very bad." This classification also included "bad" cytogenetics, which was defined as "the presence of other abnormalities without good or very bad cytogenetic features."

heterogeneous at the molecular level, with true del(16q) that are not misinterpreted inv(16) lacking an underlying *CBFB-MYH11* fusion.[67]

A normal karyotype is identified in ~40% to 45% of AML cases presenting in adults aged 16 to 60 years and, overall, these patients have an intermediate prognosis. However, as discussed later and elsewhere,[68,69] cytogenetically normal AML (CN-AML) is highly heterogeneous at the molecular level, and mutation screening is now widely applied to refine risk stratification in this group (see later discussion). Several cytogenetic abnormalities have been universally considered to confer a poor prognosis [eg, −5/del(5q), −7, and inv(3) or t(3;3)]. However, there has been little consensus as to the outcome of various structural and numerical abnormalities, including cases with rare recurring cytogenetic abnormalities (ie, with individual incidence <2%), which together account for approximately 10% of AML and have variably been considered to predict an intermediate or adverse prognosis (see **Table 1**). Another major source of variability is in the definition of a complex karyotype, with most groups applying this term to karyotypes comprising at least 3 unrelated abnormalities [in most instances excluding t(15;17), t(8;21), and inv(16) or t(16;16)], whereas in the original UK Medical Research Council classification, a higher cutoff of greater than or equal to 5 abnormalities was adopted[70] but later revised to greater than or equal to 4 abnormalities.[53]

There are significant differences in the risk-group classifications of some of the rarer cytogenetic entities, which could reflect differences in the age profiles of the patients studied, as well as problems in obtaining reliable outcome data because of small sample sizes. However, it is also possible that interstudy and intrastudy differences in treatment could have played a part, affecting the outcome of particular cytogenetically defined subsets of AML.

Despite the challenges, it would be helpful if greater standardization in risk stratification in AML could be achieved, to facilitate development of optimized treatment approaches and reporting of outcome data, thereby enabling more reliable comparison of results from different international trial groups. Establishing robust outcome data for particular cytogenetic subgroups is clinically important, taking into account the results of a recent meta-analysis that has suggested that a relapse risk in excess of 35% can provide a useful working threshold to identify patients in whom allogeneic transplant may confer a survival benefit.[71] Therefore, patients with favorable risk AML [ie, those with t(15;17)/*PML-RARA* and CBF leukemia with t(8;21)/*RUNX1-RUNX1T1* or inv(16)/t(16;16)/*CBFB-MYH11*] are no longer routinely subject to transplantation in first CR, which confers no overall survival advantage.[72]

Refinement of Cytogenetic Classification in Younger Adults with AML

In an attempt to reconcile differences between several existing cytogenetic classification systems used to direct therapy in younger adults, the UK Medical Research Council (MRC) examined outcomes for a large number (>50) of cytogenetic entities within a cohort of 5876 patients (median age 44 years) who received comparable therapy in successive clinical trials, with prolonged follow-up (median 7.3 years).[53] In multivariable analysis taking into account age, presenting white blood cell count (WBC) and type of AML (de novo vs secondary), the t(15;17), t(8;21), and inv(16) or t(16;16) were robustly confirmed as powerful independent predictors of favorable outcome, irrespective of the presence of additional cytogenetic abnormalities ($P<10^{-12}$). In patients with inv(16), the presence of additional abnormalities, particularly trisomy 22, was associated with a significantly better outcome,[53] in accordance with previous studies.[65,66] This finding may relate to differences in presenting WBC, which is significantly higher in patients with inv(16) as the sole abnormality and cannot be explained by differences in the frequency of *KIT* mutations, which constitute an adverse prognostic factor in patients with inv(16) or t(16;16).[73,74] The multivariable analysis conducted by the MRC group did not reveal any novel cytogenetic entities conferring a favorable outcome. However, a large number of abnormalities that independently predicted an adverse prognosis were identified (see **Table 1**). Apart from −5/del(5q), −7/del(7q), and inv(3) or t(3;3), which are well recognized as conferring adverse risk, the study also confirmed that t(9;22)(q34;q11), which had hitherto been the subject of small case series,[75] also predicts a poor prognosis (**Fig. 1**). There have been conflicting data for the outcomes of patients with translocations involving 11q23, which have been considered to confer a poor prognosis, with the possible exception of those with the t(9;11). In the MRC series, better outcome was observed in patients with the t(9;11)(p22;q23) and t(11;19)(q23;p13), although involvement of *MLLT1* and *ELL* was not distinguished; whereas patients with t(6;11)(q27;q23) and t(10;11)(p12;q23) involving *MLLT4* and *MLLT10*, respectively, or other 11q23 abnormalities were found to have a significantly poorer outcome in multivariable analysis. Although the t(6;9)(p23;q34) is widely considered to predict a poor outcome in AML,[76] which may in part reflect its frequent association with internal tandem duplication (ITD) in the juxtamembrane domain of the *FLT3* gene encoding Fms like tyrosine kinase 3 (*FLT3*-ITD),[76,77] and was also associated with a high relapse rate in the MRC series (62% at 10 years), the effect was not sufficiently strong to emerge in the multivariable analysis.[53] The MRC study also sought to establish the most robust cutoff to

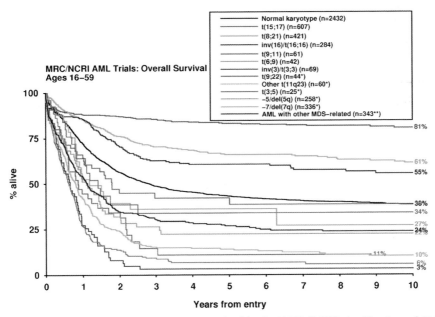

Fig. 1. Outcome of cytogenetic entities recognized in the WHO (2008) classification of AML. Overall survival is shown for 5876 adults with AML (median age 43 years, range 16–59 years) treated in successive Medical Research Council (MRC)/National Cancer Research Institute trials (MRC AML10, AML12, AML15). (*Reprinted from* Grimwade D, Hills RK, Moorman AV, et al. Refinement of cytogenetic classification in acute myeloid leukemia: determination of prognostic significance of rare recurring chromosomal abnormalities amongst 5,876 younger adult patients treated in the UK Medical Research Council trials. Blood 2010; 116(3):354–65; with permission.)

define a karyotype as complex. For this analysis, cytogenetic entities that, in their own right, conferred a favorable or adverse prognosis in the multivariable analysis were excluded, and the impact of complexity was considered solely in the context of standard risk cytogenetic abnormalities. In contrast with previous studies that used cutoffs of 3 or 5 abnormalities to define a complex karyotype, the MRC study suggests that the presence of at least 4 unrelated abnormalities provides the most appropriate cutoff, defining a group with significantly poorer prognosis.[53]

The Dutch HOVON (Haemato Oncology Foundation for Adults in the Netherlands) group also recently revisited the cytogenetic classification of AML and distinguished a subgroup of patients with a so-called monosomal karyotype (MK) that is characterized by a particularly poor prognosis.[78] Patients with non-CBF AML were defined as having a monosomal karyotype from the loss of an autosomal chromosome (ie, excluding −Y and −X) in combination with at least 1 other autosomal monosomy (eg, 44,XY,−7,−18) or 1 or more structural abnormality (eg, 45,XY,inv(3)(q21q26),−7). Monosomal karyotypes almost invariably include at least 1 chromosomal abnormality that would independently be associated with adverse risk. Moreover, because up to 75% of complex karyotypes are hypodiploid (ie, have ≤45 chromosomes) and several pseudodiploid (46 chromosomes) and hyperdiploid complex karyotypes (≥47 chromosomes) also include at least 1 monosomy,[79] most patients with a complex karyotype are considered to have a monosomal karyotype. Overall, approximately half of patients defined as having an adverse karyotype according to standard classification systems have a monosomal karyotype, and several studies have confirmed that the subgroup with MK+ AML have a particularly poor prognosis.[53,80] However, there are preliminary data to suggest that their outcome could be improved by allogeneic transplantation in first remission.[81]

Prognostic Significance of Cytogenetics in Pediatric AML

There have been few large studies considering the impact of cytogenetics on outcome in pediatric AML. The Pediatric Oncology Group (POG) considered a cohort of 478 patients aged less than 21 years, reporting the best outcomes in those with inv(16), t(8;21) and normal karyotype.[82] Patients with the t(15;17), most of whom did not receive ATRA, and those with various 11q23 abnormalities had a poor prognosis. The findings of a more recent, similarly sized study (454 patients <18 years of age) published by the Berlin-Frankfurt-Münster (BFM) group were in accordance with most adult series, showing the best outcomes in patients with inv(16), t(8;21), and t(15;17). Significantly poorer outcomes were observed in patients with monosomy 7 and 11q23 aberrations [apart from t(9;11) as the sole abnormality and the t(11;19)].[83] The largest study to date was conducted by the UK MRC group and considered the prognostic significance of 22 cytogenetically defined subgroups within a cohort of 729 children aged 0 to 15 years.[84] In this study, in which patients with APL were excluded, the best outcomes were observed in the CBF AML, with 10-year overall survivals of ∼80%. In contrast with the POG and BFM studies, patients with 11q23 abnormalities (n = 104) had an intermediate prognosis (61% OS at 10 years), with no evidence of heterogeneity according to the translocation partner. Although this study did not analyze the prognostic significance of secondary aberrations accompanying 11q23 abnormalities, a recent large international effort identified trisomy 8 as independently favorable, and trisomy 19 as adverse, prognostic factors in pediatric 11q23/*MLL*-rearranged AML, whereas complex karyotype was found to be an unfavorable prognosticator in univariable analysis only.[85] In a series analyzed by Harrison and colleagues,[84] several abnormalities that have been associated with adverse risk in adult patients (eg, −5, 3q abnormalities and complex karyotype) were not predictive of a worse outcome. However, significantly poorer survivals were observed in pediatric AML with 5q abnormalities, t(6;9), monosomy 7, trisomy 13, and 12p abnormalities, including translocations involving *ETV6*, with 36% of patients alive at 10 years.[84]

Prognostic Significance of Cytogenetics in Older Adults with AML

The outcome of AML presenting in older adults is poorer (7%–15% 5-year survival for adults >60 years old), compared with when the disease presents in younger individuals. Nevertheless, cytogenetics are still predictive in this age group. The largest study to date was conducted by the MRC group, studying 1065 patients (aged >55 years) treated in the AML11 trial.[86] The best outcome was observed in patients with APL with the t(15;17) and those with CBF leukemia, with a superior CR rate (72%) associated with low rates of resistant disease. However, overall survival rates were poorer than those observed in younger adults with the same cytogenetic abnormalities (only 34% OS at 5 years). Although the relapse rate in patients with APL with the t(15;17) was low (26% at 5 years), the relapse rates in the patients with CBF leukemia were substantially higher (>80% relapse risk at 5 years) compared with younger patients, which may reflect differences in disease biology as well being a consequence of less intensive therapy. Older patients with a complex karyotype (defined as 5 or more abnormalities) had an extremely poor prognosis, with few achieving CR (26%) because of high rates of resistant disease (56%). The small proportion of elderly patients achieving remission almost invariably relapsed, leading to overall survival rates of only 2% at 5 years.[86] Similar data have been published by other groups,[87–89] raising the question of whether elderly patients with high-risk cytogenetics might be most appropriately offered palliative nonintensive treatment approaches or supportive care. In contrast, recent preliminary data indicate that at least some patients aged 60 to 70 years who achieve a CR may benefit from reduced-intensity allogeneic transplantation.[90] Moreover, alternative, novel therapies are also being investigated in older adults with AML.[91] In the MRC series, patients with normal karyotypes or noncomplex cytogenetic aberrations had marginally better outcomes, with 5-year survivals of 15% and 10%, respectively. It is likely that the slightly better outcome in CN-AML occurring in older patients may reflect the influence of cases with *NPM1* gene mutation (see later discussion). The Cancer and Leukemia Group B (CALGB) and German AML Study Groups have both reported on the prognostic impact of cytogenetics in older adults,[87,88] also finding evidence for a better outcome in patients with the t(15;17) and CBF leukemia, and similarly reporting that patients with a complex karyotype have a dismal prognosis. Most recently, the GOELAMS (Groupe Ouest Est d'Etude des Leucémies et Autres Maladies du Sang) group showed in a study involving 186 older adults (>60 years) with unfavorable cytogenetic abnormalities that presence of a monosomal karyotype (found in 59%) predicted a particularly poor prognosis.[92]

LIMITATIONS OF CYTOGENETICS FOR RISK STRATIFICATION OF AML

Although cytogenetic analysis is routinely used to guide treatment approach, particularly in children and younger adults with AML, there are several important caveats. In particular, cytogenetic analysis can fail in up to 10% of cases, requiring the use of FISH and molecular screening to distinguish prognostically relevant subsets of disease. It is also important to appreciate that approximately 5% of patients harboring one of the fusion genes associated with favorable risk AML (ie, *PML-RARA*, *RUNX1-RUNX1T1*, or *CBFB-MYH11*) as shown by molecular screening using reverse transcriptase (RT) polymerase chain reaction (PCR), would be misclassified by conventional cytogenetic analysis because of a lack of the classic chromosomal abnormality.[16,67,93] In such situations, the fusion gene may be formed by an insertion event (the involved chromosomes can seem normal), simple variant translocations (involving one of the respective chromosomes at the usual breakpoint and an alternative partner chromosome), or more complex rearrangements. It is also important to appreciate that small insertion events leading, for example, to the *PML-RARA* fusion in APL can be missed by FISH using standard probes that are too large to reliably detect subtle fusion signals.[16] As reflected in the latest WHO classification, cases of APL or CBF leukemia with cryptic fusions are considered to be biologically identical to those in which the classic abnormality is identifiable by standard cytogenetic analysis.[10] There is evidence to suggest that the outcome of patients with APL with the *PML-RARA* identified solely on molecular screening is comparable with those with the classic t(15;17), responding similarly to molecularly targeted therapies.[94] A small study suggested that patients with cytogenetically cryptic *RUNX1-RUNX1T1* gene fusions may have a poorer prognosis, but this remains to be substantiated[95]; particularly because gene expression profiling lends further support to the notion that cases in which the *RUNX1-RUNX1T1* fusion results from insertion events are biologically comparable with those with the t(8;21).[96] Highest pickup rates for molecular screening may occur in patients with an underlying *CBFB-MYH11* fusion, because the inv(16) is a subtle cytogenetic lesion that can be missed, particularly in the absence of central cytogenetic review.[97] Molecular screening has also been used to identify cases of AML with cryptic cytogenetic abnormalities associated with poor risk, particularly those with rearrangements of 3q26 leading to upregulation of the *EVI1* gene[98] or a cryptic t(5;11)(q35;p15) resulting in a *NUP98/NSD1* fusion gene.[99] Moreover, application of genome-wide single-nucleotide polymorphism (SNP) microarray analyses can identify acquired submicroscopic lesions of potential prognostic relevance, namely copy number alterations and regions of uniparental disomy (UPD).[100–103]

In the last 15 years there have been major advances in identifying gene mutations underlying the pathogenesis of AML, which have proved particularly useful in distinguishing subsets of patients with normal karyotype with markedly differing outcomes.[68,104,105] The first prognostically important lesion to be identified was *FLT3*-ITD,[106,107] which predicts a significantly increased risk of relapse and a poorer clinical outcome.[108] The prognosis is particularly poor for patients with high *FLT3*-ITD allelic ratio,[77,109] which may stem from homozygous mutations resulting from acquired uniparental disomy,[110] and for patients with coexisting mutations of the Wilms tumor gene (*WT1*).[111–114] Other abnormalities that have been consistently shown to confer a poorer prognosis include mutations in the *RUNX1* gene[115–117] and partial tandem duplications of the *MLL* gene (*MLL*-PTD),[118–121] although recent data indicate that intensive consolidation therapy that includes autologous transplant in the first CR may improve the outcome for patients with CN-AML with the latter rearrangement.[122]

Major steps forward were the discoveries of mutations in the genes encoding CCAAT/enhancer protein α (*CEBPA*) and nucleophosmin (*NPM1*), which serve to identify subsets of patients with AML with favorable prognosis.[123,124] Mutations in the *CEBPA* gene, which encodes a myeloid transcription factor, were first described in 2001 and occur in ~10% of CN-AML.[125] Mutations cluster in both the amino-terminal and carboxy-terminal regions, with the former leading to expression of a - truncated isoform of CEBPA (p30) and loss of the full-length protein (p42).[126] Carboxy-terminal mutations affect regions involved in mediating dimerization and DNA binding. In most patients with *CEBPA* mutations, both alleles are involved, combining an upstream mutation in one allele with a downstream mutation in the other.[125,126] Analysis of patient samples has shown that CEBPA mutations can be inherited through the germline, with progression to AML in later life being associated with acquisition of additional mutations, which can include involvement of the other CEBPA allele.[127,128] Significant insights into the biology of CEBPA mutations have been provided by murine models, which have shown how loss of p42 expression (mimicking biallelic N-terminal CEBPA mutations) or compound heterozygous mutations affecting amino-terminal and carboxy-terminal regions in combination affect hematopoiesis and give rise to AML.[129,130] Although early studies reported that CEBPA mutation predicts a favorable outcome in AML,[121,131–133] it has subsequently been shown that this effect is accounted for by the subset of patients with biallelic mutations, especially those who lack FLT3-ITD.[134–138]

Mutations in NPM1, discovered by Falini and colleagues[124] in 2005, represent the commonest molecular lesion identified in AML to date, occurring in one-third of cases, including 50% to 60% of those with CN-AML. More than 20 different mutations have been described that involve the C-terminal region of the protein and lead to loss of tryptophan residues and generation of a nuclear export signal that act in concert to cause delocalization of nucleophosmin from the nucleoli to the cytoplasm.[139] Nucleophosmin mutation is considered to be a primary lesion in the pathogenesis of AML, being stable over the disease course,[140,141] and has recently been shown to enhance self-renewal of hematopoietic progenitors, associated with expanded myelopoiesis leading to the development of AML in a murine model.[142] Patients with AML harboring an NPM1 mutation in the absence of FLT3-ITD have consistently been shown to have a favorable prognosis.[143–146] NPM1 mutations were also recently shown to be strong, independent predictors of better outcome in older patients, especially those aged 70 years and older.[147] Although several studies have focused on CN-AML,[68] patients with cytogenetic abnormalities that would be considered as standard risk and who harbor an NPM1 mutation have also been reported to have a better outcome in the absence of FLT3-ITD; however, those with FLT3-ITD in the absence of the protective effect of NPM1 mutation have a poor prognosis.[53,148]

FUTURE PERSPECTIVE

In the last 15 years, there have been significant advances in identifying genetic lesions underlying AML that distinguish subgroups of patients with markedly differing outcome, and which are increasingly being used to shape treatment approach. In the late 1990s, cytogenetic analysis was the major tool used for predicting outcome and guiding therapy, with the favorable risk group comprising the t(15;17), t(8;21), and inv(16) or t(16;16) accounting for a quarter of AML arising in children and younger adults. Approximately 15% of younger adults were classified as having adverse risk AML, whereas most (ie, ~60%) were classified as standard risk. As a result of a series of breakthroughs in understanding the molecular basis of AML, coupled with systematic analysis of large cohorts of uniformly treated patients, it has been possible to further refine outcome prediction, distinguishing subsets of patients who would formerly have been classed as standard risk, but who have markedly different prognoses. Patients with biallelic CEBPA mutations or NPM1 mutation who lack FLT3-ITD, and who, respectively, account for 3% and 18% of younger adults with AML (**Fig. 2**), have a comparable outcome with patients with CBF leukemia (**Fig. 3**), and hence are likely to represent further groups of patients who are unlikely to benefit from routine use of allogeneic transplant in first CR. Conversely, improved molecular knowledge and more reliable information concerning rarer recurring cytogenetic

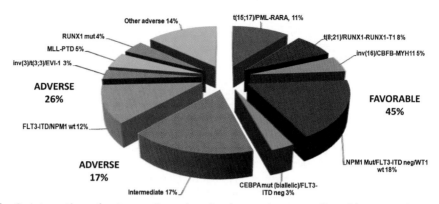

Fig. 2. Integration of cytogenetic and molecular markers to refine risk groups in AML. (*Reprinted from* Smith ML, Hills RK, Grimwade D. Independent prognostic variables in acute myeloid leukaemia. Blood Rev 2011;25(1):39–51; with permission.)

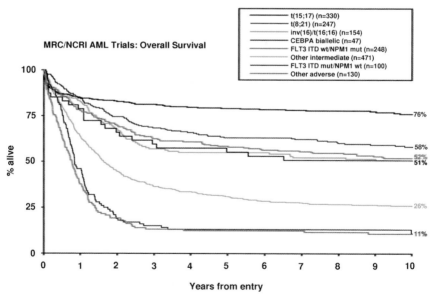

Fig. 3. Outcome of younger adults with AML according to cytogenetic and molecular abnormalities. Overall survival for younger adults treated in the MRC AML10 and AML12 trials reported previously[137,146] for whom cytogenetic data were available. Cases were classified in hierarchical fashion with t(15;17), t(8;21), and inv(16)/t(16;16) at the top of the hierarchy, then *CEBPA* biallelic mutations, $NPM1^{mut}/ITD^{neg}$, $NPM1^{wt}/ITD^{pos}$, other intermediate and other adverse. (*Reprinted from* Grimwade D, Hills RK, Moorman AV, et al. Refinement of cytogenetic classification in acute myeloid leukemia: determination of prognostic significance of rare recurring chromosomal abnormalities amongst 5,876 younger adult patients treated in the UK Medical Research Council trials. Blood 2010;116(3):354–65; with permission.)

aberrations has led to reclassification of a significant proportion of patients as adverse risk, which includes those with FLT3-ITD, RUNX1 mutation, MLL-PTD, or EVI1 overexpression and who lack a favorable cytogenetic abnormality. Patients with such adverse risk features are now routinely considered for allogeneic transplant, although the extent to which this improves outcome of these poor-risk patients remains to be firmly established. To address this, it is important to develop standardized approaches to reporting of clinical trial data that take into account cytogenetic and molecular genetic risk factors. The first such scheme to be developed by an international panel was recently published by the European LeukemiaNet.[62] However, as additional molecular lesions are identified (eg, mutations in TET2, ASXL1, IDH1 and IDH2, DNMT3A; see review by Abdel-Wahab and Levine elsewhere in this issue), particularly as a result of recent high-throughput sequencing initiatives,[149,150] the subgroups of patients with particular constellations of abnormalities represent ever-diminishing proportions of the total population, rendering it challenging, or statistically impossible, to determine their prognostic significance with any reliability, unless very large numbers of patients are analyzed, which would require extensive international collaboration. These issues have been highlighted by recent studies investigating the prognostic significance of mutations in the isocitrate dehydrogenase 1 and 2 genes (IDH1 and IDH2, respectively) (see review by Abdel-Wahab and Levine elsewhere in this issue). Although some data are conflicting,[105] it seems that clinical outcome may not only differ according to which of the 2 genes is mutated but also according to the location of the mutation within the gene. Recent studies suggest that prognostic impact of R140 and R172 mutations in IDH2 differs, with R172 mutations conferring poor prognosis[151–153] and R140 mutations being either not prognostic[151] or associated with a favorable outcome.[152,153]

It is hoped that establishing the mutational profile through high-throughput sequencing of a sizeable panel of AML cases will ultimately provide insights into different pathways that can potentially cooperate to induce leukemic transformation. High-throughput approaches may also provide some insights into predisposing factors to the development of particular types of leukemia. For example, a genome-wide association study has implicated variants in the PRDM1 gene at 6q21 in the development of second neoplasms in children treated with radiotherapy for Hodgkin disease,[154] whereas whole-genome sequencing applied in a case of therapy-related AML arising from early-onset BRCA1/2 mutation–negative breast and ovarian cancer revealed a novel TP53 cancer susceptibility mutation.[155]

Another active area of research concerns the role played in AML biology by micro-RNAs, a new class of noncoding RNAs hybridizing to target messenger RNAs and regulating their translation into proteins. Recent studies identified distinctive patterns of silencing and/or increased expression of multiple microRNAs (ie, microRNA expression signatures) to be associated with specific cytogenetic [eg, CBF AML with t(8;21) and inv(16) or t(16;16); APL with t(15;17); and AML with 11q23/MLL rearrangements], and molecular (eg, CN-AML with NPM1 and CEBPA mutations) AML subsets.[156] Moreover, both the microRNA expression signature[157] and expression levels of a single microRNA (miR-181a)[158] have been shown to have prognostic significance in patients with CN-AML. Undoubtedly, further associations between microRNA expression and treatment outcome in particular cytogenetic and/or molecular subsets of AML will be uncovered in the future.

Recent studies have also provided insights into DNA repair mechanisms operating in hematopoietic stem/progenitor cells that may render them susceptible to development of chromosomal abnormalities that give rise to AML.[159,160] Some insights into molecular mechanisms underlying formation of leukemia-associated chromosomal abnormalities may be gained through characterization of therapy-related leukemias, with several studies showing that chromosomal breakpoints are preferential sites of DNA damage induced by topoisomerase II that are aberrantly repaired to generate balanced translocations [eg, t(15;17) and t(11q23)] occurring in patients exposed to chemotherapeutic agents that target the enzyme.[161–164] Exposure to environmental toxins and agents targeting topoisomerase II has been implicated in the development of infant leukemia with translocations involving the *MLL* locus[165] (reviewed in Ref.[166]). Recent evidence lends further support for topoisomerase II in the etiology of chromosomal translocations, inducing DNA damage in the *TMPRSS2* and *ERG* loci in response to androgen signaling, leading to formation of fusion genes involved in prostate cancer.[167]

A further key focus of current research relates to improving understanding of the biology of the leukemic stem cell (LSC) compartment, defining how LSCs differ from their normal bone marrow counterparts and how they interact with the marrow microenvironment. Advances in this area, such as recent identification of protein bromodomain containing 4 (Brd4) as being critically required for maintaining LSC populations and preventing terminal myeloid differentiation,[168] or demonstration that a small molecule inhibitor of Brd4 and other members of bromodomain and extra terminal (BET) family of proteins (Brd2, Brd3 and Brdt) has potent efficacy against human and murine leukemic cell lines with, respectively, *MLL-AFF1* (formerly known as *AF4*) and *Mll-Mllt3* fusion genes,[169] offer prospects for development of novel targeted therapies, which are urgently required to help improve the dismal prognosis of older patients in whom AML predominates, as well as the subset of younger patients with poor-risk disease. Better characterization of the phenotypic features of LSCs complemented by a comprehensive catalog of the mutations that are bona fide primary lesions in AML pathogenesis will provide greater scope than is currently possible to using flow cytometric and quantitative PCR-based methods to track treatment responses. This ability may allow development of more individualized treatment approaches and better informed decisions concerning the role of allogeneic transplant. In this respect, APL has provided considerable grounds for hope; this form of AML was recognized as rapidly fatal when the underlying t(15;17) was first identified in the late 1970s, but has become the most prognostically favorable disease subset following the discovery of targeted therapies, guided by molecular monitoring. A key question is whether similar therapeutic opportunities can be identified that similarly transform the outcome of other cytogenetically and molecularly defined subsets of AML in the future.

ACKNOWLEDGMENTS

We are indebted to Alan Burnett, Nigel Russell, Robert Hills, Rosemary Gale, David Linch, and members of the UK National Cancer Research Institute (NCRI) AML Working Group for their assistance in providing relevant data. DG gratefully acknowledges the National Institute for Health Research (NIHR) for support for molecular diagnostics and assessment of minimal residual disease in the UK NCRI AML17 trial. This paper presents independent research funded by the National Institute for Health Research (NIHR) under its Programme Grants for Applied Research Programme (Grant Reference Number RP-PG-0108-10093). The views expressed are those of the authors and not necessarily those of the NHS, the NIHR or the Department of Health. In addition, DG is grateful for research funding from Leukemia & Lymphoma Research of Great Britain, the Guy's and

St Thomas' Charity, and the MRD Workpackage (WP12) of the European Leukemia-Net. KM thanks Clara D. Bloomfield for her constant help and encouragement, and gratefully acknowledges support from The Coleman Leukemia Research Foundation.

REFERENCES

1. Rowley JD. Identification of a translocation with quinacrine fluorescence in a patient with acute leukemia. Ann Genet 1973;16(2):109–12.
2. Rowley JD, Golomb HM, Dougherty C. 15/17 translocation, a consistent chromosomal change in acute promyelocytic leukaemia. Lancet 1977;1(8010): 549–50.
3. Caspersson T, Zech L, Johansson C. Differential binding of alkylating fluorochromes in human chromosomes. Exp Cell Res 1970;60(3):315–9.
4. Seabright M. A rapid banding technique for human chromosomes. Lancet 1971; 2(7731):971–2.
5. Mitelman F, Johansson B, Mertens F, editors, Mitelman database of chromosome aberrations and gene fusions in cancer. 2011. Available: http://cgap.nci. nih.gov/Chromosomes/Mitelman. Accessed August 2, 2011.
6. Mrózek K, Heinonen K, Bloomfield CD. Clinical importance of cytogenetics in acute myeloid leukaemia. Best Pract Res Clin Haematol 2001;14(1):19–47.
7. Grimwade D. The clinical significance of cytogenetic abnormalities in acute myeloid leukaemia. Best Pract Res Clin Haematol 2001;14(3):497–529.
8. Mrózek K, Heerema NA, Bloomfield CD. Cytogenetics in acute leukemia. Blood Rev 2004;18(2):115–36.
9. Smith ML, Hills RK, Grimwade D. Independent prognostic variables in acute myeloid leukaemia. Blood Rev 2011;25(1):39–51.
10. Swerdlow SH, Campo E, Harris NL, et al, editors. WHO classification of tumours of haematopoietic and lymphoid tissues. Lyon (France): IARC; 2008.
11. Vardiman JW, Thiele J, Arber DA, et al. The 2008 revision of the World Health Organization (WHO) classification of myeloid neoplasms and acute leukemia: rationale and important changes. Blood 2009;114(5):937–51.
12. de Thé H, Chomienne C, Lanotte M, et al. The t(15;17) translocation of acute promyelocytic leukaemia fuses the retinoic acid receptor α gene to a novel transcribed locus. Nature 1990;347(6293):558–61.
13. Borrow J, Goddard AD, Sheer D, et al. Molecular analysis of acute promyelocytic leukemia breakpoint cluster region on chromosome 17. Science 1990; 249(4976):1577–80.
14. Goddard AD, Borrow J, Freemont PS, et al. Characterization of a zinc finger gene disrupted by the t(15;17) in acute promyelocytic leukemia. Science 1991;254(5036):1371–4.
15. Brown NJ, Ramalho M, Pedersen EW, et al. PML nuclear bodies in the pathogenesis of acute promyelocytic leukemia: active players or innocent bystanders? Front Biosci 2009;14:1684–707.
16. Grimwade D, Biondi A, Mozziconacci M-J, et al. Characterization of acute promyelocytic leukemia cases lacking the classic t(15;17): results of the European Working Party. Blood 2000;96(4):1297–308.
17. Chen Z, Brand NJ, Chen A, et al. Fusion between a novel *Krüppel*-like zinc finger gene and the retinoic acid receptor-α locus due to a variant t(11;17) translocation associated with acute promyelocytic leukaemia. EMBO J 1993;12(3): 1161–7.

18. Redner RL, Rush EA, Faas S, et al. The t(5;17) variant of acute promyelocytic leukemia expresses a nucleophosmin-retinoic acid receptor fusion. Blood 1996;87(3):882–6.

19. Wells RA, Catzavelos C, Kamel-Reid S. Fusion of retinoic acid receptor α to NuMA, the nuclear mitotic apparatus protein, by a variant translocation in acute promyelocytic leukaemia. Nat Genet 1997;17(1):109–13.

20. Kondo T, Mori A, Darmanin S, et al. The seventh pathogenic fusion gene *FIP1L1-RARA* was isolated from a t(4;17)-positive acute promyelocytic leukemia. Haematologica 2008;93(9):1414–6.

21. Yamamoto Y, Tsuzuki S, Tsuzuki M, et al. BCOR as a novel fusion partner of retinoic acid receptor alpha in a t(X;17)(p11;q12) variant of acute promyelocytic leukemia. Blood 2010;116(20):4274–83.

22. Catalano A, Dawson MA, Somana K, et al. The *PRKAR1A* gene is fused to *RARA* in a new variant acute promyelocytic leukemia. Blood 2007;110(12):4073–6.

23. Arnould C, Philippe C, Bourdon V, et al. The signal transducer and activator of transcription STAT5b gene is a new partner of retinoic acid receptor alpha in acute promyelocytic-like leukaemia. Hum Mol Genet 1999;8(9):1741–9.

24. Grimwade D, Mistry AR, Solomon E, et al. Acute promyelocytic leukemia: a paradigm for differentiation therapy. Cancer Treat Res 2010;145:219–35.

25. Licht JD, Chomienne C, Goy A, et al. Clinical and molecular characterization of a rare syndrome of acute promyelocytic leukemia associated with translocation (11;17). Blood 1995;85(4):1083–94.

26. Dong S, Tweardy DJ. Interactions of STAT5b-RARα, a novel acute promyelocytic leukemia fusion protein, with retinoic acid receptor and STAT3 signaling pathways. Blood 2002;99(8):2637–46.

27. Guidez F, Parks S, Wong H, et al. RARα-PLZF overcomes PLZF-mediated repression of *CRABPI*, contributing to retinoid resistance in t(11;17) acute promyelocytic leukemia. Proc Natl Acad Sci U S A 2007;104(47):18694–9.

28. Zhang XW, Yan XJ, Zhou ZR, et al. Arsenic trioxide controls the fate of the PML-RARα oncoprotein by directly binding PML. Science 2010;328(5975):240–3.

29. Such E, Cervera J, Valencia A, et al. A novel *NUP98/RARG* gene fusion in acute myeloid leukemia resembling acute promyelocytic leukemia. Blood 2011;117(1):242–5.

30. Goyama S, Mulloy JC. Molecular pathogenesis of core binding factor leukemia: current knowledge and future prospects. Int J Hematol 2011;94(2):126–33.

31. Martens JHA, Stunnenberg HG. The molecular signature of oncofusion proteins in acute myeloid leukemia. FEBS Lett 2010;584(12):2662–9.

32. De Braekeleer E, Férec C, De Braekeleer M. *RUNX1* translocations in malignant hemopathies. Anticancer Res 2009;29(4):1031–7.

33. Guastadisegni MC, Lonoce A, Impera L, et al. *CBFA2T2* and *C20orf112*: two novel fusion partners of *RUNX1* in acute myeloid leukemia. Leukemia 2010;24(8):1516–9.

34. Slovak ML, Bedell V, Popplewell L, et al. 21q22 balanced chromosome aberrations in therapy-related hematopoietic disorders: report from an international workshop. Genes Chromosomes Cancer 2002;33(4):379–94.

35. Ottone T, Hasan SK, Montefusco E, et al. Identification of a potential "hotspot" DNA region in the *RUNX1* gene targeted by mitoxantrone in therapy-related acute myeloid leukemia with t(16;21) translocation. Genes Chromosomes Cancer 2009;48(3):213–21.

36. Meyer C, Kowarz E, Hofmann J, et al. New insights to the *MLL* recombinome of acute leukemias. Leukemia 2009;23(8):1490–9.

37. Smith E, Lin C, Shilatifard A. The super elongation complex (SEC) and MLL in development and disease. Genes Dev 2011;25(7):661–72.
38. Rubnitz JE, Raimondi SC, Tong X, et al. Favorable impact of the t(9;11) in childhood acute myeloid leukemia. J Clin Oncol 2002;20(9):2302–9.
39. Mrózek K, Heinonen K, Lawrence D, et al. Adult patients with de novo acute myeloid leukemia and t(9;11)(p22;q23) have a superior outcome to patients with other translocations involving band 11q23: a Cancer and Leukemia Group B study. Blood 1997;90(11):4532–8.
40. Beverloo HB, Le Coniat M, Wijsman J, et al. Breakpoint heterogeneity in t(10;11) translocation in AML-M4/M5 resulting in fusion of *AF10* and *MLL* is resolved by fluorescent *in situ* hybridization analysis. Cancer Res 1995; 55(19):4220–4.
41. Klaus M, Schnittger S, Haferlach T, et al. Cytogenetics, fluorescence in situ hybridization, and reverse transcriptase polymerase chain reaction are necessary to clarify the various mechanisms leading to an *MLL-AF10* fusion in acute myelocytic leukemia with 10;11 rearrangement. Cancer Genet Cytogenet 2003; 144(1):36–43.
42. Bloomfield CD, Archer KJ, Mrózek K, et al. 11q23 balanced chromosome aberrations in treatment-related myelodysplastic syndromes and acute leukemia: report from an international workshop. Genes Chromosomes Cancer 2002; 33(4):362–78.
43. Felix CA, Kolaris CP, Osheroff N. Topoisomerase II and the etiology of chromosomal translocations. DNA Repair (Amst) 2006;5(9–10):1093–108.
44. Soekarman D, von Lindern M, Daenen S, et al. The translocation (6;9)(p23;q34) shows consistent rearrangement of two genes and defines a myeloproliferative disorder with specific clinical features. Blood 1992;79(11):2990–7.
45. Xu S, Powers MA. Nuclear pore proteins and cancer. Semin Cell Dev Biol 2009; 20(5):620–30.
46. Secker-Walker LM, Mehta A, Bain B. Abnormalities of 3q21 and 3q26 in myeloid malignancy: a United Kingdom Cancer Cytogenetic Group study. Br J Haematol 1995;91(2):490–501.
47. Morishita K, Parker DS, Mucenski ML, et al. Retroviral activation of a novel gene encoding a zinc finger protein in IL-3-dependent myeloid leukemia cell lines. Cell 1988;54(6):831–40.
48. Du Y, Jenkins NA, Copeland NG. Insertional mutagenesis identifies genes that promote the immortalization of primary bone marrow progenitor cells. Blood 2005;106(12):3932–9.
49. Stein S, Ott MG, Schultze-Strasser S, et al. Genomic instability and myelodysplasia with monosomy 7 consequent to *EVI1* activation after gene therapy for chronic granulomatous disease. Nat Med 2010;16(2):198–204.
50. Mercher T, Le Coniat MB, Monni R, et al. Involvement of a human gene related to the *Drosophila spen* gene in the recurrent t(1;22) translocation of acute megakaryocytic leukemia. Proc Natl Acad Sci U S A 2001;98(10):5776–9.
51. Ma Z, Morris SW, Valentine V, et al. Fusion of two novel genes, *RBM15* and *MKL1*, in the t(1;22)(p13;q13) of acute megakaryoblastic leukemia. Nat Genet 2001;28(3):220–1.
52. Cheng E-C, Luo Q, Bruscia EM, et al. Role for MKL1 in megakaryocytic maturation. Blood 2009;113(12):2826–34.
53. Grimwade D, Hills RK, Moorman AV, et al. Refinement of cytogenetic classification in acute myeloid leukemia: determination of prognostic significance of rare recurring chromosomal abnormalities amongst 5,876 younger adult

patients treated in the UK Medical Research Council trials. Blood 2010; 116(3):354–65.

54. Mrózek K, Heinonen K, Theil KS, et al. Spectral karyotyping in patients with acute myeloid leukemia and a complex karyotype shows hidden aberrations, including recurrent overrepresentation of 21q, 11q, and 22q. Genes Chromosomes Cancer 2002;34(2):137–53.

55. Galván AB, Mallo M, Arenillas L, et al. Does monosomy 5 really exist in myelodysplastic syndromes and acute myeloid leukemia? Leuk Res 2010;34(9): 1242–5.

56. Yoneda-Kato N, Look AT, Kirstein MN, et al. The t(3;5)(q25.1;q34) of myelodysplastic syndrome and acute myeloid leukemia produces a novel fusion gene, NPM-MLF1. Oncogene 1996;12(2):265–75.

57. Ebert BL. Deletion 5q in myelodysplastic syndrome: a paradigm for the study of hemizygous deletions in cancer. Leukemia 2009;23(7):1252–6.

58. Ebert BL. Genetic deletions in AML and MDS. Best Pract Res Clin Haematol 2010;23(4):457–61.

59. Mrózek K, Holland KB, Pettenati MJ, et al. Prognostic significance of unbalanced chromosome abnormalities used by 2008 World Health Organization (WHO) classification to define "acute myeloid leukemia (AML) with myelodysplasia-related changes" in adults: a Cancer and Leukemia Group B (CALGB) study [abstract 2602]. Blood 2009;114(22):1021.

60. Haematological Malignancy Research Network, University of York, United Kingdom. Available at: http://www.hmrn.org/Statistics/Incidence_Wizard.aspx. Accessed July 25, 2011.

61. Chessells JM, Harrison CJ, Kempski H, et al. Clinical features, cytogenetics and outcome in acute lymphoblastic and myeloid leukaemia of infancy: report from the MRC Childhood Leukaemia Working Party. Leukemia 2002;16(5):776–84.

62. Döhner H, Estey EH, Amadori S, et al. Diagnosis and management of acute myeloid leukemia in adults: recommendations from an international expert panel, on behalf of the European LeukemiaNet. Blood 2010;115(3):453–74.

63. Schoch C, Haase D, Haferlach T, et al. Fifty-one patients with acute myeloid leukemia and translocation t(8;21)(q22;q22): an additional deletion in 9q is an adverse prognostic factor. Leukemia 1996;10(8):1288–95.

64. Byrd JC, Mrózek K, Dodge RK, et al. Pretreatment cytogenetic abnormalities are predictive of induction success, cumulative incidence of relapse, and overall survival in adult patients with de novo acute myeloid leukemia: results from Cancer and Leukemia Group B (CALGB 8461). Blood 2002;100(13):4325–36.

65. Schlenk RF, Benner A, Krauter J, et al. Individual patient data-based meta-analysis of patients aged 16 to 60 years with core binding factor acute myeloid leukemia: a survey of the German Acute Myeloid Leukemia Intergroup. J Clin Oncol 2004;22(18):3741–50.

66. Marcucci G, Mrózek K, Ruppert AS, et al. Prognostic factors and outcome of core binding factor acute myeloid leukemia patients with t(8;21) differ from those of patients with inv(16): a Cancer and Leukemia Group B study. J Clin Oncol 2005;23(24):5705–17.

67. Mrózek K, Prior TW, Edwards C, et al. Comparison of cytogenetic and molecular genetic detection of t(8;21) and inv(16) in a prospective series of adults with de novo acute myeloid leukemia: a Cancer and Leukemia Group B study. J Clin Oncol 2001;19(9):2482–92.

68. Mrózek K, Marcucci G, Paschka P, et al. Clinical relevance of mutations and gene-expression changes in adult acute myeloid leukemia with normal

cytogenetics: are we ready for a prognostically prioritized molecular classification? Blood 2007;109(2):431–48.

69. Marcucci G, Haferlach T, Döhner H. Molecular genetics of adult acute myeloid leukemia: prognostic and therapeutic implications. J Clin Oncol 2011;29(5): 475–86.

70. Grimwade D, Walker H, Oliver F, et al. The importance of diagnostic cytogenetics on outcome in AML: analysis of 1,612 patients entered into the MRC AML10 trial. The Medical Research Council Adult and Children's Leukaemia Working Parties. Blood 1998;92(7):2322–33.

71. Cornelissen JJ, van Putten WLJ, Verdonck LF, et al. Results of a HOVON/SAKK donor versus no-donor analysis of myeloablative HLA-identical sibling stem cell transplantation in first remission acute myeloid leukemia in young and middle-aged adults: benefits for whom? Blood 2007;109(9):3658–66.

72. Koreth J, Schlenk R, Kopecky KJ, et al. Allogeneic stem cell transplantation for acute myeloid leukemia in first complete remission: systematic review and meta-analysis of prospective clinical trials. JAMA 2009;301(22):2349–61.

73. Care RS, Valk PJM, Goodeve AC, et al. Incidence and prognosis of c-KIT and FLT3 mutations in core binding factor (CBF) acute myeloid leukaemias. Br J Haematol 2003;121(5):775–7.

74. Paschka P, Marcucci G, Ruppert AS, et al. Adverse prognostic significance of *KIT* mutations in adult acute myeloid leukemia with inv(16) and t(8;21): a Cancer and Leukemia Group B study. J Clin Oncol 2006;24(24):3904–11.

75. Cuneo A, Ferrant A, Michaux JL, et al. Philadelphia chromosome-positive acute myeloid leukemia: cytoimmunologic and cytogenetic features. Haematologica 1996;81(5):423–7.

76. Slovak ML, Gundacker H, Bloomfield CD, et al. A retrospective study of 69 patients with t(6;9)(p23;q34) AML emphasizes the need for a prospective, multi-center initiative for rare 'poor prognosis' myeloid malignancies. Leukemia 2006; 20(7):1295–7.

77. Thiede C, Steudel C, Mohr B, et al. Analysis of FLT3-activating mutations in 979 patients with acute myelogenous leukemia: association with FAB subtypes and identification of subgroups with poor prognosis. Blood 2002; 99(12):4326–35.

78. Breems DA, Van Putten WLJ, De Greef GE, et al. Monosomal karyotype in acute myeloid leukemia: a better indicator of poor prognosis than a complex karyotype. J Clin Oncol 2008;26(29):4791–7.

79. Mrózek K. Cytogenetic, molecular genetic, and clinical characteristics of acute myeloid leukemia with a complex karyotype. Semin Oncol 2008;35(4): 365–77.

80. Medeiros BC, Othus M, Fang M, et al. Prognostic impact of monosomal karyotype in young adult and elderly acute myeloid leukemia: the Southwest Oncology Group (SWOG) experience. Blood 2010;116(13):2224–8.

81. Fang M, Storer B, Estey E, et al. Outcome of patients with acute myeloid leukemia with monosomal karyotype who undergo hematopoietic cell transplantation. Blood 2011;118(6):1490–4.

82. Raimondi SC, Chang MN, Ravindranath Y, et al. Chromosomal abnormalities in 478 children with acute myeloid leukemia: clinical characteristics and treatment outcome in a cooperative Pediatric Oncology Group study-POG 8821. Blood 1999;94(11):3707–16.

83. von Neuhoff C, Reinhardt D, Sander A, et al. Prognostic impact of specific chromosomal aberrations in a large group of pediatric patients with acute myeloid

leukemia treated uniformly according to trial AML-BFM 98. J Clin Oncol 2010; 28(16):2682–9.

84. Harrison CJ, Moorman AV, Hills RK, et al. Cytogenetics of childhood acute myeloid leukemia: 753 patients in UK Medical Research Council treatment trials, AML 10 and 12. J Clin Oncol 2010;28(16):2674–81.

85. Coenen EA, Raimondi SC, Harbott J, et al. Prognostic significance of additional cytogenetic aberrations in 733 de novo pediatric 11q23/*MLL*-rearranged AML patients: results of an international study. Blood 2011;117(26):7102–11.

86. Grimwade D, Walker H, Harrison G, et al. The predictive value of hierarchical cytogenetic classification in older adults with acute myeloid leukemia (AML): analysis of 1065 patients entered into the United Kingdom Medical Research Council AML11 trial. Blood 2001;98(5):1312–20.

87. Farag SS, Archer KJ, Mrózek K, et al. Pretreatment cytogenetics add to other prognostic factors predicting complete remission and long-term outcome in patients 60 years of age or older with acute myeloid leukemia: results from Cancer and Leukemia Group B 8461. Blood 2006;108(1):63–73.

88. Fröhling S, Schlenk RF, Kayser S, et al. Cytogenetics and age are major determinants of outcome in intensively treated acute myeloid leukemia patients older than 60 years: results from AMLSG trial AML HD98-B. Blood 2006;108(10): 3280–8.

89. Schoch C, Haferlach T, Haase D, et al. Patients with de novo acute myeloid leukaemia and complex karyotype aberrations show a poor prognosis despite intensive treatment: a study of 90 patients. Br J Haematol 2001;112(1):118–26.

90. Farag SS, Maharry K, Zhang M-J, et al. Comparison of reduced-intensity hematopoietic cell transplantation with chemotherapy in patients aged 60-70 years with acute myeloid leukemia in first remission. Biol Blood Marrow Transplant 2011. DOI: 10.1016/j.bbmt.2011.06.005.

91. Blum W, Garzon R, Klisovic RB, et al. Clinical response and *miR-29b* predictive significance in older AML patients treated with a 10-day schedule of decitabine. Proc Natl Acad Sci U S A 2010;107(16):7473–8.

92. Perrot A, Luquet I, Pigneux A, et al. Dismal prognostic value of monosomal karyotype in elderly patients with acute myeloid leukemia: a GOELAMS study of 186 patients with unfavorable cytogenetic abnormalities. Blood 2011; 118(3):679–85.

93. Grimwade D. Screening for core binding factor gene rearrangements in acute myeloid leukemia. Leukemia 2002;16(5):964–9.

94. Burnett AK, Grimwade D, Solomon E, et al. Presenting white blood cell count and kinetics of molecular remission predict prognosis in acute promyelocytic leukemia treated with all-*trans* retinoic acid: result of the randomized MRC trial. Blood 1999;93(12):4131–43.

95. Sarriera JE, Albitar M, Estrov Z, et al. Comparison of outcome in acute myelogenous leukemia patients with translocation (8;21) found by standard cytogenetic analysis and patients with AML1/ETO fusion transcript found only by PCR testing. Leukemia 2001;15(1):57–61.

96. Rücker FG, Bullinger L, Gribov A, et al. Molecular characterization of AML with ins(21;8)(q22;q22q22) reveals similarity to t(8;21) AML. Genes Chromosomes Cancer 2011;50(1):51–8.

97. Mrózek K, Carroll AJ, Maharry K, et al. Central review of cytogenetics is necessary for cooperative group correlative and clinical studies of adult acute leukemia: the Cancer and Leukemia Group B experience. Int J Oncol 2008; 33(2):239–44.

98. Lugthart S, van Drunen E, van Norden Y, et al. High *EVI1* levels predict adverse outcome in acute myeloid leukemia: prevalence of *EVI1* overexpression and chromosome 3q26 abnormalities underestimated. Blood 2008; 111(8):4329–37.
99. Hollink IHIM, van den Heuvel-Eibrink MM, Arentsen-Peters STCJM, et al. *NUP98/NSD1* characterizes a novel poor prognostic group in acute myeloid leukemia with a distinct *HOX* gene expression pattern. Blood 2011;118(13): 3645–56.
100. Walter MJ, Payton JE, Ries RE, et al. Acquired copy number alterations in adult acute myeloid leukemia genomes. Proc Natl Acad Sci U S A 2009;106(31): 12950–5.
101. Tiu RV, Gondek LP, O'Keefe CL, et al. New lesions detected by single nucleotide polymorphism array-based chromosomal analysis have important clinical impact in acute myeloid leukemia. J Clin Oncol 2009;27(31):5219–26.
102. Bullinger L, Krönke J, Schön C, et al. Identification of acquired copy number alterations and uniparental disomies in cytogenetically normal acute myeloid leukemia using high-resolution single-nucleotide polymorphism analysis. Leukemia 2010;24(2):438–49.
103. Parkin B, Erba H, Ouillette P, et al. Acquired genomic copy number aberrations and survival in adult acute myelogenous leukemia. Blood 2010;116(23): 4958–67.
104. Grimwade D, Hills RK. Independent prognostic factors for AML outcome. Hematology Am Soc Hematol Educ Program 2009;385–95.
105. Löwenberg B. Genetic markers in relation to the therapeutic management of acute myeloid leukemia. Hematology Education 2011;5:36–41.
106. Nakao M, Yokota S, Iwai T, et al. Internal tandem duplication of the flt3 gene found in acute myeloid leukemia. Leukemia 1996;10(12):1911–8.
107. Kiyoi H, Naoe T, Yokota S, et al. Internal tandem duplication of *FLT3* associated with leukocytosis in acute promyelocytic leukemia. Leukemia 1997;11(9): 1447–52.
108. Kottaridis PD, Gale RE, Linch DC. FLT3 mutations and leukaemia. Br J Haematol 2003;122(4):523–38.
109. Whitman SP, Archer KJ, Feng L, et al. Absence of the wild-type allele predicts poor prognosis in adult *de novo* acute myeloid leukemia with normal cytogenetics and the internal tandem duplication of *FLT3*: a Cancer and Leukemia Group B study. Cancer Res 2001;61(19):7233–9.
110. Fitzgibbon J, Smith LL, Raghavan M, et al. Association between acquired uniparental disomy and homozygous gene mutation in acute myeloid leukemias. Cancer Res 2005;65(20):9152–4.
111. Paschka P, Marcucci G, Ruppert AS, et al. Wilms' tumor 1 gene mutations independently predict poor outcome in adults with cytogenetically normal acute myeloid leukemia: a Cancer and Leukemia Group B study. J Clin Oncol 2008; 26(28):4595–602.
112. Virappane P, Gale R, Hills R, et al. Mutation of the Wilms' tumor 1 gene is a poor prognostic factor associated with chemotherapy resistance in normal karyotype acute myeloid leukemia: the United Kingdom Medical Research Council Adult Leukaemia Working Party. J Clin Oncol 2008;26(33):5429–35.
113. Renneville A, Boissel N, Zurawski V, et al. Wilms tumor 1 gene mutations are associated with a higher risk of recurrence in young adults with acute myeloid leukemia: a study from the Acute Leukemia French Association. Cancer 2009; 115(16):3719–27.

114. Gaidzik VI, Schlenk RF, Moschny S, et al. Prognostic impact of *WT1* mutations in cytogenetically normal acute myeloid leukemia: a study of the German-Austrian AML Study Group. Blood 2009;113(19):4505–11.

115. Tang J-L, Hou H-A, Chen C-Y, et al. *AML1/RUNX1* mutations in 470 adult patients with de novo acute myeloid leukemia: prognostic implication and interaction with other gene alterations. Blood 2009;114(26):5352–61.

116. Schnittger S, Dicker F, Kern W, et al. *RUNX1* mutations are frequent in de novo AML with noncomplex karyotype and confer an unfavorable prognosis. Blood 2011;117(8):2348–57.

117. Gaidzik VI, Bullinger L, Schlenk RF, et al. *RUNX1* mutations in acute myeloid leukemia: results from a comprehensive genetic and clinical analysis from the AML study group. J Clin Oncol 2011;29(10):1364–72.

118. Caligiuri MA, Strout MP, Lawrence D, et al. Rearrangement of *ALL1* (*MLL*) in acute myeloid leukemia with normal cytogenetics. Cancer Res 1998;58(1):55–9.

119. Schnittger S, Kinkelin U, Schoch C, et al. Screening for MLL tandem duplication in 387 unselected patients with AML identify a prognostically unfavorable subset of AML. Leukemia 2000;14(5):796–804.

120. Döhner K, Tobis K, Ulrich R, et al. Prognostic significance of partial tandem duplications of the *MLL* gene in adult patients 16 to 60 years old with acute myeloid leukemia and normal cytogenetics: a study of the Acute Myeloid Leukemia Study Group Ulm. J Clin Oncol 2002;20(15):3254–61.

121. Schlenk RF, Döhner K, Krauter J, et al. Mutations and treatment outcome in cytogenetically normal acute myeloid leukemia. N Engl J Med 2008;358(18): 1909–18.

122. Whitman SP, Ruppert AS, Marcucci G, et al. Long-term disease-free survivors with cytogenetically normal acute myeloid leukemia and *MLL* partial tandem duplication: a Cancer and Leukemia Group B study. Blood 2007;109(12): 5164–7.

123. Pabst T, Mueller BU, Zhang P, et al. Dominant-negative mutations of *CEBPA*, encoding CCAAT/enhancer binding protein-α (C/EBPα), in acute myeloid leukemia. Nat Genet 2001;27(3):263–70.

124. Falini B, Mecucci C, Tiacci E, et al. Cytoplasmic nucleophosmin in acute myelogenous leukemia with a normal karyotype. N Engl J Med 2005;352(3): 254–66.

125. Nerlov C. C/EBPα mutations in acute myeloid leukaemias. Nat Rev Cancer 2004; 4(5):394–400.

126. Pabst T, Mueller BU. Complexity of CEBPA dysregulation in human acute myeloid leukemia. Clin Cancer Res 2009;15(17):5303–7.

127. Smith ML, Cavenagh JD, Lister TA, et al. Mutation of *CEBPA* in familial acute myeloid leukemia. N Engl J Med 2004;351(23):2403–7.

128. Pabst T, Eyholzer M, Haefliger S, et al. Somatic *CEBPA* mutations are a frequent second event in families with germline *CEBPA* mutations and familial acute myeloid leukemia. J Clin Oncol 2008;26(31):5088–93.

129. Kirstetter P, Schuster MB, Bereshchenko O, et al. Modeling of C/EBPα mutant acute myeloid leukemia reveals a common expression signature of committed myeloid leukemia-initiating cells. Cancer Cell 2008;13(4):299–310.

130. Bereshchenko O, Mancini E, Moore S, et al. Hematopoietic stem cell expansion precedes the generation of committed myeloid leukemia-initiating cells in C/EBPα mutant AML. Cancer Cell 2009;16(5):390–400.

131. Preudhomme C, Sagot C, Boissel N, et al. Favorable prognostic significance of *CEBPA* mutations in patients with de novo acute myeloid leukemia: a study

from the Acute Leukemia French Association (ALFA). Blood 2002;100(8): 2717–23.

132. Fröhling S, Schlenk RF, Stolze I, et al. *CEBPA* mutations in younger adults with acute myeloid leukemia and normal cytogenetics: prognostic relevance and analysis of cooperating mutations. J Clin Oncol 2004;22(4):624–33.
133. Marcucci G, Maharry K, Radmacher MD, et al. Prognostic significance of, and gene and microRNA expression signatures associated with, *CEBPA* mutations in cytogenetically normal acute myeloid leukemia with high-risk molecular features: a Cancer and Leukemia Group B study. J Clin Oncol 2008;26(31): 5078–87.
134. Wouters BJ, Löwenberg B, Erpelinck-Verschueren CAJ, et al. Double *CEBPA* mutations, but not single *CEBPA* mutations, define a subgroup of acute myeloid leukemia with a distinctive gene expression profile that is uniquely associated with a favorable outcome. Blood 2009;113(13):3088–91.
135. Pabst T, Eyholzer M, Fos J, et al. Heterogeneity within AML with CEBPA mutations; only CEBPA double mutations, but not single CEBPA mutations are associated with favourable prognosis. Br J Cancer 2009;100(8):1343–6.
136. Renneville A, Boissel N, Gachard N, et al. The favorable impact of CEBPA mutations in patients with acute myeloid leukemia is only observed in the absence of associated cytogenetic abnormalities and FLT3 internal duplication. Blood 2009;113(21):5090–3.
137. Green CL, Koo KK, Hills RK, et al. Prognostic significance of *CEBPA* mutations in a large cohort of younger adult patients with acute myeloid leukemia: impact of double *CEBPA* mutations and the interaction with *FLT3* and *NPM1* mutations. J Clin Oncol 2010;28(16):2739–47.
138. Taskesen E, Bullinger L, Corbacioglu A, et al. Prognostic impact, concurrent genetic mutations, and gene expression features of AML with *CEBPA* mutations in a cohort of 1182 cytogenetically normal AML patients: further evidence for *CEBPA* double mutant AML as a distinctive disease entity. Blood 2011;117(8): 2469–75.
139. Falini B. Acute myeloid leukemia with mutated nucleophosmin (*NPM1*): molecular, pathological, and clinical features. Cancer Treat Res 2010;145:149–68.
140. Schnittger S, Kern W, Tschulik C, et al. Minimal residual disease levels assessed by *NPM1* mutation-specific RQ-PCR provide important prognostic information in AML. Blood 2009;114(11):2220–31.
141. Krönke J, Schlenk RF, Jensen K-O, et al. Monitoring of minimal residual disease in *NPM1*-mutated acute myeloid leukemia: a study from the German-Austrian Acute Myeloid Leukemia Study Group. J Clin Oncol 2011;29(19): 2709–16.
142. Vassiliou GS, Cooper JL, Rad R, et al. Mutant nucleophosmin and cooperating pathways drive leukemia initiation and progression in mice. Nat Genet 2011; 43(5):470–5.
143. Schnittger S, Schoch C, Kern W, et al. Nucleophosmin gene mutations are predictors of favorable prognosis in acute myelogenous leukemia with a normal karyotype. Blood 2005;106(12):3733–9.
144. Döhner K, Schlenk RF, Habdank M, et al. Mutant nucleophosmin (*NPM1*) predicts favorable prognosis in younger adults with acute myeloid leukemia and normal cytogenetics: interaction with other gene mutations. Blood 2005; 106(12):3740–6.
145. Verhaak RGW, Goudswaard CS, van Putten W, et al. Mutations in nucleophosmin (*NPM1*) in acute myeloid leukemia (AML): association with other gene

abnormalities and previously established gene expression signatures and their favorable prognostic significance. Blood 2005;106(12):3747–54.

146. Gale RE, Green C, Allen C, et al. The impact of *FLT3* internal tandem duplication mutant level, number, size, and interaction with *NPM1* mutations in a large cohort of young adult patients with acute myeloid leukemia. Blood 2008; 111(5):2776–84.

147. Becker H, Marcucci G, Maharry K, et al. Favorable prognostic impact of *NPM1* mutations in older patients with cytogenetically normal de novo acute myeloid leukemia and associated gene- and microRNA-expression signatures: a Cancer and Leukemia Group B study. J Clin Oncol 2010;28(4): 596–604.

148. Haferlach C, Mecucci C, Schnittger S, et al. AML with mutated *NPM1* carrying a normal or aberrant karyotype show overlapping biologic, pathologic, immunophenotypic, and prognostic features. Blood 2009;114(14):3024–32.

149. Mardis ER, Ding L, Dooling DJ, et al. Recurring mutations found by sequencing an acute myeloid leukemia genome. N Engl J Med 2009;361(11):1058–66.

150. Ley TJ, Ding L, Walter MJ, et al. *DNMT3A* mutations in acute myeloid leukemia. N Engl J Med 2010;363(25):2424–33.

151. Marcucci G, Maharry K, Wu Y-Z, et al. *IDH1* and *IDH2* gene mutations identify novel molecular subsets within de novo cytogenetically normal acute myeloid leukemia: a Cancer and Leukemia Group B study. J Clin Oncol 2010;28(14): 2348–55.

152. Green CL, Evans CM, Zhao L, et al. The prognostic significance of *IDH2* mutations in AML depends on the location of the mutation. Blood 2011;118(2): 409–12.

153. Boissel N, Nibourel O, Renneville A, et al. Differential prognosis impact of *IDH2* mutations in cytogenetically normal acute myeloid leukemia. Blood 2011; 117(13):3696–7.

154. Best T, Li D, Skol AD, et al. Variants at 6q21 implicate *PRDM1* in the etiology of therapy-induced second malignancies after Hodgkin's lymphoma. Nat Med 2011;17(8):941–3.

155. Link DC, Schuettpelz LG, Shen D, et al. Identification of a novel *TP53* cancer susceptibility mutation through whole-genome sequencing of a patient with therapy-related AML. JAMA 2011;305(15):1568–76.

156. Marcucci G, Mrózek K, Radmacher MD, et al. The prognostic and functional role of microRNAs in acute myeloid leukemia. Blood 2011;117(4):1121–9.

157. Marcucci G, Radmacher MD, Maharry K, et al. MicroRNA expression in cytogenetically normal acute myeloid leukemia. N Engl J Med 2008;358(18):1919–28.

158. Schwind S, Maharry K, Radmacher MD, et al. Prognostic significance of expression of a single microRNA, miR-181a, in cytogenetically normal acute myeloid leukemia: a Cancer and Leukemia Group B study. J Clin Oncol 2010;28(36): 5257–64.

159. Mohrin M, Bourke E, Alexander D, et al. Hematopoietic stem cell quiescence promotes error-prone DNA repair and mutagenesis. Cell Stem Cell 2010;7(2): 174–85.

160. Milyavsky M, Gan OI, Trottier M, et al. A distinctive DNA damage response in human hematopoietic stem cells reveals an apoptosis-independent role for p53 in self-renewal. Cell Stem Cell 2010;7(2):186–97.

161. Lovett BD, Strumberg D, Blair IA, et al. Etoposide metabolites enhance DNA topoisomerase II cleavage near leukemia-associated *MLL* translocation breakpoints. Biochemistry 2001;40(5):1159–70.

162. Mistry AR, Felix CA, Whitmarsh RJ, et al. DNA topoisomerase II in therapy-related acute promyelocytic leukemia. N Engl J Med 2005;352(15):1529–38.
163. Hasan SK, Mays AN, Ottone T, et al. Molecular analysis of t(15;17) genomic breakpoints in secondary acute promyelocytic leukemia arising after treatment of multiple sclerosis. Blood 2008;112(8):3383–90.
164. Mays AN, Osheroff N, Xiao Y, et al. Evidence for direct involvement of epirubicin in the formation of chromosomal translocations in t(15;17) therapy-related acute promyelocytic leukemia. Blood 2010;115(2):326–30.
165. Alexander FE, Patheal SL, Biondi A, et al. Transplacental chemical exposure and risk of infant leukemia with *MLL* gene fusion. Cancer Res 2001;61(6): 2542–6.
166. Hall GW. Childhood myeloid leukaemias. Best Pract Res Clin Haematol 2001; 14(3):573–91.
167. Haffner MC, Aryee MJ, Toubaji A, et al. Androgen-induced TOP2B-mediated double-strand breaks and prostate cancer gene rearrangements. Nat Genet 2010;42(8):668–75.
168. Zuber J, Shi J, Wang E, et al. RNAi screen identifies Brd4 as a therapeutic target in acute myeloid leukaemia. Nature 2011;478(7370):524–8.
169. Dawson MA, Prinjha RK, Dittmann A, et al. Inhibition of BET recruitment to chromatin as an effective treatment for MLL-fusion leukaemia. Nature 2011; 478(7370):529–33.
170. Slovak ML, Kopecky KJ, Cassileth PA, et al. Karyotypic analysis predicts outcome of preremission and postremission therapy in adult acute myeloid leukemia: a Southwest Oncology Group/Eastern Cooperative Oncology Group study. Blood 2000;96(13):4075–83.
171. Suciu S, Mandelli F, de Witte T, et al. Allogeneic compared with autologous stem cell transplantation in the treatment of patients younger than 46 years with acute myeloid leukemia (AML) in first complete remission (CR1): an intention-to-treat analysis of the EORTC/GIMEMA AML-10 trial. Blood 2003;102(4):1232–40.
172. Schoch C, Schnittger S, Klaus M, et al. AML with 11q23/*MLL* abnormalities as defined by the WHO classification: incidence, partner chromosomes, FAB subtype, age distribution, and prognostic impact in an unselected series of 1897 cytogenetically analyzed AML cases. Blood 2003;102(7):2395–402.

Prognostic Factors in Adult Acute Leukemia

Chezi Ganzel, MD*, Jacob M. Rowe, MD

KEYWORDS

- Acute myeloid leukemia • Acute lymphoblastic leukemia
- Adult acute leukemia • Cytogenetics • Mutations

ACUTE MYELOID LEUKEMIA

The recognized prognostic factors in acute myeloid leukemia (AML) have dramatically evolved over the past few years, becoming progressively more complex. Generally, the impact and significance of the older prognostic factors, such as morphology, immunophenotyping, and cytochemistry, which deal with the structure of the malignant cell, are subsiding as new factors dominate, such as cytogenetics and molecular determinants. Despite this evolution, the treatment of AML has not markedly changed except for the increasing use of allogeneic bone marrow transplantation because of an ever-increasing unrelated donor pool and the use of reduced-intensity conditioning for older patients and those with comorbidities. Therefore, currently, the most important implication of the prognostication is in the decision whether to send patients to allogeneic transplant in the first complete remission (CR).

Patient-Related Prognostic Factors

Age

Age is a major prognostic factor in most of the hematological malignancies, including AML. Older patients have a poorer performance status and more comorbidities. Their leukemia is more frequently secondary to an antecedent hematological disorder or is therapy-related and the malignant cells commonly have unfavorable cytogenetics and express the multidrug resistance glycoprotein 1 (MDR1).[1] The Swedish National Acute Leukemia Registry is the largest population-based unselected series that demonstrated that, regardless of management, age is a continuum and also has a strong poor prognostic impact within the group of older patients.[2] Despite the importance of age as a prognostic factor, age alone should not be a barrier to treating patients. Performance status and comorbidities are of paramount consideration.

Disclosures: The authors have nothing to disclose.
Department of Hematology, Shaare Zedek Medical Center, PO Box 3235, Jerusalem 91031, Israel
* Corresponding author.
E-mail address: ganzelct@yahoo.com

Hematol Oncol Clin N Am 25 (2011) 1163–1187
doi:10.1016/j.hoc.2011.09.017   hemonc.theclinics.com

Performance status

Performance status was historically considered an important prognostic factor in AML.[3] In a recent retrospective analysis from the Medical Research Council (MRC) in Great Britain of more than 1000 patients aged more than 60 years, performance status was found, by multivariate analysis, to be 1 of 5 independent factors that significantly influence prognosis. This finding was subsequently validated by data from another large MRC trial.[4]

Comorbidities

One of the most common explanations for the poor prognosis of older patients is their comorbidities. A retrospective study from the MD Anderson Cancer Center examined the validity of the hematopoietic cell transplantation comorbidity index (HCTCI) in patients with AML aged more than 60 years. This scoring system includes pulmonary, cardiac, hepatic, and renal impairments, as well as psychiatric disturbances, infectious disease, obesity, and a history of a solid tumor. They found that the HCTCI was predictive of an early death rate and overall survival (OS).[5]

Socioeconomic status

A Swedish study, using a cohort of more than 9000 patients with AML in Sweden between 1973 and 2005, observed that white-collar workers had a lower mortality than other socioeconomic status groups ($P = .005$).[6] Possible explanations for this observation are biologic differences in tumor characteristics, differences in the health care provider's attitude toward management, and different frequencies among patients undergoing an allogeneic transplant. In addition, lifestyle factors, such as nutritional status, physical activity, obesity, among others, that are influenced by socioeconomic status may also have an impact on patients' tolerance.[6]

Race and gender

A retrospective analysis by the Cancer and Leukemia Group B (CALGB) of 2300 whites and 270 African American patients with de novo AML found a lower CR rate ($P = .001$) and worse OS ($P = .004$) among African American men compared with whites and African American women.[7] A superior prognosis for women was also observed in white populations. The large Swedish study demonstrated a lower relative risk of death ($P = .02$) in women compared with men.[6]

Disease-Related Prognostic Factors

White blood cell count

A high white blood cell (WBC) count at diagnosis expresses a high blast count and high tumor burden. Not surprisingly, this variable was historically considered an important poor prognostic factor. It is unknown whether the prognostic effect of a high WBC count is a result of a high tumor burden or is a surrogate for leukemias that have distinct entities with different pathophysiology and clinical characteristics. For example, a high leukocyte count may be associated with a molecular change, like the FLT3-ITD mutation, and the molecular aberration is likely to be responsible for the poor prognosis and not the WBC itself. Furthermore, a precise cutoff defining a high WBC has not been established. Different investigators have preferred different cutoffs of WBC: 20,000/μL,[8] 30,000/μL,[9] 50,000/μL,[10] or 100,000/μL.[11–13] When the WBC exceeds 100,000/μL, the term hyperleukocytosis is usually used and patients are at an increased risk of developing clinical symptoms of leukostasis. Dutcher and colleagues[14] showed that among patients with AML, those with hyperleukocytosis have a lower CR rate, disease-free survival (DFS), and OS and a high rate of early mortality as opposed to Greenwood and colleagues,[9] who demonstrated that only early mortality was affected by hypoleukocytosis without influence on the other prognostic parameters. In contrast to the importance of a high WBC count at diagnosis, leukopenia at diagnosis does not seem to have any prognostic significance in AML.[15]

Immunophenotyping

Many studies have attempted to find an association between immunophenotyping and prognosis. Some reported on single antigen expression that correlate with poor prognosis and others identified clusters of antigens to be associated to the prognosis. Examples of antigens with a poor prognosis, demonstrated in more than one study include the following: CD7,[16,17] CD11b,[16,18] CD14,[16,17] CD34[19,20] and HLA-DR.[19,21] Li and colleagues[17] demonstrated, in a cohort of more than 800 patients with AML, that the poor-risk antigens correlate not only with poor prognosis but also with unfavorable-risk cytogenetics. This finding confirms that antigens on the leukemic cells may not independently influence the prognosis. They are associated markers for the more important genetic changes.

Other factors, such as thrombocytopenia, organomegaly, and an elevated lactate dehydrogenase, have been proposed in some publications as poor prognostic factors, but these findings are clearly not consistently observed.

Cytogenetics

Cytogenics came into the forefront in AML in the 1970s, when some of the seminal early predictions of the impact on prognosis in AML were reported.[22,23] Since that time, several refinements have been made because of improved karyotypic resolution. As a result, karyotypic analysis has become indispensable in the management of patients with AML and are now an inherent part of the analysis of data in any large clinical trial in AML. Several classifications have been reported, all following a similar broader outline that, nevertheless, includes important differences.[24–26] Currently, cytogenetics are considered the single most important factor in the management of patients with AML. An abnormal karyotype is found in about 60% of patients with AML.[27] Several studies in recent years have attempted to divide patients with AML into prognostic groups according to their karyotype. Most of the data from the different studies are consistent and the variations are summarized in **Table 1**.[27]

Only 3 types of karyotypes are considered as having a favorable outcome after intensive chemotherapy. These karyotypes are the following: t(15;17) in APL, inv(16)/t(16;16), and t(8:21), which are genomic aberrations that are characterized at the molecular stage by the interruption of genes encoding subunits of the core-binding factor (CBF).[24,26,28,29] On the other hand, some types of karyotypes represent adverse prognostic outcomes that are associated with greater resistance to any form of aggressive chemotherapy. These karyotypes include abnormalities of (3q), monosomy 5 or 7, del (5q) or (7q), t(9;22), and a complex karyotype. There are other, less-frequent karyotypes lacking information because of the small number of patients in any group. Patients with a normal karyotype or with aberrations that are not included in the previous groups are considered an intermediate prognostic group. Recently, Grimwade and colleagues[29] summarized the largest cytogenetic cohort of patients with AML containing cytogenetic and clinical information of 5876 younger adults (aged 16–59 years) who were treated in several MRC trials between 1988 and 2009. This study adds information about rare recurring cytogenetic abnormalities and several combinations of aberrations (**Table 2**). In a multivariate analysis, the poorer outcome observed in this study was in patients with the following: abn(3q) excluding t(3;5)(q25;q34); inv(3)(q21q26)/t(3;3)(q21;q26); add(5q)/del(5q); -5,-7,add(7q)/del(7q); t(6;11)(q27;q23); t(10;11)(p11˜13;q23); other t(11q23), excluding t(9;11)(p21˜22;q23)

Table 1
Variation in cytogenetic risk group classification across clinical trial group

	Original MRC[24]	SWOG/ECOG[26]	CALGB[28]	GIMEMA AML10[35]	GERMAN AMLCG[155]	HOVON/SAKK[37]	Refined MRC[29]
Favorable	t(15;17) t(8;21) inv(16)/t(16;16)	t(15;17) t(8;21)(lacking del(9q), complex (ie, ≥3 unrel abn) inv(16)/t(16;16)/del(16q)	t(15;17) t(8;21) inv(16)/t(16;16)	t(15;17) t(8;21) inv(16)/t(16;16)	t(15;17) t(8;21) inv(16)/t(16;16)	t(15;17) t(8;21) inv/del(16) & lacking unfav abn	t(15;17) t(8;21) inv(16)/t(16;16)
Intermediate	Normal other noncomplex abn(3q) -5/del(5q) -7 complex [≥5 unrel abn]	Normal +6, +8, -Y, del(12p), abn(3q), (9q), (11q), (21q) abn(17p) -5/del(5q) -7/del(7q) t(6;9) t(9;22) complex [≥3 unrel abn]	Normal other noncomplex inv(3)/t(3;3) -7 t(6;9) t(6;11) t(11;19) +8 complex [≥3 unrel abn]	Normal -Y Other	Normal other noncomplex inv(3)/t(3;3) -5/del(5q) -7/del (7q) abn(11q23) del(12p) abn(17p) complex [≥3 unrel abn]	Normal other noncomplex abn(3q) -5/del(5q) -7/del (7q) abn(11q23) t(6;9) t(9;22) complex [≥3 unrel abn]	Normal other noncomplex abn(3q) [excluding t(3;5)] inv(3)/t(3;3) add(5q)/del(5q),/-5, -7/add(7q), t(6;11) t(10;11) t(9;22) -17, abn(17p) with other changes complex [≥3 unrel abn]
Adverse	Excluding those with favorable changes		Excluding those with favorable changes				

Abbreviations: abn, abnormal; SWOG, South West Oncology Group; unfav abn, unfavorable abnormality; unrel abn, unrelated abnormality.
Data from Grimwade D, Hills RK. Independent prognostic factors for AML outcome. Hematology Am Soc Hematol Educ Program 2009:385–95.

Table 2
Summary of most of the known prognostic factors in AML

	Standard	Intermediate	Unfavorable	Uncertain
A. Patient related				
Age			>50 >65 >75	
Performance status			Poor	
Comorbidities			Multiple	
Socioeconomic status	White collar			
Race and gender			African American men	
B. Disease related				
WBC count			More than 20/ 30/ 50/ 100,000/μL	
Immunophenotype			CD7/ 11b/ 14/34, HLA-DR	
Cytogenetics (according the MRC)	t(15;17)(q22;q21), t(8;21)(q22;q22), inv(16)(p13q22)/ t(16;16)(p13;q22) Regardless of additional cytogenetics	Entities not classified as favorable or unfavorable	abn(3q) [excluding t(3;5)(q25;q34)], inv(3)(q21q26)/ t(3;3)(q21;q26), add(5q)/del(5q), -5, -7,add(7q)/del(7q), t(6;11)(q27;q23), t(10;11)(p1Ῑ13;q23), other t(11q23) [excluding t(9;11) (p2Ῑ22;q23) and t(11;19)(q23;p13)], t(9;22)(q34;q11), -17, and abn(17p), Complex (≥4 unrelated abnormalities) Excluding cases with favorable karyotype	
Molecular diagnosis:				
CBF AML			T(8;21) + KIT mut	inv(16) + KIT mut
Normal karyotype			FLT3-ITD	FLT3-TKD
	NPM1 mut FLT3 wt		TET2	IDH1+IDH2
	CEBPA dm FLT3 wt		DNMT3A	NRAS+KRAS
			TP53 mut	WT1
			MDR1 overexposed	MLL-PTD
Secondary AML (in addition to karyotype)		t-AML in int. cytogenetic group	t-AML in unfavorable group	t-AML in favorable group

(continued on next page)

Table 2 (continued)				
	Standard	Intermediate	Unfavorable	Uncertain
C. Response related				
Day 14–16 marrow	<10% blasts		≥10% blasts	
			In a cellular BM	
PB blast clearance	Early			
MRD	Negative		Positive	

Prognostic factors in AML listed are not exclusive but in most cases included those reported by more than one group.
Abbreviations: abn, abnormal; BM, bone marrow; dm, double mutation (biallelic); int, intermediate; mut, mutated; PB, peripheral blood; wt, wild type.

and t(11;19)(q23;p13); t(9;22)(q34;q11); -17; and abn(17p). Another uncertainty that this study tried to resolve was the definition of a complex karyotype, which, among published studies, ranged between 3[26,28] and 5 aberrations.[24,30] In this study, patients with 4 or more cytogenetic abnormalities, which are not included in the standard (favorable) and poor prognostic ones, were considered as having a complex karyotype with a poor prognosis. It is likely that the unfavorable prognostic group needs to be further subdivided into smaller groups. An important report from the Dutch Hovon group was the first to report on the unfavorable prognosis of patients with the monosomal karyotype, which was defined as 2 or more monosomies or a single monosomy in the presence of structural abnormalities, having an extremely poor prognosis.[31,32] These data were subsequently confirmed by other groups evaluating a large cohort of patients with AML and correlating with cytogenetic abnormalities.[33]

Another type of combination with conflicting reports is the favorable karyotype, such as inv(16), together with additional abnormalities. The data here are limited because of the small numbers of patients in the different studies. The huge cohort of the MRC suggested that additional cytogenetic aberrations do not adversely impact the favorable prognosis of patients with t(15;17), inv(16)/t(16;16), and t(8;21) treated on current intensive protocols. Furthermore, in patients with inv(16), the presence of additional chromosomal changes, such +22, have been reported to predict a better outcome.[29]

The standard or favorable karyotype group accounts for about 20% of young patients with AML (aged <55 years) and about 7% of older patients, although the absolute incidence of patients with the favorable karyotype is not decreased with older age. The CR rate of these patients is high (about 90%), the 5-year OS is about 45% to 65%, and the relapse rate is low.[24,26,28,30] On the other hand, the unfavorable cytogenetic group consists of about 15% to 20% of patients with AML, depending on the age and the different study definitions. The CR rate is less than 50% and the 5-year OS is less than 20%.[24,26,30]

The practical implication of assigning patients to prognostic groups relates to the decision regarding which patients should be referred for allogeneic transplant in the first CR. In terms of DFS, the MRC study[34] demonstrated a benefit for transplant mainly in the intermediate group, but the European Organization for Research and Treatment of Cancer - Gruppo Italiano Malattie Ematologiche Maligne dell'Adulto (EORTC-GIMEMA)[35] found benefit only in the unfavorable group. A meta-analysis, which took into consideration these 2 studies together with the Dutch-Belgian Hemato-Oncology Cooperative Group - Swiss Group for Clinical Cancer Research (HOVON-SAKK) and

Bordeaux Grenoble Marseille Toulouse Cooperative Group (BGMT)[36] studies, showed a benefit for allogeneic transplant with both intermediate and high-risk groups. The benefit was not only in DFS but also in OS.[37] Despite these conclusions of the meta-analysis, the intermediate risk group, especially the huge subgroup of normal karyotype, still comprises a large heterogeneous group of patients. The need for the refinement of prognostic subgroups has led to the use of molecular markers, which allows for better discrimination of the prognostic impact (**Fig. 1**).

MOLECULAR MARKERS
CBF AMLs

The long-term OS of CBF AMLs is better than other AMLs but is still only about 45%.[38] Thus, the common name of this group as favorable is a misnomer. Defining the patients with the worst prognosis will facilitate sending these patients to allogeneic transplant early and improving their outcome.

KIT mutations

The KIT gene encodes a 145-kD transmembrane glycoprotein, which is a member of the type III receptor tyrosine kinase family. Following ligand binding, the receptor activates downstream signaling pathways involved in proliferation and differentiation. Gain-of-function mutations can cause ligand-independent activation of KIT. In CBF AML, KIT mutations cluster most frequently within exon 17, which encodes the KIT activation loop in the kinase domain, and in exon 8, which encodes a region in the extracellular portion of the KIT receptor that is thought to play a role in receptor dimerization.[39] The incidence of KIT mutation is between 20% to 40% in both t(8;21) and inv(16) in different studies.[39–41] Some studies examined the prognostic implication of KIT mutation but with different conclusions. In patients with t(8;21), the cumulative incidence of relapse is higher in patients with KIT mutation compared with wild type (WT). Most studies,[40–43] but not all of them,[39] also showed decreased OS in patients with a mutation. In patients with inv(16), some have reported that OS had an adverse impact among the mutated patients,[39] whereas other studies failed to demonstrate any prognostic impact.[40,43]

Normal Karyotype

About 40% of AMLs have a normal karyotype and belong to the intermediate prognostic group. Several molecular markers can help to subcategorize this heterogeneous group (see **Table 2**).

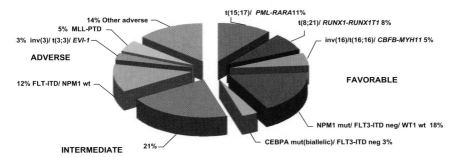

Fig. 1. Distribution of cytogenetically and molecularly defined risk group in AML.[97] (*Reproduced from* American Society of Hematology (ASH), Smith ML, Hills RK, Grimwade D. Independent prognostic variables in acute myeloid leukaemia. Blood Rev 2011;25(1):39–51; with permission.)

Mutations

FLT3 mutations FLT3 is another member of the type III receptor tyrosine kinase family. It is expressed normally in early progenitors in the bone marrow and has an important part in hematopoiesis.[44] FLT3 is expressed at high levels in 70% to 100% of patients with AML.[45] The most common mutations are the internal tandem duplications (ITD) that occur in about 25% of AMLs.[46] These mutations disrupt the autoinhibitory function of the juxtamembrane domain of the receptor.[47] Patients with these mutations present frequently with a high WBC count,[48,49] and most of them have normal cytogenetics.[50] Although the CR rate of patients with these mutations is not significantly different from those with the WT,[49,51] the DFS and OS are reduced.[48,51,52] High FLT3 mutant levels tend to worsen the prognosis.[50,53] Another type of FLT3 mutations, although less frequent, were described in the tyrosine kinase domain. These mutations are also associated with a high WBC count[54] and are most frequent in patients with a normal karyotype, but reports on their prognostic impact is conflicting. Different studies showed positive,[54] negative,[55,56] or no[57] impact on prognosis. This variability can be related to different combinations of aberrations[57] or to different incidence of biallelic disease.[58]

Nucleophosmin mutations Nucleophosmin (NPM1) is a nucleolar protein that shuttles between the nucleus and the cytoplasm. It has several functions, including regulation of the transport and import of different particles through the nuclear membrane[59] and interaction with p53 in controlling cell proliferation and apoptosis.[44] NPM1 mutations seem to be founder genetic alterations.[60] These mutations are responsible for the aberrant expression of the nucleolar nucleophosmin in the cytoplasm of the leukemic cells. For this reason, these aberrations can be recognized not only by molecular assays but also by immunohistochemical staining and flow cytometry.[60] The mutations can be found in about one-third of adult AML and about 50% of AMLs with normal karyotype.[61] Several studies demonstrated the favorable effect of NPM1 mutations on prognosis. Some demonstrated this in patients with both FLT3-ITD mutations and FLT3-WT, creating 3 different prognostic groups: NPM1+/FLT3-WT (favorable), NPM1-/FLT3-WT or NPM1+/FLT3-ITD (intermediate), and NPM1-/FLT3-ITD (unfavorable) (**Fig. 2**).[53] Others confirmed its favorable effect only in patients with FLT3-WT and not in patients with FLT3-ITD.[62,63] The NPM1 mutations, as founder aberrations, are stable throughout the course of the disease and can be used as markers for MRD assessment and for the detection of early relapse.[64]

CEBPA mutations CEBPA (CCAAT/enhancer-binding protein alpha) encodes a transcription factor essential for neutrophil development. CEBPA mutations create an imbalance between proliferation and differentiation of hematopoietic progenitors.[65] In patients with a normal karyotype, biallelic mutations have significant advantage in both CR rate[65] and OS.[65,66] The picture of monoallelic mutations is much less clear. Some reported a survival advantage over WT,[65] and others found both conditions to be the same.[66] No study found monoallelic mutations to be an independent favorable prognostic factor in multivariate analysis.[65,66] In patients with monoallelic mutations, the presence of FLT3-ITD mutations is still an independent unfavorable prognostic factor (see **Fig. 2**).[65] There are some reports of patients with germ line mutations, part of them with familial AML.[65,67]

Other mutations Many other mutations have been described with different importance and varying significance. Mutations of the isocitrate dehydrogenase 1 and 2 genes (IDH1 and IDH2) were described in about 10% to 15% of patients with AML with normal karyotype,[68–71] but their prognostic impact is not clear. IDH1 mutations

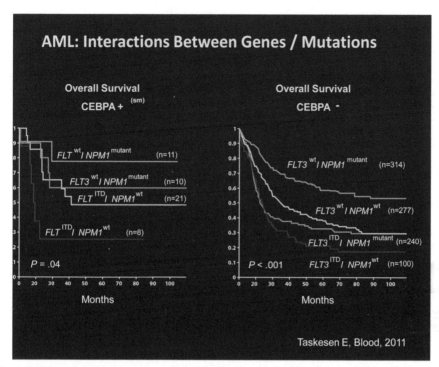

Fig. 2. Kaplan-Meier survival curves for overall survival in AML with and without the CEBPα mutation. All 4 genotypes have improved overall survival with even a single CEBPα mutation (*left graph*). (*Reproduced from* American Society of Hematology, Taskesen E, Bullinger L, Corbacioglu A. Prognostic impact, concurrent genetic mutations, and gene expression features of AML with CEBPA double mutant AML as a distinctive disease entity. Blood 2011;117:2469–75; with permission.)

may be associated with unfavorable outcomes[70,71] or do not have any prognostic impact.[72] In IDH2, the variation of descriptions is wider with claims for unfavorable,[71] favorable,[73] and no[72,74] prognostic impact. RAS mutations (NRAS and KRAS) can be seen in between 12% and 27% of patients with AML[75] and do not have clear outcome implication.[72,76–79] There are data to suggest that patients with RAS mutations benefit most from postremission high-dose cytarabine.[75,80] Wilms tumor gene mutation occurs in about 10% of patients with normal karyotype AML.[81,82] Here again, its prognostic impact is controversial; although studies of the MRC and CALGB demonstrated association with poorer outcome,[81,82] a German group did not find any prognostic impact.[83] Partial tandem duplications of the mixed lineage leukemia gene (MLL-PTD) were found in about 10% of normal karyotype AMLs.[84] Most of the studies showed association between these aberrations and unfavorable outcomes[85,86] but not all of them.[84] TET2 mutations are a common event in a spectrum of myeloid malignancies, including MDS, myeloproliferative disorder, and acute leukemia.[87] A recent study found unfavorable prognosis in patients with AML with TET2 mutations.[88] DNMT3A mutations are associated with poor outcomes.[89] Mutations in TP53 can be seen mainly in patients with complex karyotype and are quite rare in normal karyotype AMLs,[90] and, not surprisingly, they predict for an unfavorable outcome.[91]

Overexpression

Overexpression of some genes has been demonstrated to have significant prognostic impact in patients with normal karyotype AML. Important examples are the Brain and Acute Leukemia Cytoplasmic gene (BAALC),[92] Meningioma1 gene,[93,94] and Ectopic Virus Integration 1 gene.[95,96] The interpretation of such quantitative tests is complex and it holds within it questions of standardization and establishment of reference values.[97]

Multidrug resistance Overexpression of some genes is responsible for high levels of resistance proteins that disturb the influence of chemotherapeutic agents on the malignant cells. The most important one is the MDR1. This gene encodes for a P-glycoprotein, which is a drug efflux protein that decreases anthracyclines accumulation in the cells resulting in the development of anthracyclines-resistant cells. MDR1 expression increases with age[98] and has a significant independent adverse influence on both CR rate and OS.[99,100] This influence is also relevant when looking on a subgroup of patients with AML with intermediate-risk cytogenetics.[100] Overexpression of other drug-resistance genes, such as as MRP1 and lung resistance protein gene, has less significant prognostic influence on patients with AML.[98,100]

Secondary AML

Secondary AML is a broad definition that includes AMLs secondary to an antecedent stem cell disorder, like MDS or myeloproliferative neoplasm, or secondary to past chemotherapeutic/radiotherapeutic treatment (t-AML). These leukemias are thought to have a worse prognosis. The main reason is that most of the secondary AMLs have cytogenetic abnormalities associated with a poor outcome.[30] Whether the outcome of secondary AML is a result of the unfavorable cytogenetics only or is also independently related to the history of the disease has been a controversial issue. The German AML Cooperative Group (AMLCG) compared karyotype and survival between patients with t-AML and those with primary AML. They found that in the t-AML, the percentage of patients with unfavorable karyotype was higher than in the de novo patients. The median OS was significantly shorter in the t-AML group. Favorable and unfavorable cytogenetics had a significant survival impact in the t-AML group.[101] In an update of this study, it was reported that in the favorable and unfavorable group, the t-AMLs do worse than their parallels in the de novo group. In contrast, in the intermediate karyotype group, there was no significant difference between the groups.[102] Another study reported that CBF t-AMLs have similar results and the same characteristics as de novo patients,[103] but more recent studies from the MD Anderson Cancer Center found that the CBF t-AML have worse outcomes than the de novo ones.[104,105]

Regarding AML secondary to MDS, the German AMLCG demonstrated that dysplasia by itself has no independent prognostic impact under the conditions of intensive induction therapy but is related in many cases to an unfavorable karyotype.[106]

Response-Related Prognostic Factors

Early response

A different approach for the prediction of an individual outcome is by evaluation of early response parameters. The amount of residual leukemic blasts in bone marrow on the sixteenth day from the beginning of the induction therapy was demonstrated, in the German AMLCG, to predict for a long-term outcome, even in patients who achieved CR.[107] Others showed that the number of blasts (less or more than 5%) on day 14 can predict CR but not long-term outcomes.[108] There is also evidence for an association between the high number of plasma cells in day 14 marrow and residual leukemia.[109] An Italian group attempted to substitute early bone marrow examination by following the clearance of the leukemic blasts from the peripheral blood using daily flow cytometry. They found correlation between the clearance rate and the day 14 marrow.[110]

Cytogenetic CR

Achievement of CR is a requirement, although not sufficient, for cure.[111] The CALGB demonstrated that patients with abnormal karyotype at diagnosis, in whom the bone marrow was converted to normal karyotype at first CR, have significantly better outcomes.[112]

MRD

MRD is a developing and promising risk-assessment system. The model of MRD in AML came from APL, in which real-time quantitative polymerase chain reaction (RQ-PCR) for PML-RARA transcript level, after consolidation, became the follow-up standard of care.[113] Basically, there are 2 main methods of MRD assessment based on PCR amplification of molecular abnormalities and flow cytometric detection of abnormal immunophenotypes. RQ-PCR is now considered the preferred PCR method because it is less prone to contamination, allows the kinetics of disease response and relapse to be defined, and enables poor quality samples that could have given rise to false negative results according to older PCR assays to be identified based on the level of endogenous control gene transcripts (eg, *ABL*).[113] The PCR method is based on amplification of fusion transcripts as AML1-ETO, CBFbeta/MYH11 and MLL-AF9 with the limitation that only about one-third of patients with AML have these transcripts.[114] Patients with persistent high levels of fusion transcripts at the end of consolidation or reappearance of transcripts after molecular remission are prone to early relapse.[115–117] Other options are based on the detection of overexpressed genes, like WT1, or mutated genes, like FLT3-ITD and NPM1. The European Leukemia study demonstrated that greater WT1 transcript reduction after induction can predict the relapse risk,[118] although the background of normal bone marrow cells may limit the reliability of this assay.[114] NPM1 MRD level was shown, by multivariate analysis, to be an important prognostic factor[118] but FLT3-ITD is more controversial as an MRD marker because of the observation that this marker may not be stable during the course of disease.[114,119,120] The other method of MRD detection uses flow cytometry for identifying the aberrant expression pattern of cellular markers on the leukemic cells. In about 75% of patients with AML there is abnormal immunophenotype.[114] Because the immunophenotype can distinguish the leukemic cells from the normal bone marrow cells, the sensitivity of the test improves, in the range of between 1 leukemic cell among 1000 to 10,000 normal cells.[114] An Italian study demonstrated that a bone marrow with more than 3.5×10^{-4} residual leukemic cells after consolidation is considered MRD positive and carries a poor prognosis.[121] The limitations of this method are the option of immunophenotypic changes that may occur during the course of the disease and that the results depend on the investigator interpretation.[114]

Scores

Because of the large number of prognostic factors in AML, many groups tried to compose prognostic scores that take into account some factors together. For example, a Korean group developed a model based on MDR status and cytogenetics.[122] An Italian group developed a prognostic scoring for cytogenetically normal patients that rely on age of more than 50 years, secondary AML, and a WBC greater than 20,000/ml. A European group recently published an integrative prognostic risk score for normal karyotype AMLs based on age; WBC; and several molecular markers, like NPM1, FLT3-ITD, BAALC, WT1, and others.[123] The main problem of these and of many other models is that they were not prospectively validated in large cohorts.

ACUTE LYMPHOBLASTIC LEUKEMIA

As in AML, it is important to distinguish between pretreatment prognostic factors and those that only become apparent after therapy has been given.

At Presentation

Many of the historic prognostic factors have been superseded by cytogenetics and molecular determinants, in a manner similar to AML. Thus, morphology[124] and cyto-chemistry,[125] so dominant in the 1970s, now have no prognostic significance in acute lymphoblastic leukemia (ALL). Even immunophenotyping, which was the dominant determining factor for several decades since the 1980s, is rapidly becoming less important for prognostication, even if it remains crucial for the initial diagnosis, for the detection of MRD and for the application of specific and targeted therapies. Thus, although B- and T-lineage patients are often treated differently, the level of maturity within B-lineage is no longer important for prognosis.[126,127] Among T-lineage patients, data from sequential trials by the German Acute Lymphoblastic Leukemia Group suggest that within T-lineage patients there seems to be a significant prognostic difference depending on the level of maturity.[128] These data were confirmed in the large analysis of 356 uniformly treated patients from the international ALL study conducted jointly by the MRC in Britain and the Eastern Cooperative Oncology Group (ECOG) in the United States whereby patients with the cortical thymocyte stage, characterized by the expression of CD1a, have a significantly improved outcome compared with patients who were CD1a- (64% vs 39%, $P = .01$). In this same study, patients with T-ALL with CD1a-, who were also negative for CD13, had a better OS than those who were CD13+ (61% vs 35%, $P = .001$).[129] At the same time, among B-lineage patients, several reports have recognized the presence of CD20 as having a significant adverse prognostic impact.[130,131]

Age has withstood the test of time and remains the most important prognostic factor in ALL that is unlikely to be superseded by any of the new molecular determinants. Not only are there enormous differences in childhood and adult ALL but age also critically affects the prognosis within adult groups. Although most clinical studies have used an arbitrary cutoff of 35 or 40 years,[132–134] the prognostic significance of age is in fact a continuum between the age of 20 and 60 years (**Fig. 3**) and similarly in older patients.

As in AML, the pretreatment prognosis is moving rapidly to an almost complete dependence on cytogenetics and molecular markers.

Until fairly recently, the practical use of cytogenetics in ALL, especially in adults, was limited to the presence of the Philadelphia chromosome. This limited use was partly because of the relative infrequency of ALL in adults and the limited information on the importance of recurring cytogenetic abnormalities other than the Philadelphia chromosome.

The Philadelphia chromosome, t(9;22)(q44;q11), remains the most frequent and clinically significant abnormality in adult ALL, with an incidence that increases to 50% among older adults with B-lineage ALL.[135] The importance of this information

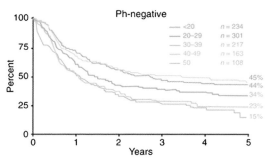

Fig. 3. Overall survival by age for Philadelphia-chromosome negative ALL, ages 15 to 60 years. MRC UKALLXII//ECOG 2993 trial. (*Reproduced from* American Society of Hematology, Rowe JM, Buck G, Burnett AK, et al. Induction therapy for adults with acute lymphoblastic leukemia: results of more than 1500 patients from the international ALL trial: MRC UKALL XII/ECOG E2993. Blood 2005;106:3760–7; with permission.)

in adults is crucial, not only for a prognostic reason but also because of the availability of novel tyrosine kinase inhibitors, which have dramatically altered the prognosis of such patients.[136] Although the presence of the Philadelphia chromosome in a 75-year-old individual previously spelled impending doom, now, in such a patient, the presence of the Philadelphia chromosome actually predicts for a better outcome with a high likelihood of a good initial response because of the availability of specific therapy with one of the tyrosine kinase inhibitors.

There have been many recurring cytogenetic abnormalities reported, but in several of the publications it has not been easy to determine the absolute independent prognostic significance because of the small number in most reports.[137–140] The analysis of cytogenetics of patients treated on the MRC UKALL XII/ECOG 2993 study provided the largest prospective analysis and report of prognostic factors in adult ALL and has propelled cytogenetics into the forefront of the classification of ALL (**Table 3**).[141] A complex karyotype, previously intuitively thought to predict for a poor outcome, for the first time, was demonstrated to be a completely independent prognostic factor in ALL.

Most of the prognostic factors in adults are similar to the prognostic value in childhood ALL, although with markedly differing frequencies, but there are some

Table 3
Cytogenetic, molecular, and immunologic markers of prognostic significance in adult ALL

Cytogenetics	Molecular Markers	Immunologic Surface Markers	Significance
t(9;22) (q24; q11.2)	BCR-ABL fusion	Early T-cell	Poor prognosis
t(4;11) (q21; q23)	MLL-AF4		
t(8;14) (q24.1; q32)	BAALC gene	CD20	
Low hypodiploidy/ near triploidy	IKAROS gene		
Complex karyotype			
t(1;19) (q21; p13.3)	NOTCH1		Conflicting data
	FBXW7		
High hyperdiploidy Del (9q)			Better prognosis

exceptions. Most important here is the del(9p) that had a significantly improved outcome in the large MRC/ECOG study in contrast to childhood ALL whereby 9p abnormalities are often considered with more unfavorable prognostic factors, especially among B-lineage ALL.[142] The reliability of data from the MRC/ECOG study is partly caused by the large numbers in this trial and, just as importantly, by the fact that this was not a risk-adapted strategy. Rather, because all patients were either biologically selected or randomly assigned to a transplant, regardless of the risk group, all patients received the identical postremission therapy, thus, allowing for a degree of confidence that the abnormalities detected in this study have a prognostic significance that is independent of the therapy that was given.

Molecular markers have clearly become a potent prognostic tool in ALL and also provide for potential targeted therapies. Probably the most common molecular markers in T-ALL are the activating mutations of NOTCH1,[143,144] although the prognostic implications of the NOTCH1 pathway are still uncertain, with conflicting data reported among 2 of the major groups.[145,146] It must be noted that it is always difficult to separate out the different therapies used in the various trials that may have potentially overcome the prognostic significance of any molecular marker, thus, accounting for discrepancies between these reports. Another important molecular marker is the BAALC gene, which is present in early hematopoietic progenitor cells and has been demonstrated to be associated with a poor outcome in adults with T-cell ALL[147] and among B-lineage patients.[148] Importantly, this prognostic factor identifies a high-risk group of B-lineage patients that is independent of BCR-ABL or MLL-AF4.

Response-Based Prognostic Factors

Multiple studies have reported on the importance of achieving a complete response within 4 weeks of therapy,[149] although this could not be confirmed in the MRC/ECOG study.[134] However, such markers are being superseded by the importance of achieving a complete molecular response rather than just a morphologic CR. The assessment of MRD provides for more individualized prognostication because it reflects the biology of the disease, the pharmacokinetics, and the pharmacodynamics in individual patients. Although the measurement of MRD is rapidly moving into the forefront of prognostication in ALL, there is still considerable confusion around the optimal method used for such measurement and, most importantly, the optimal timing for the evaluation of MRD and assigning the appropriate medical relevance. The most widely used technique is the PCR of immunoglobulin and TCR gene rearrangement. The sensitivity of this method is about 0.01% to 0.001%, which means the detection of one leukemic cell in 10,000 to 100,000 normal cells. Other methodologies use either multiparameter flow cytometry or a PCR analysis of fusion genes, although the latter is limited to patients who have a defined genetic abnormality, such as BCR-ABL.

The most important data for the use of MRD in adults comes from the German ALL Group, which defined 3 risk groups according to MRD. The lower-risk group had a rapid MRD decline or negative MRD at both days 11 and 24, when the relapse rate at 3 years was 0%. The high-risk group had a positive MRD until week 16; in such patients, the 3-year relapse rate was 94%. Most patients, more than two-thirds, composed the intermediate risk group, with a 3-year relapse rate of 47%.[150] Cleary the greatest uncertainty rests with this large intermediate group, and, as in AML, attempts are being made for a better predictive value using an integrated use of MRD with pretreatment molecular markers, such as IKZF1.[151] Although the MRD alone in the intermediate group could identify only 46% of relapses and IKZF1 predicted 54%, the integrated use predicted almost 80% of relapses with 93% specificity.[151]

The importance of MRD for ALL cannot be overemphasized, and it is likely that molecular response to treatment will redefine many pretreatment prognostic factors in ALL, both in childhood and adult ALL.[152]

Pharmacogenetics

Just as the measurement of MRD provides for individualized information for the response to therapy, the results within each group also depend on drug pharmacogenetics, which relates to drug metabolism and excretion, and the pharmacodynamics, which are affected by the direct efficacy of the drug on the leukemia cell and the toxicity of the normal cells. There is an enormous variation among individual patients, which is influenced by drug metabolism, enzyme levels, and various transportation mechanisms. There are multiple studies of genetic mechanisms, including single-nucleotide polymorphisms and other genomic alterations,[153,154] that directly affect drug metabolism. Although not of clinical use now, the increasing ability for genetic profiling and proteomic analysis is likely to have a major impact in the next decade and it is hoped that it will further help in the design and prediction of patient response to therapy.

SUMMARY

The prognostic factors in acute leukemia have undergone a major change over the past decade and are likely to be further refined in the coming years. While age is the single most important prognostic factor in both AML and in ALL, recurring cytogenetic abnormalities and molecular markers have become crucial for the prognosis of patients and for new directions in the development of targeted therapies. No less important is the development of a personalized approach for therapy as determined by the response to therapy using increasingly sensitive technologies. The assessment of MRD is rapidly superseding other prognostic factors in ALL and, somewhat lacking behind, coming into its own in AML. The next decade should see further refinement of response-driven prognostication, to include epigenetics as well as pharmacogenetics and pharmacodynamics of individual drugs used and the responses to them. It is hoped that these refinements and better predictors of response will also lead to a significantly improved overall outcome of patients with both AML and ALL.

ACKNOWLEDGMENTS

The assistance of Sarah Farkash in the preparation of this article is gratefully acknowledged.

REFERENCES

1. Hiddemann W, Kern W, Schoch C, et al. Management of acute myeloid leukemia in elderly patients. J Clin Oncol 1999;17(11):3569–76.
2. Juliusson G, Antunovic P, Derolf A, et al. Age and acute myeloid leukemia: real world data on decision to treat and outcomes from the Swedish Acute Leukemia Registry. Blood 2009;113(18):4179–87.
3. Johnson PR, Hunt LP, Yin JA. Prognostic factors in elderly patients with acute myeloid leukaemia: development of a model to predict survival. Br J Haematol 1993;85(2):300–6.
4. Wheatley K, Brookes CL, Howman AJ, et al. Prognostic factor analysis of the survival of elderly patients with AML in the MRC AML11 and LRF AML14 trials. Br J Haematol 2009;145(5):598–605.

5. Giles FJ, Borthakur G, Ravandi F, et al. The haematopoietic cell transplantation comorbidity index score is predictive of early death and survival in patients over 60 years of age receiving induction therapy for acute myeloid leukaemia. Br J Haematol 2007;136(4):624–7.
6. Kristinsson SY, Derolf AR, Edgren G, et al. Socioeconomic differences in patient survival are increasing for acute myeloid leukemia and multiple myeloma in Sweden. J Clin Oncol 2009;27(12):2073–80.
7. Sekeres MA, Peterson B, Dodge RK, et al. Differences in prognostic factors and outcomes in African Americans and whites with acute myeloid leukemia. Blood 2004;103(11):4036–42.
8. Malagola M, Skert C, Vignetti M, et al. A simple prognostic scoring system for newly diagnosed cytogenetically normal acute myeloid leukemia: retrospective analysis of 530 patients. Leuk Lymphoma. [Epub ahead of print].
9. Greenwood MJ, Seftel MD, Richardson C, et al. Leukocyte count as a predictor of death during remission induction in acute myeloid leukemia. Leuk Lymphoma 2006;47(7):1245–52.
10. Vaughan WP, Kimball AW, Karp JE, et al. Factors affecting survival of patients with acute myelocytic leukemia presenting with high WBC counts. Cancer Treat Rep 1981;65(11–12):1007–13.
11. Hug V, Keating M, McCredie K, et al. Clinical course and response to treatment of patients with acute myelogenous leukemia presenting with a high leukocyte count. Cancer 1983;52(5):773–9.
12. Chen CC, Yang CF, Yang MH, et al. Pretreatment prognostic factors and treatment outcome in elderly patients with de novo acute myeloid leukemia. Ann Oncol 2005;16(8):1366–73.
13. Lowenberg B, Suciu S, Archimbaud E, et al. Use of recombinant GM-CSF during and after remission induction chemotherapy in patients aged 61 years and older with acute myeloid leukemia: final report of AML-11, a phase III randomized study of the Leukemia Cooperative Group of European Organisation for the Research and Treatment of Cancer and the Dutch Belgian Hemato-Oncology Cooperative Group. Blood 1997;90(8):2952–61.
14. Dutcher JP, Schiffer CA, Wiernik PH. Hyperleukocytosis in adult acute nonlymphocytic leukemia: impact on remission rate and duration, and survival. J Clin Oncol 1987;5(9):1364–72.
15. Arellano M, Bernal-Mizrachi L, Pan L, et al. Prognostic significance of leukopenia at the time of diagnosis in acute myeloid leukemia. Clin Lymphoma Myeloma Leuk 2011;5:427–32.
16. Mason KD, Juneja SK, Szer J. The immunophenotype of acute myeloid leukemia: is there a relationship with prognosis? Blood Rev 2006;20(2):71–82.
17. Li X, Li J, Du W, et al. Relevance of immunophenotypes to prognostic subgroups of age, WBC, platelet count, and cytogenetics in de novo acute myeloid leukemia. APMIS 2011;119(1):76–84.
18. Bradstock K, Matthews J, Benson E, et al. Prognostic value of immunophenotyping in acute myeloid leukemia. Australian Leukaemia Study Group. Blood 1994;84(4):1220–5.
19. Chang H, Salma F, Yi QL, et al. Prognostic relevance of immunophenotyping in 379 patients with acute myeloid leukemia. Leuk Res 2004;28(1):43–8.
20. Casasnovas RO, Slimane FK, Garand R, et al. Immunological classification of acute myeloblastic leukemias: relevance to patient outcome. Leukemia 2003;17(3):515–27.

21. Callea V, Morabito F, Martino B, et al. Diagnostic and prognostic relevance of the immunophenotype in acute myelocytic leukemia. Tumori 1991;77(1):28–31.
22. Sakurai M, Sandberg AA. Prognosis of acute myeloblastic leukemia: chromosomal correlation. Blood 1973;41(1):93–104.
23. Arthur DC, Berger R, Golomb HM, et al. The clinical significance of karyotype in acute myelogenous leukemia. Cancer Genet Cytogenet 1989;40(2):203–16.
24. Grimwade D, Walker H, Oliver F, et al. The importance of diagnostic cytogenetics on outcome in AML: analysis of 1,612 patients entered into the MRC AML 10 trial. The Medical Research Council Adult and Children's Leukaemia Working Parties. Blood 1998;92(7):2322–33.
25. Grimwade D. The clinical significance of cytogenetic abnormalities in acute myeloid leukaemia. Best Pract Res Clin Haematol 2001;14(3):497–529.
26. Slovak ML, Kopecky KJ, Cassileth PA, et al. Karyotypic analysis predicts outcome of preremission and postremission therapy in adult acute myeloid leukemia: a Southwest Oncology Group/Eastern Cooperative Oncology Group Study. Blood 2000;96(13):4075–83.
27. Grimwade D, Hills RK. Independent prognostic factors for AML outcome. Hematology Am Soc Hematol Educ Program 2009;385–95.
28. Byrd JC, Mrozek K, Dodge RK, et al. Pretreatment cytogenetic abnormalities are predictive of induction success, cumulative incidence of relapse, and overall survival in adult patients with de novo acute myeloid leukemia: results from Cancer and Leukemia Group B (CALGB 8461). Blood 2002;100(13): 4325–36.
29. Grimwade D, Hills RK, Moorman AV, et al. Refinement of cytogenetic classification in acute myeloid leukemia: determination of prognostic significance of rare recurring chromosomal abnormalities among 5876 younger adult patients treated in the United Kingdom Medical Research Council trials. Blood 2010; 116(3):354–65.
30. Grimwade D, Walker H, Harrison G, et al. The predictive value of hierarchical cytogenetic classification in older adults with acute myeloid leukemia (AML): analysis of 1065 patients entered into the United Kingdom Medical Research Council AML11 trial. Blood 2001;98(5):1312–20.
31. Breems DA, Lowenberg B. Acute myeloid leukemia with monosomal karyotype at the far end of the unfavorable prognostic spectrum. Haematologica 2011; 96(4):491–3.
32. Breems DA, Van Putten WL, De Greef GE, et al. Monosomal karyotype in acute myeloid leukemia: a better indicator of poor prognosis than a complex karyotype. J Clin Oncol 2008;26(29):4791–7.
33. Medeiros BC, Othus M, Fang M, et al. Prognostic impact of monosomal karyotype in young adult and elderly acute myeloid leukemia: the Southwest Oncology Group (SWOG) experience. Blood 2010;116(13):2224–8.
34. Burnett AK, Wheatley K, Goldstone AH, et al. The value of allogeneic bone marrow transplant in patients with acute myeloid leukaemia at differing risk of relapse: results of the UK MRC AML 10 trial. Br J Haematol 2002;118(2): 385–400.
35. Suciu S, Mandelli F, de Witte T, et al. Allogeneic compared with autologous stem cell transplantation in the treatment of patients younger than 46 years with acute myeloid leukemia (AML) in first complete remission (CR1): an intention-to-treat analysis of the EORTC/GIMEMAAML-10 trial. Blood 2003;102(4):1232–40.
36. Jourdan E, Boiron JM, Dastugue N, et al. Early allogeneic stem-cell transplantation for young adults with acute myeloblastic leukemia in first complete

remission: an intent-to-treat long-term analysis of the BGMT experience. J Clin Oncol 2005;23(30):7676–84.

37. Cornelissen JJ, van Putten WL, Verdonck LF, et al. Results of a HOVON/SAKK donor versus no-donor analysis of myeloablative HLA-identical sibling stem cell transplantation in first remission acute myeloid leukemia in young and middle-aged adults: benefits for whom? Blood 2007;109(9):3658–66.

38. Appelbaum FR, Kopecky KJ, Tallman MS, et al. The clinical spectrum of adult acute myeloid leukaemia associated with core binding factor translocations. Br J Haematol 2006;135(2):165–73.

39. Paschka P, Marcucci G, Ruppert AS, et al. Adverse prognostic significance of KIT mutations in adult acute myeloid leukemia with inv(16) and t(8;21): a Cancer and Leukemia Group B Study. J Clin Oncol 2006;24(24):3904–11.

40. Cairoli R, Beghini A, Grillo G, et al. Prognostic impact of c-KIT mutations in core binding factor leukemias: an Italian retrospective study. Blood 2006;107(9): 3463–8.

41. Schnittger S, Kohl TM, Haferlach T, et al. KIT-D816 mutations in AML1-ETO-positive AML are associated with impaired event-free and overall survival. Blood 2006;107(5):1791–9.

42. Jiao B, Wu CF, Liang Y, et al. AML1-ETO9a is correlated with C-KIT overexpression/mutations and indicates poor disease outcome in t(8;21) acute myeloid leukemia-M2. Leukemia 2009;23(9):1598–604.

43. Park SH, Chi HS, Min SK, et al. Prognostic impact of c-KIT mutations in core binding factor acute myeloid leukemia. Leuk Res 2011;35(10):1376–83.

44. Foran JM. New prognostic markers in acute myeloid leukemia: perspective from the clinic. Hematology Am Soc Hematol Educ Program 2010;2010:47–55.

45. Gilliland DG, Griffin JD. The roles of FLT3 in hematopoiesis and leukemia. Blood 2002;100(5):1532–42.

46. Levis M, Small D. FLT3: ITDoes matter in leukemia. Leukemia 2003;17(9): 1738–52.

47. Levis M. FLT3/ITD AML and the law of unintended consequences. Blood 2011; 117(26):6987–90.

48. Frohling S, Schlenk RF, Breitruck J, et al. Prognostic significance of activating FLT3 mutations in younger adults (16 to 60 years) with acute myeloid leukemia and normal cytogenetics: a study of the AML Study Group Ulm. Blood 2002; 100(13):4372–80.

49. Schnittger S, Schoch C, Dugas M, et al. Analysis of FLT3 length mutations in 1003 patients with acute myeloid leukemia: correlation to cytogenetics, FAB subtype, and prognosis in the AMLCG study and usefulness as a marker for the detection of minimal residual disease. Blood 2002;100(1):59–66.

50. Thiede C, Steudel C, Mohr B, et al. Analysis of FLT3-activating mutations in 979 patients with acute myelogenous leukemia: association with FAB subtypes and identification of subgroups with poor prognosis. Blood 2002; 99(12):4326–35.

51. Kottaridis PD, Gale RE, Frew ME, et al. The presence of a FLT3 internal tandem duplication in patients with acute myeloid leukemia (AML) adds important prognostic information to cytogenetic risk group and response to the first cycle of chemotherapy: analysis of 854 patients from the United Kingdom Medical Research Council AML 10 and 12 trials. Blood 2001;98(6):1752–9.

52. Altucci L, Rossin A, Hirsch O, et al. Rexinoid-triggered differentiation and tumor-selective apoptosis of acute myeloid leukemia by protein kinase A-mediated desubordination of retinoid X receptor. Cancer Res 2005;65(19):8754–65.

53. Gale RE, Green C, Allen C, et al. The impact of FLT3 internal tandem duplication mutant level, number, size, and interaction with NPM1 mutations in a large cohort of young adult patients with acute myeloid leukemia. Blood 2008;111(5): 2776–84.

54. Mead AJ, Linch DC, Hills RK, et al. FLT3 tyrosine kinase domain mutations are biologically distinct from and have a significantly more favorable prognosis than FLT3 internal tandem duplications in patients with acute myeloid leukemia. Blood 2007;110(4):1262–70.

55. Whitman SP, Ruppert AS, Radmacher MD, et al. FLT3 D835/I836 mutations are associated with poor disease-free survival and a distinct gene-expression signature among younger adults with de novo cytogenetically normal acute myeloid leukemia lacking FLT3 internal tandem duplications. Blood 2008; 111(3):1552–9.

56. Yanada M, Matsuo K, Suzuki T, et al. Prognostic significance of FLT3 internal tandem duplication and tyrosine kinase domain mutations for acute myeloid leukemia: a meta-analysis. Leukemia 2005;19(8):1345–9.

57. Bacher U, Haferlach C, Kern W, et al. Prognostic relevance of FLT3-TKD mutations in AML: the combination matters–an analysis of 3082 patients. Blood 2008; 111(5):2527–37.

58. Mead AJ, Gale RE, Hills RK, et al. Conflicting data on the prognostic significance of FLT3/TKD mutations in acute myeloid leukemia might be related to the incidence of biallelic disease. Blood 2008;112(2):444–5 [author reply: 445].

59. Falini B, Mecucci C, Tiacci E, et al. Cytoplasmic nucleophosmin in acute myelogenous leukemia with a normal karyotype. N Engl J Med 2005;352(3): 254–66.

60. Falini B, Martelli MP, Bolli N, et al. Acute myeloid leukemia with mutated nucleophosmin (NPM1): is it a distinct entity? Blood 2011;117(4):1109–20.

61. Falini B, Mecucci C, Saglio G, et al. NPM1 mutations and cytoplasmic nucleophosmin are mutually exclusive of recurrent genetic abnormalities: a comparative analysis of 2562 patients with acute myeloid leukemia. Haematologica 2008; 93(3):439–42.

62. Dohner K, Schlenk RF, Habdank M, et al. Mutant nucleophosmin (NPM1) predicts favorable prognosis in younger adults with acute myeloid leukemia and normal cytogenetics: interaction with other gene mutations. Blood 2005; 106(12):3740–6.

63. Schlenk RF, Dohner K, Krauter J, et al. Mutations and treatment outcome in cytogenetically normal acute myeloid leukemia. N Engl J Med 2008;358(18): 1909–18.

64. Kronke J, Schlenk RF, Jensen KO, et al. Monitoring of minimal residual disease in NPM1-mutated acute myeloid leukemia: a study from the German-Austrian acute myeloid leukemia study group. J Clin Oncol 2011; 29(19):2709–16.

65. Taskesen E, Bullinger L, Corbacioglu A, et al. Prognostic impact, concurrent genetic mutations, and gene expression features of AML with CEBPA mutations in a cohort of 1182 cytogenetically normal AML patients: further evidence for CEBPA double mutant AML as a distinctive disease entity. Blood 2011;117(8): 2469–75.

66. Dufour A, Schneider F, Metzeler KH, et al. Acute myeloid leukemia with biallelic CEBPA gene mutations and normal karyotype represents a distinct genetic entity associated with a favorable clinical outcome. J Clin Oncol 2010;28(4): 570–7.

67. Smith ML, Cavenagh JD, Lister TA, et al. Mutation of CEBPA in familial acute myeloid leukemia. N Engl J Med 2004;351(23):2403–7.
68. Mardis ER, Ding L, Dooling DJ, et al. Recurring mutations found by sequencing an acute myeloid leukemia genome. N Engl J Med 2009;361(11):1058–66.
69. Patel KP, Ravandi F, Ma D, et al. Acute myeloid leukemia with IDH1 or IDH2 mutation: frequency and clinicopathologic features. Am J Clin Pathol 2011; 135(1):35–45.
70. Schnittger S, Haferlach C, Ulke M, et al. IDH1 mutations are detected in 6.6% of 1414 AML patients and are associated with intermediate risk karyotype and unfavorable prognosis in adults younger than 60 years and unmutated NPM1 status. Blood 2010;116(25):5486–96.
71. Marcucci G, Maharry K, Wu YZ, et al. IDH1 and IDH2 gene mutations identify novel molecular subsets within de novo cytogenetically normal acute myeloid leukemia: a Cancer and Leukemia Group B study. J Clin Oncol 2010;28(14): 2348–55.
72. Rockova V, Abbas S, Wouters BJ, et al. Risk stratification of intermediate-risk acute myeloid leukemia: integrative analysis of a multitude of gene mutation and gene expression markers. Blood 2011;118(4):1069–76.
73. Chou WC, Lei WC, Ko BS, et al. The prognostic impact and stability of isocitrate dehydrogenase 2 mutation in adult patients with acute myeloid leukemia. Leukemia 2011;25(2):246–53.
74. Thol F, Damm F, Wagner K, et al. Prognostic impact of IDH2 mutations in cyto-genetically normal acute myeloid leukemia. Blood 2010;116(4):614–6.
75. Neubauer A, Maharry K, Mrozek K, et al. Patients with acute myeloid leukemia and RAS mutations benefit most from postremission high-dose cy-tarabine: a Cancer and Leukemia Group B study. J Clin Oncol 2008;26(28): 4603–9.
76. Kiyoi H, Naoe T, Nakano Y, et al. Prognostic implication of FLT3 and N-RAS gene mutations in acute myeloid leukemia. Blood 1999;93(9):3074–80.
77. Bacher U, Haferlach T, Schoch C, et al. Implications of NRAS mutations in AML: a study of 2502 patients. Blood 2006;107(10):3847–53.
78. Bowen DT, Frew ME, Hills R, et al. RAS mutation in acute myeloid leukemia is associated with distinct cytogenetic subgroups but does not influence outcome in patients younger than 60 years. Blood 2005;106(6):2113–9.
79. Neubauer A, Dodge RK, George SL, et al. Prognostic importance of mutations in the ras proto-oncogenes in de novo acute myeloid leukemia. Blood 1994;83(6): 1603–11.
80. Ahmad EI, Gawish HH, Al Azizi NM, et al. The prognostic impact of K-RAS muta-tions in adult acute myeloid leukemia patients treated with high-dose cytarabine. Onco Targets Ther 2011;4:115–21.
81. Virappane P, Gale R, Hills R, et al. Mutation of the Wilms' tumor 1 gene is a poor prognostic factor associated with chemotherapy resistance in normal karyotype acute myeloid leukemia: the United Kingdom Medical Research Council Adult Leukaemia Working Party. J Clin Oncol 2008;26(33):5429–35.
82. Paschka P, Marcucci G, Ruppert AS, et al. Wilms' tumor 1 gene mutations inde-pendently predict poor outcome in adults with cytogenetically normal acute myeloid leukemia: a cancer and leukemia group B study. J Clin Oncol 2008; 26(28):4595–602.
83. Damm F, Heuser M, Morgan M, et al. Single nucleotide polymorphism in the mutational hotspot of WT1 predicts a favorable outcome in patients with cytoge-netically normal acute myeloid leukemia. J Clin Oncol 2010;28(4):578–85.

84. Whitman SP, Ruppert AS, Marcucci G, et al. Long-term disease-free survivors with cytogenetically normal acute myeloid leukemia and MLL partial tandem duplication: a Cancer and Leukemia Group B study. Blood 2007;109(12):5164–7.

85. Schnittger S, Kinkelin U, Schoch C, et al. Screening for MLL tandem duplication in 387 unselected patients with AML identify a prognostically unfavorable subset of AML. Leukemia 2000;14(5):796–804.

86. Dohner K, Tobis K, Ulrich R, et al. Prognostic significance of partial tandem duplications of the MLL gene in adult patients 16 to 60 years old with acute myeloid leukemia and normal cytogenetics: a study of the Acute Myeloid Leukemia Study Group Ulm. J Clin Oncol 2002;20(15):3254–61.

87. Mulligham CG. TET2 mutations in myelodysplasia and myeloid malignancies. Nat Genet 2009;41(7):766–7.

88. Chou WC, Chou SC, Liu CY, et al. TET2 mutation is an unfavorable prognostic factor in acute myeloid leukemia patients with intermediate-risk cytogenetics. Blood 2011;118(4):3803–10.

89. Ley TJ, Ding L, Walter MJ, et al. DNMT3A mutations in acute myeloid leukemia. N Engl J Med 2010;363(25):2424–33.

90. Haferlach C, Dicker F, Herholz H, et al. Mutations of the TP53 gene in acute myeloid leukemia are strongly associated with a complex aberrant karyotype. Leukemia 2008;22(8):1539–41.

91. Bowen D, Groves MJ, Burnett AK, et al. TP53 gene mutation is frequent in patients with acute myeloid leukemia and complex karyotype, and is associated with very poor prognosis. Leukemia 2009;23(1):203–6.

92. Santamaria C, Chillon MC, Garcia-Sanz R, et al. BAALC is an important predictor of refractoriness to chemotherapy and poor survival in intermediate-risk acute myeloid leukemia (AML). Ann Hematol 2010;89(5):453–8.

93. Heuser M, Beutel G, Krauter J, et al. High meningioma 1 (MN1) expression as a predictor for poor outcome in acute myeloid leukemia with normal cytogenetics. Blood 2006;108(12):3898–905.

94. Langer C, Marcucci G, Holland KB, et al. Prognostic importance of MN1 transcript levels, and biologic insights from MN1-associated gene and microRNA expression signatures in cytogenetically normal acute myeloid leukemia: a Cancer and Leukemia Group B study. J Clin Oncol 2009;27(19):3198–204.

95. Lugthart S, van Drunen E, van Norden Y, et al. High EVI1 levels predict adverse outcome in acute myeloid leukemia: prevalence of EVI1 overexpression and chromosome 3q26 abnormalities underestimated. Blood 2008;111(8):4329–37.

96. Groschel S, Lugthart S, Schlenk RF, et al. High EVI1 expression predicts outcome in younger adult patients with acute myeloid leukemia and is associated with distinct cytogenetic abnormalities. J Clin Oncol 2010;28(12):2101–7.

97. Smith ML, Hills RK, Grimwade D. Independent prognostic variables in acute myeloid leukaemia. Blood Rev 2011;25(1):39–51.

98. Leith CP, Kopecky KJ, Chen IM, et al. Frequency and clinical significance of the expression of the multidrug resistance proteins MDR1/P-glycoprotein, MRP1, and LRP in acute myeloid leukemia: a Southwest Oncology Group study. Blood 1999;94(3):1086–99.

99. Wuchter C, Leonid K, Ruppert V, et al. Clinical significance of P-glycoprotein expression and function for response to induction chemotherapy, relapse rate and overall survival in acute leukemia. Haematologica 2000;85(7):711–21.

100. Schaich M, Soucek S, Thiede C, et al. MDR1 and MRP1 gene expression are independent predictors for treatment outcome in adult acute myeloid leukaemia. Br J Haematol 2005;128(3):324–32.

101. Schoch C, Kern W, Schnittger S, et al. Karyotype is an independent prognostic parameter in therapy-related acute myeloid leukemia (t-AML): an analysis of 93 patients with t-AML in comparison to 1091 patients with de novo AML. Leukemia 2004;18(1):120–5.

102. Kern W, Haferlach T, Schnittger S, et al. Prognosis in therapy-related acute myeloid leukemia and impact of karyotype. J Clin Oncol 2004;22(12):2510–1.

103. Quesnel B, Kantarjian H, Bjergaard JP, et al. Therapy-related acute myeloid leukemia with t(8;21), inv(16), and t(8;16): a report on 25 cases and review of the literature. J Clin Oncol 1993;11(12):2370–9.

104. Borthakur G, Lin E, Jain N, et al. Survival is poorer in patients with secondary core-binding factor acute myelogenous leukemia compared with de novo core-binding factor leukemia. Cancer 2009;115(14):3217–21.

105. Gustafson SA, Lin P, Chen SS, et al. Therapy-related acute myeloid leukemia with t(8;21) (q22;q22) shares many features with de novo acute myeloid leukemia with t(8;21)(q22;q22) but does not have a favorable outcome. Am J Clin Pathol 2009;131(5):647–55.

106. Haferlach T, Schoch C, Loffler H, et al. Morphologic dysplasia in de novo acute myeloid leukemia (AML) is related to unfavorable cytogenetics but has no independent prognostic relevance under the conditions of intensive induction therapy: results of a multiparameter analysis from the German AML Cooperative Group studies. J Clin Oncol 2003;21(2):256–65.

107. Kern W, Haferlach T, Schoch C, et al. Early blast clearance by remission induction therapy is a major independent prognostic factor for both achievement of complete remission and long-term outcome in acute myeloid leukemia: data from the German AML Cooperative Group (AMLCG) 1992 Trial. Blood 2003; 101(1):64–70.

108. Hussein K, Jahagirdar B, Gupta P, et al. Day 14 bone marrow biopsy in predicting complete remission and survival in acute myeloid leukemia. Am J Hematol 2008;83(6):446–50.

109. Al-Shughair N, Al-Dawsari G, Gyger M, et al. Clinical significance of plasmacytosis in the day+14 bone marrow of patients with acute myeloid leukaemia undergoing induction chemotherapy. J Clin Pathol 2007;60(5):520–3.

110. Gianfaldoni G, Mannelli F, Baccini M, et al. Clearance of leukaemic blasts from peripheral blood during standard induction treatment predicts the bone marrow response in acute myeloid leukaemia: a pilot study. Br J Haematol 2006;134(1): 54–7.

111. Cheson BD, Bennett JM, Kopecky KJ, et al. Revised recommendations of the International Working Group for Diagnosis, Standardization of Response Criteria, Treatment Outcomes, and Reporting Standards for Therapeutic Trials in Acute Myeloid Leukemia. J Clin Oncol 2003;21(24):4642–9.

112. Marcucci G, Mrozek K, Ruppert AS, et al. Abnormal cytogenetics at date of morphologic complete remission predicts short overall and disease-free survival, and higher relapse rate in adult acute myeloid leukemia: results from Cancer and Leukemia Group B study 8461. J Clin Oncol 2004;22(12): 2410–8.

113. Sanz MA, Grimwade D, Tallman MS, et al. Management of acute promyelocytic leukemia: recommendations from an expert panel on behalf of the European LeukemiaNet. Blood 2009;113(9):1875–91.

114. Shook D, Coustan-Smith E, Ribeiro RC, et al. Minimal residual disease quantitation in acute myeloid leukemia. Clin Lymphoma Myeloma 2009;9(Suppl 3): S281–5.

115. Perea G, Lasa A, Aventin A, et al. Prognostic value of minimal residual disease (MRD) in acute myeloid leukemia (AML) with favorable cytogenetics [t(8;21) and inv(16)]. Leukemia 2006;20(1):87–94.
116. Weisser M, Haferlach C, Hiddemann W, et al. The quality of molecular response to chemotherapy is predictive for the outcome of AML1-ETO-positive AML and is independent of pretreatment risk factors. Leukemia 2007;21(6):1177–82.
117. Freeman SD, Jovanovic JV, Grimwade D. Development of minimal residual disease-directed therapy in acute myeloid leukemia. Semin Oncol 2008;35(4):388–400.
118. Cilloni D, Renneville A, Hermitte F, et al. Real-time quantitative polymerase chain reaction detection of minimal residual disease by standardized WT1 assay to enhance risk stratification in acute myeloid leukemia: a European LeukemiaNet study. J Clin Oncol 2009;27(31):5195–201.
119. Kottaridis PD, Gale RE, Langabeer SE, et al. Studies of FLT3 mutations in paired presentation and relapse samples from patients with acute myeloid leukemia: implications for the role of FLT3 mutations in leukemogenesis, minimal residual disease detection, and possible therapy with FLT3 inhibitors. Blood 2002;100(7):2393–8.
120. Shih LY, Huang CF, Wu JH, et al. Internal tandem duplication of FLT3 in relapsed acute myeloid leukemia: a comparative analysis of bone marrow samples from 108 adult patients at diagnosis and relapse. Blood 2002;100(7):2387–92.
121. Maurillo L, Buccisano F, Del Principe MI, et al. Toward optimization of postremission therapy for residual disease-positive patients with acute myeloid leukemia. J Clin Oncol 2008;26(30):4944–51.
122. Kim DH, Lee NY, Baek JH, et al. Prognostic scoring model based on multi-drug resistance status and cytogenetics in adult patients with acute myeloid leukemia. Leuk Lymphoma 2006;47(3):461–7.
123. Damm F, Heuser M, Morgan M, et al. Integrative prognostic risk score in acute myeloid leukemia with normal karyotype. Blood 2011;117(17):4561–8.
124. Pantazopoulos N, Sinks LF. Morphological criteria for prognostication of acute lymphoblastic leukaemia. Br J Haematol 1974;27(1):25–30.
125. Hayhoe FG. Cytochemistry of the acute leukaemias. Histochem J 1984;16(10):1051–9.
126. Hunault M, Harousseau JL, Delain M, et al. Better outcome of adult acute lymphoblastic leukemia after early genoidentical allogeneic bone marrow transplantation (BMT) than after late high-dose therapy and autologous BMT: a GOELAMS trial. Blood 2004;104(10):3028–37.
127. Litzow MR, Buck G, Dewald G, et al. Outcome of 1,229 adult Philadelphia chromosome negative B acute lymphoblastic leukemia (B-ALL) patients (pts) from the International UKALLXII/E2993 trial: no difference in results between B cell immunophenotypic subgroups. Blood 2010;116:524a.
128. Hoelzer D, Thiel E, Arnold R, et al. Successful subtype oriented treatment strategies in adult T-ALL; results of 744 patients treated in three consecutive GMALL studies. Blood 2009;114:324a.
129. Marks DI, Paietta EM, Moorman AV, et al. T-cell acute lymphoblastic leukemia in adults: clinical features, immunophenotype, cytogenetics, and outcome from the large randomized prospective trial (UKALL XII/ECOG 2993). Blood 2009;114(25):5136–45.
130. Thomas DA, O'Brien S, Jorgensen JL, et al. Prognostic significance of CD20 expression in adults with de novo precursor B-lineage acute lymphoblastic leukemia. Blood 2009;113(25):6330–7.

131. Maury S, Huguet F, Leguay T, et al. Adverse prognostic significance of CD20 expression in adults with Philadelphia chromosome-negative B-cell precursor acute lymphoblastic leukemia. Haematologica 2010;95(2):324–8.

132. Hoelzer D, Thiel E, Loffler H, et al. Prognostic factors in a multicenter study for treatment of acute lymphoblastic leukemia in adults. Blood 1988;71(1):123–31.

133. Copelan EA, McGuire EA. The biology and treatment of acute lymphoblastic leukemia in adults. Blood 1995;85(5):1151–68.

134. Rowe JM, Buck G, Burnett AK, et al. Induction therapy for adults with acute lymphoblastic leukemia: results of more than 1500 patients from the international ALL trial: MRC UKALL XII/ECOG E2993. Blood 2005;106(12):3760–7.

135. Faderl S, Jeha S, Kantarjian HM. The biology and therapy of adult acute lymphoblastic leukemia. Cancer 2003;98(7):1337–54.

136. Fielding AK. How I treat Philadelphia chromosome-positive acute lymphoblastic leukemia. Blood 2010;116(18):3409–17.

137. Faderl S, Kantarjian HM, Talpaz M, et al. Clinical significance of cytogenetic abnormalities in adult acute lymphoblastic leukemia. Blood 1998;91(11):3995–4019.

138. Cytogenetic abnormalities in adult acute lymphoblastic leukemia: correlations with hematologic findings outcome. A collaborative study of the Group Francais de Cytogenetique Hematologique. Blood 1996;87(8):3135–42.

139. Wetzler M, Dodge RK, Mrozek K, et al. Prospective karyotype analysis in adult acute lymphoblastic leukemia: the Cancer and Leukemia Group B experience. Blood 1999;93(11):3983–93.

140. Mancini M, Scappaticci D, Cimino G, et al. A comprehensive genetic classification of adult acute lymphoblastic leukemia (ALL): analysis of the GIMEMA 0496 protocol. Blood 2005;105(9):3434–41.

141. Moorman AV, Harrison CJ, Buck GA, et al. Karyotype is an independent prognostic factor in adult acute lymphoblastic leukemia (ALL): analysis of cytogenetic data from patients treated on the Medical Research Council (MRC) UKALLXII/Eastern Cooperative Oncology Group (ECOG) 2993 trial. Blood 2007;109(8):3189–97.

142. Heerema NA, Sather HN, Sensel MG, et al. Association of chromosome arm 9p abnormalities with adverse risk in childhood acute lymphoblastic leukemia: a report from the Children's Cancer Group. Blood 1999;94(5):1537–44.

143. Weng AP, Ferrando AA, Lee W, et al. Activating mutations of NOTCH1 in human T cell acute lymphoblastic leukemia. Science 2004;306(5694):269–71.

144. Ferrando AA. The role of NOTCH1 signaling in T-ALL. Hematology Am Soc Hematol Educ Program 2009;353–61.

145. Asnafi V, Buzyn A, Le Noir S, et al. NOTCH1/FBXW7 mutation identifies a large subgroup with favorable outcome in adult T-cell acute lymphoblastic leukemia (T-ALL): a Group for Research on Adult Acute Lymphoblastic Leukemia (GRAALL) study. Blood 2009;113(17):3918–24.

146. Mansour MR, Sulis ML, Duke V, et al. Prognostic implications of NOTCH1 and FBXW7 mutations in adults with T-cell acute lymphoblastic leukemia treated on the MRC UKALLXII/ECOG E2993 protocol. J Clin Oncol 2009;27(26):4352–6.

147. Baldus CD, Martus P, Burmeister T, et al. Low ERG and BAALC expression identifies a new subgroup of adult acute T-lymphoblastic leukemia with a highly favorable outcome. J Clin Oncol 2007;25(24):3739–45.

148. Kuhnl A, Gokbuget N, Stroux A, et al. High BAALC expression predicts chemo-resistance in adult B-precursor acute lymphoblastic leukemia. Blood 2010; 115(18):3737–44.
149. Hoelzer D, Thiel E, Loffler H, et al. Intensified therapy in acute lymphoblastic and acute undifferentiated leukemia in adults. Blood 1984;64(1):38–47.
150. Bruggemann M, Raff T, Flohr T, et al. Clinical significance of minimal residual disease quantification in adult patients with standard-risk acute lymphoblastic leukemia. Blood 2006;107(3):1116–23.
151. Waanders E, van der Velden VH, van der Schoot CE, et al. Integrated use of minimal residual disease classification and IKZF1 alteration status accurately predicts 79% of relapses in pediatric acute lymphoblastic leukemia. Leukemia 2011;25(2):254–8.
152. Rowe JM. Prognostic factors in adult acute lymphoblastic leukaemia. Br J Haematol 2010;150(4):389–405.
153. Chang KL, O'Donnell MR, Slovak ML, et al. Primary myelodysplasia occurring in adults under 50 years old: a clinicopathologic study of 52 patients. Leukemia 2002;16(4):623–31.
154. Hulot JS, Villard E, Maguy A, et al. A mutation in the drug transporter gene ABCC2 associated with impaired methotrexate elimination. Pharmacogenet Genomics 2005;15(5):277–85.
155. Haferlach T, Kern W, Schoch C, et al. A new prognostic score for patients with acute myeloid leukemia based on cytogenetics and early blast clearance in trials of the German AML Cooperative Group. Haematologica 2004;89(4): 408–18.

Induction and Postremission Strategies in Acute Myeloid Leukemia: State of the Art and Future Directions

Todd L. Rosenblat, MD[a,b], Joseph G. Jurcic, MD[a,b,*]

KEYWORDS

• Acute myeloid leukemia • Induction • Consolidation
• Postremission therapy

Acute myeloid leukemia (AML) represents a group of heterogeneous neoplasms with acquired genetic abnormalities that result in impaired differentiation and increased proliferation of hematopoietic cells. AML is a rare disease with an incidence rate in the United States of approximately 3.5 per 100,000 persons.[1] Among individuals aged 65 years and older, the incidence increases dramatically to more than 16 per 100,000 persons. Despite modest improvements in the outcome of younger patients over the past decade, overall treatment results remain disappointing, particularly for older individuals. Data from the Surveillance, Epidemiology, and End Results program of the National Cancer Institute indicate that the 5-year survival rate for patients less than age 65 years, diagnosed from 2001 to 2007, is approximately 40%. In contrast, the 5-year survival rate for patients 65 years and older is only 5%.[1] New understanding of the molecular pathogenesis of this disease has led to the identification of diagnostic and prognostic markers and to the refinement of karyotype-based risk classification, discussed elsewhere in this issue. These insights are now beginning to guide therapeutic strategies and provide novel targets for drug discovery.

The authors have nothing to disclose.
[a] Leukemia Service, Department of Medicine, Weill Cornell Medical College, Memorial Sloan-Kettering Cancer Center, 1275 York Avenue, New York, NY 10065, USA
[b] Weill Cornell Medical College, New York, NY 10065, USA
* Corresponding author. Leukemia Service, Department of Medicine, Weill Cornell Medical College, Memorial Sloan-Kettering Cancer Center, 1275 York Avenue, New York, NY 10065.
E-mail address: jurcicj@mskcc.org

Hematol Oncol Clin N Am 25 (2011) 1189–1213
doi:10.1016/j.hoc.2011.09.007
0889-8588/11/$ – see front matter © 2011 Elsevier Inc. All rights reserved.

INDUCTION THERAPY FOR YOUNGER ADULTS

Elimination of morphologic evidence of leukemic blasts and restoration of normal hematopiesis are the goals of induction therapy. For the past two decades, the combination of anthracycline or anthracycline-like drugs with cytarabine has remained the standard of care for patients aged 60 years or less. With 3 days of daunorubicin (at least 60 mg/m^2/d), idarubicin (10–12 mg/m^2/d), or mitoxantrone (10–12 mg/m^2/d), and 7 days of cytarabine (100–200 mg/m^2/d continuous intravenous infusion), complete remission (CR) is obtained in 60% to 80% of patients less than 60 years of age.[2] Most centers use one of the previously mentioned combinations, sometimes with the addition of etoposide, although this has been shown to have a limited benefit in patients less than age 55 years.[3] AML is still considered one of the few true oncologic emergencies; prompt initiation of therapy seems to be crucial. In one retrospective study, treatment delays beyond 5 days from diagnosis resulted in a decreased response rate and overall survival (OS) in patients less than 55 years of age.[4]

To improve response rates and OS, investigators have explored several modifications to standard induction approaches. Studies comparing idarubicin and mitoxantrone with daunorubicin at doses of 45 to 60 mg/m^2 have failed to show a clear survival benefit.[5–9] More recently, dose intensification of daunorubicin (90 vs 45 mg/m^2) was reported to result in a higher CR rate and OS in patients younger than 60 years of age, particularly those with favorable- or intermediate-risk disease (**Fig 1**).[10] The Acute Leukemia French Association (ALFA) compared high-dose daunorubicin (80 mg/m^2 for 3 days) with idarubicin (12 mg/m^2 for 3 or 4 days) combined with intermediate-dose cytarabine for induction in patients 50 to 70 years of age.[11] Although the CR rate was significantly higher using the 3-day schedule of idarubicin, no differences in event-free survival (EFS) or OS were observed among the three groups. Similarly, the Japan Adult Leukemia Study Group compared high-dose daunorubicin (50 mg/m^2 for 5 days) with idarubicin (12 mg/m^2 for 3 days) in combination with standard-dose cytarabine and found no differences in CR or OS rates.[12]

Given that high-dose cytarabine (HiDAC) can overcome resistance to standard doses of cytarabine, its use has been evaluated in induction with cumulative doses of 18 to 24 g/m^2. This approach did not improve OS and generally was associated with increased toxicity.[13–17] The Dutch-Belgian Cooperative Trial Group for Hemato-Oncology (HOVON) and the Swiss Group for Clinical Cancer research (SAKK) recently compared intermediate-dose cytarabine (200 mg/m^2 for 7 days by continuous infusion in cycle 1 and 1000 mg/m^2 over 3 hours twice daily for 6 days in cycle 2) with HiDAC (1000 mg/m^2 twice daily for 5 days in cycle 1 and 2000 mg/m^2 twice daily over 6 hours for 4 days in cycle 2) during induction.[18] No differences in remission rate, relapse rate, EFS, or OS were seen; however, the high-dose regimen was associated with increased toxicity. A subgroup analysis of this trial and data from the Southwest Oncology Group (SWOG)[19] suggest that treatment with higher doses of cytarabine may confer a survival benefit for patients with a highly unfavorable monosomal karyotype. Nevertheless, these results provide evidence for a plateau in the dose-response for cytarabine and argue against the use of HiDAC during induction outside the setting of a clinical trial.

Similarly, the use of additional cytotoxic agents (etoposide, fludarabine, topotecan, and thioguanine) during induction has not shown a clear advantage.[3,20–23] Neither cyclosporine[24] nor valspodar (PSC-833),[25] which act as modulators of multidrug resistance by inhibiting P-glycoprotein–mediated cellular export of anthracyclines, improved results compared with standard therapy. During induction and consolidation, myeloid growth factors may be given to reduce the duration of neutropenia. Although the safety of these agents in AML has been clearly established in multiple trials, benefits

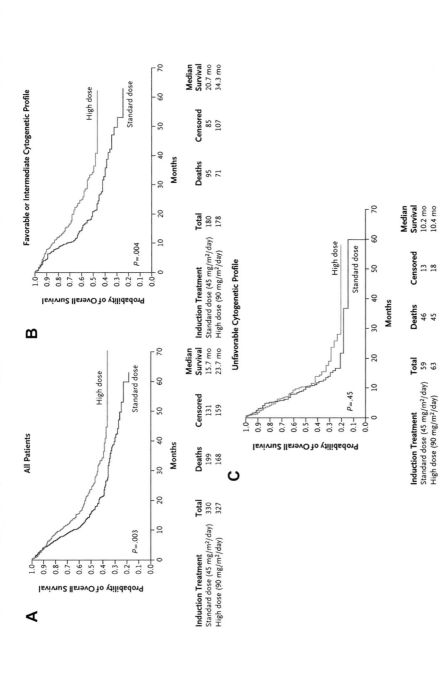

Fig. 1. Kaplan-Meier estimates of OS after high-dose (90 mg/m²) or standard-dose (45 mg/m²) daunorubicin. Data from the intention-to-treat analysis are shown for all patients (*A*), those with a favorable or an intermediate cytogenetic profile (*B*), and those with an unfavorable cytogenetic profile (*C*). (*From* Fernandez HF, Sun Z, Yao X, et al. Anthracycline dose intensification in acute myeloid leukemia. N Engl J Med 2009;361:1256; with permission.)

are limited.[26,27] In general, the use of myeloid growth factors is recommended primarily in older individuals, where the risk of periinduction mortality because of infectious complications is greatest; however, their use should also be considered in younger patients with severe infection after induction. The use of granulocyte colony-stimulating factor (G-CSF) and granulocyte macrophage (GM)-CSF as sensitizing agents has also been evaluated because of the potential to act as priming agents by moving leukemia cells into a phase of the cell cycle more susceptible to cytotoxic chemotherapy. Conflicting results have been reported, and no clear benefit has been established. The HOVAN/SAKK group found that priming with G-CSF resulted in a significant improvement in disease-free survival (DFS) and superior OS in intermediate-risk disease. The CR rate, however, was unaffected.[28] The ALFA group found that priming with GM-CSF improved CR and EFS rates but had no effect on OS.[29] In contrast, a study by the AML Cooperative Group found that G-CSF priming had no impact on relapse-free survival or OS.[30]

Two large studies tested the addition of antibody-directed chemotherapy with gemtuzumab ozogamicin (GO) to standard induction chemotherapy. GO consists of a recombinant humanized anti-CD33 monoclonal antibody conjugated to calicheamicin, a potent antitumor antibiotic. Within the acidic environment of lysosomes after internalization, calicheamicin dissociates from the antibody and migrates to the nucleus, where it causes double-stranded DNA breaks. As a single agent, GO produced remissions in 26% of older patients with AML in first relapse.[31] When combined with standard chemotherapy, dose reductions of GO were necessary to avoid hepatic toxicity. A randomized trial conducted by SWOG compared induction with daunorubicin, cytarabine, and GO with daunorubicin and cytarabine alone.[32] The trial was stopped early after an interim analysis showed an increase in periinduction mortality in the GO arm (5.8% vs 0.8%). The early death rate in the control arm, however, was significantly lower than expected. Additionally, no differences in CR rate (66% vs 69%), relapse-free survival, DFS, or OS were seen between the two groups. In a larger study conducted by the United Kingdom National Cancer Research Institute (NCRI) (formerly the Medical Research Council), patients were randomized to receive one of three chemotherapy regimens (daunorubicin and cytarabine; cytarabine, daunorubicin, and etoposide; or fludarabine, cytarabine, G-CSF, and idarubicin), with or without a single dose of GO.[33] Although there was no difference in response or survival among the arms, in prespecified risk groups, there was a significant survival benefit in patients with favorable cytogenetics. Moreover, an internally validated prognostic index (based on age, presenting leukocyte count, performance status, and presence of secondary AML) identified 70% of patients with intermediate-risk cytogenetics who benefited with a 10% improvement in survival at 5 years. Although marketing authorization of GO was withdrawn in the United States because of concerns about safety and lack of efficacy in the pivotal SWOG trial, the NCRI study suggests that it may have a role in induction therapy for selected patients.

POSTREMISSION THERAPY FOR YOUNGER PATIENTS

Several postremission treatment strategies have been studied to eradicate minimal residual disease in patients with AML who achieve a CR but remain at risk for relapse. These include intensive conventional chemotherapy, autologous or allogeneic hematopoietic cell transplantation (HCT), and prolonged low-dose maintenance therapy. The choice of postremission strategy for an individual patient depends on cytogenetic and molecular risk factors, availability of a suitable allogeneic stem cell donor, and predicted treatment-related mortality (TRM).

Intensive Chemotherapy

A pivotal study by the Cancer and Leukemia Group B (CALGB) examined three dose levels of cytarabine given for four cycles as postremission therapy. This study clearly demonstrated that outcomes after HiDAC (3 g/m^2 every 12 hours on days 1, 3, and 5) were superior to intermediate-dose (400 mg/m^2 continuous infusion for 5 days) or standard-dose cytarabine (100 mg/m^2 continuous infusion for 5 days) in patients less than age 60 years.[34] A subgroup analysis demonstrated that this benefit was most pronounced in patients with core-binding factor (CBF; ie, t[8;21][q22;q22], inv[16][p13.1;q22], t[16;16][p13.1;q22]) AML and, to a lesser extent, in patients with a normal karyotype.[35] Although the benefit of HiDAC consolidation has been demonstrated in younger patients, the optimal dose, schedule, and number of cycles has not been established definitively. Retrospective studies by the CALGB suggested that three cycles or more of HiDAC was superior to only one cycle.[36,37] The NCRI, however, reported a similar OS rate with only one course of HiDAC in consolidation for patients with favorable-risk cytogenetics.[38] Moreover, results of a US Intergroup study that included only one cycle of postremission HiDAC were similar to outcomes in other studies where three or four cycles of HiDAC were used.[39] More recently, the NCRI reported that outcomes after consolidation with two or three courses of cytarabine at doses of 1.5 or 3 g/m^2 for six doses were equivalent.[33] These results, however, may be confounded by the use of variable induction regimens and the administration of GO to some patients during consolidation.

For younger patients with CBF leukemia, three or four cycles of HiDAC consolidation remains appropriate postremission therapy, resulting in an OS rate of 60% to 75%.[36,37,40–42] A survival benefit has not been demonstrated for patients with CBF leukemia with autologous or allogeneic HCT in first CR (CR1).[43–48] Despite this, there may be a subset of CBF leukemia patients with additional risk factors for relapse, including *KIT* mutations and elevated WBC in t(8;21), who may benefit from allogeneic HCT in CR1 if expected TRM is sufficiently low.[47,49] HiDAC consolidation may also be appropriate for at least a subgroup younger patients with normal cytogenetics and mutated nucleophosmin gene (*NPM1*) without the fms-related tyrosine kinase 3 gene (*FLT3*) internal tandem duplication (ITD) mutation. In a retrospective study, the German-Austrian AML Study Group reported a similar outcome for patients with or without a suitable related stem cell donor who had a normal karyotype and were *NPM1*$^+$ and *FLT3*-ITD$^-$.[50] More recent data, however, suggest that the favorable prognostic impact of the *NPM1* mutation occurs primarily in patients without mutations in isocitrate dehydrogenase 1 (*IDH1*) and *IDH2* genes.[51] Even further, additional data suggest that the location of the mutation in *IDH2* influences patient outcome. When there are concomitant mutations in *NPM1* and *IDH2* at R140, the prognosis is favorable, whereas an *IDH2* mutation at R172 is associated with a poor outcome.[52] The therapeutic implications of these recently described molecular abnormalities are unclear. Additional studies are required to determine which patients with *NPM1* mutations may benefit from allogeneic HCT in CR1 and which will have superior outcomes with postremission chemotherapy alone. Intensive consolidation may also be appropriate for patients with a normal karyotype who have a mutated CCAAT/enhancer binding protein α (*CEBPA*) gene. It has recently been shown that the improved prognosis in *CEBPA*$^+$ patients is only seen with the double mutation. A single *CEBPA* mutation, even without the presence of a *FLT3*-ITD mutation, does not seem to confer the same favorable long-term outcomes.[53]

Allogeneic Hematopoietic Stem Cell Transplantation

Allogeneic HCT is highly effective therapy for AML because of the immunologically mediated graft-versus-leukemia effect and the intensive antileukemic effects of conditioning regimens.[54] With this in mind, it is not surprising that the relapse rate for patients with AML in CR1 is lowest with allogeneic HCT. However, this strong antileukemic effect is balanced by a higher TRM rate compared with chemotherapy alone. In patients with AML in CR1, multiple prospective trials have failed to show an improvement in OS with allogeneic HCT.[39,55,56] In patients with intermediate- and high-risk AML, however, a clear OS advantage was shown in several metaanalyses that prospectively assigned allogeneic HCT versus consolidation chemotherapy or autologous HCT in an intent-to-treat donor versus no-donor fashion.[44,45]

Patients with AML and normal cytogenetics lacking the specific good-risk genetic mutations discussed previously are often treated with standard HiDAC consolidation; however, the risk of relapse remains high in this patient population. The OS benefit of allogeneic HCT has been shown in AML with normal cytogenetics, particularly in the absence of a mutated NMP1 without FLT3-ITD or mutated CEBPA.[44,45,50] For patients who have normal cytogenetics and FLT3-ITD mutation, an allogeneic HCT transplant in CR1 should be considered.[50] More recently, mutations in *TET2* were described in patients with AML with a frequency of approximately 12%. *TET2* abnormalities were associated with decreased OS compared with *TET2* wild-type patients.[57] The therapeutic implications of this finding, however, are still unknown.

Outcomes for patients with unfavorable cytogenetics after standard chemotherapy consolidation or autologous HCT are poor.[35,38,39] The worst prognosis has been reported for patients with one or more autosomal monosomies. Breems and colleagues[58] reported a 4-year OS of 12% with a single monosomy and a 4-year OS of 3% for patients with two or more monosomies. In contrast, patients with non-CBF cytogenetic abnormalities had a 4-year OS of 27%. Based on results from individual trials and meta-analyses, allogeneic HCT in CR1 with a matched, related donor is recommended for patients with poor-risk cytogenetics.[44,45,59]

The use of a matched unrelated donor (MUD) for allogeneic HCT in CR1 is not as clearly defined, because most published trials are retrospective comparisons. The only study to address this issue prospectively is the German AML 01/99 trial. Patients with high-risk disease, defined as having unfavorable cytogenetics or residual disease on day 15 postinduction, were treated with allogeneic HCT from a matched sibling if available, a MUD HCT if such a donor could be identified, or autologous HCT otherwise.[60] Survival at 4 years was 68% for patients with an HLA-matched sibling donor, 56% for patients with a MUD, and 23% for patients allocated to autologous HCT. A retrospective analysis reported by the Fred Hutchinson Cancer Research Center showed that 5-year survival rates were equivalent between matched sibling and unrelated allografts in CR1 at 63% and 61%, respectively, for all risk groups.[61] These data suggest that indications for HCT in AML using a matched related or 10 of 10 MUD should be similar. Further large-scale studies are still required to confirm this finding. The Center for International Blood and Marrow Transplant Research, however, demonstrated only a 30% 5-year survival for poor-risk patients with AML in CR1 after transplant with a MUD.[62] Nevertheless, given the high risk for relapse for patients with unfavorable cytogenetics, allogeneic HCT from either a matched sibling or MUD should be pursued in CR1.

There are emerging data that HCT using alternative sources of hematopoietic stem cells may be useful in younger patients with high-risk AML. Although there are limited data regarding umbilical cord blood transplantation for AML in CR1, this modality may represent a reasonable option for patients without a matched related or unrelated donor. Initially, the widespread use of this approach was restricted by stem cell dose requirements. Double cord blood transplantation, however, seems to lessen the risk of graft rejection and improve early survival, making this approach more broadly applicable to adult patients. Investigators from the University of Minnesota and the Fred Hutchinson Cancer Research Center showed that leukemia-free survival for HCT recipients from double umbilical cord blood, matched related donors, MUD, and mismatched unrelated donors was similar (**Fig. 2**).[63] The use of a genetically haploidentical donor for HCT is another possible approach for poor-risk patients without a suitable matched sibling or unrelated donor. The European Blood and Marrow Transplant Group reported results after haploidentical HCT in high-risk patients that are similar to those after MUD transplantation.[64]

Autologous Hematopoietic Stem Cell Transplantation

Autologous HCT after intensive chemotherapy is considered a reasonable option for postremission therapy in favorable- and intermediate-risk cytogenetic groups. In patients with poor-risk cytogenetics, however, its use cannot be recommended.[39,55,65,66] Although a benefit in DFS has been reported in some randomized studies, OS was not improved. This is related in part to the higher TRM in studies where bone marrow was used as the source of hematopoietic stem cells. The data are further confounded by the intensity of prior therapy and patient selection. For example, in a recent Eastern Cooperative Oncology Group (ECOG) study, patients with favorable- and intermediate-risk disease received postremission therapy

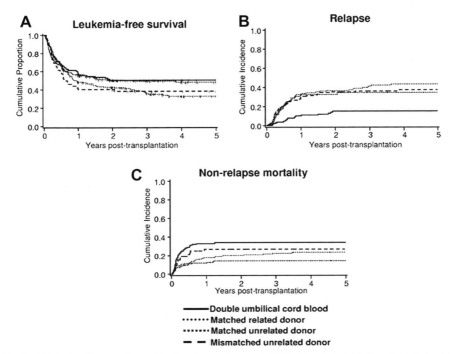

Fig. 2. Clinical outcomes for patients who underwent HCT with a 4–6/6 HLA-matched double umbilical cord blood (dUCB) graft (n = 128); an HLA-matched related donor (MRD) (n = 204); an HLA-matched unrelated donor (MUD) (n = 152); or a one-antigen mismatched unrelated adult donor (MMUD) (n = 52). (A) Leukemia-free survival was similar for all groups. (B) Risk of relapse was lower in recipients of dUCB (15%) compared with MRD (43%); MUD (37%); and MMUD (35%). (C) Nonrelapse mortality was higher for dUCB (34%); MRD (24%); and MUD (14%). (Adapted from Brunstein CG, Gutman JA, Weisdorf DJ, et al. Allogeneic hematopoietic cell transplantation for hematologic malignancy: relative risks and benefits of double umbilical cord blood. Blood 2010;116:469; with permission.)

consisting of two courses of HiDAC followed by a course of GO and autologous HCT or autologous HCT alone. Only 49% of patients received the planned therapy, with disease progression as the most common reason for patients not proceeding to HCT. An intention-to-treat analysis demonstrated 4-year DFS and OS of approximately 35% and 41%, respectively, with no benefit from GO. Nevertheless, in favorable-risk AML, patients receiving induction that included high-dose daunorubicin who underwent autologous HCT, 4-year DFS and OS rates were 60% and 80%, respectively. For intermediate-risk patients, 4-year DFS and OS were 40% and 49%, respectively (**Fig. 3**).[67] These data suggest that autologous HCT may play a role in postremission therapy for a selected subgroup of patients with AML.

Maintenance Therapy

Although several trials have demonstrated an increase in DFS with maintenance therapy after intensive induction, an OS benefit has not been shown.[68–70] Therefore, for younger patients, maintenance chemotherapy cannot replace more intensive post-remission strategies. Immunotherapeutic approaches for maintenance therapy have also been proposed. Although several randomized studies failed to show an advantage for interleukin-2 as maintenance,[71,72] a recent study showed that interleukin-2 and histamine dichloride given after the completion of consolidation therapy conferred a leukemia-free survival advantage compared with no maintenance therapy.[73] Novel vaccination strategies are also under investigation for maintenance therapy. Wilms' tumor antigen (WT1) and proteinase 3 (PR1) peptide vaccines have elicited immune responses and produced remissions in patients with AML.[74–77] Cellular therapies, such as autologous dendritic cell vaccination targeting WT1, also hold promise for postremission immunotherapy.[78] Nevertheless, maintenance is currently not recommended outside of a clinical trial for non-APL AML.

TREATMENT OF OLDER PATIENTS WITH AML

Both patient-specific and disease-related factors contribute to the extraordinarily poor prognosis of older adults with AML. A report compiled from five SWOG trials highlighted important clinical and biologic features for younger and older patients with AML and their effect on outcome after intensive induction therapy.[79] Although the incidence of patients with favorable cytogenetic abnormalities fell from 16% in those younger than 56 years to 4% in those older than age 75 years, the proportion of patients with unfavorable cytogenetics rose from 33% in younger patients to 50% in the older group. Similarly, the CR rate decreased from 64% in younger patients to 33% for patients older than age 75 years. The median OS durations for patients younger than age 56 and older than age 75 years were 18.8 months and 3.5 months, respectively. Although a higher rate of poor-risk cytogenetics contributed to a worse outcome for older patients, within each cytogenetic risk group, treatment outcome deteriorated with advancing age. Because of the poor prognosis of older patients with AML, many physicians are reluctant to offer intensive therapy. An analysis of Medicare recipients with AML older than age 65 years showed that because of these factors, only 30% were offered any form of intravenous chemotherapy.[80] Nevertheless, intensive chemotherapy appears to confer a survival benefit to patients who are appropriate candidates. In a retrospective analysis of data from the Swedish Acute Leukemia Registry, outcomes were strongly dependent on age and performance status, but early death rates were lower with intensive therapy than with palliation across all age groups.[81]

   The development of prognostic models may allow clinicians to identify patients who may benefit from intensive induction chemotherapy and those who should be treated

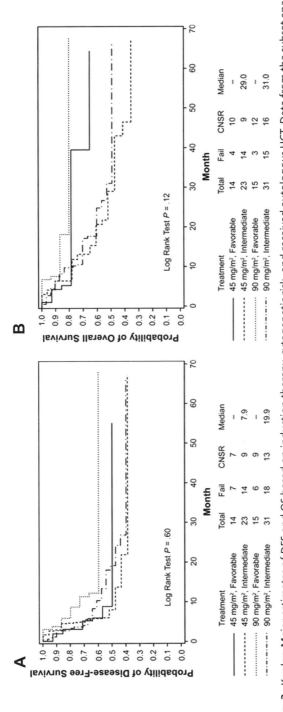

Fig. 3. Kaplan-Meier estimates of DFS and OS based on induction therapy, cytogenetic risk, and received autologous HCT. Data from the subset analysis are shown for DFS (*A*) and OS (*B*) for patients who received protocol-prescribed autologous HCT based on the induction therapy with standard-dose (45 mg/m²) or high-dose (90 mg/m²) daunorubicin and on cytogenetic risk group. (*From* Fernandez HF, Sun Z, Litzow MR, et al. Autologous transplantation gives encouraging results for young adults with favorable–risk acute myeloid leukemia, but is not improved with gemtuzumab ozogamicin. Blood 2011;117:5311; with permission.)

using alternative approaches.[82,83] A multivariate analysis performed by investigators at the MD Anderson Cancer Center (MDACC) in patients aged 65 years and older yielded several independent poor prognostic factors, including age 75 years or older, unfavorable karyotype, poor performance status, longer duration of antecedent hematologic disorders, and abnormal organ function. Those with no adverse risk factors had expected remission rates higher than 60%, induction mortality rates of 10%, and 1-year survival rates higher than 50%. Patients with one or two risk factors had expected CR rates of 50%, induction mortality rates of 30%, and 1-year survival rates of 30%. Patients with three or more risk factors had CR rates of less than 20%, induction mortality rates of 50%, and 1-year survival rates of less than 10%.[84] In a similar model, the MDACC group showed that most patients aged 70 years and older do not benefit from intensive induction therapy.[85] Such predictive models, however, must be refined and validated by independent groups before integration into the design of clinical trials for new treatment regimens.

Intensive Chemotherapy

Although many strategies have been investigated to improve the outcome of induction therapy for older adults, a combination of an anthracycline and cytarabine remains the most commonly used regimen for individuals who are candidates for intensive therapy, just as in younger patients. A classic Phase III study conducted by ECOG in patients older than 55 years showed no difference in outcomes with the use of daunorubicin, idarubicin, or mitoxantrone combined with cytarabine.[86] As with many studies in younger patients, no benefit was seen with GM-CSF priming in this trial. Although no anthracycline is clearly superior, a recent study by the HOVON, AMLSG, and SAKK groups showed that the use of higher-dose daunorubicin (90 mg/m^2 for 3 days) is feasible in patients up to age 65 years and results in improved EFS and OS compared with conventional-dose daunorubicin (45 mg/m^2).[87] Despite a high incidence of multidrug resistance in older patients,[77] the strategy of P-glycoprotein inhibition also seems of limited use in older patients with AML. SWOG investigators showed that zosuquidar, a highly selective P-glycoprotein inhibitor that does not significantly affect anthracycline clearance, did not improve OS when given with cytarabine and daunorubicin in patients older than age 60 years.[88] The use of myeloid growth factors to reduce infectious complications and periinduction mortality during induction has only modest benefits. Both CALGB and ECOG conducted studies in which GM-CSF or placebo was given after the completion of daunorubicin and cytarabine to older patients with AML.[89,90] The median duration of Grade 4 neutropenia was reduced by 2 to 4 days; however, the ECOG study showed a decreased incidence of infection-related mortality. G-CSF or placebo was studied in a similar fashion after standard induction chemotherapy. The duration of neutropenia was shortened by 6 days, but no difference in early mortality or OS was seen.[91]

Except in patients with favorable-risk disease, postremission therapy provides only marginal benefit to older patients with AML. In addition to the good-risk cytogenetic and molecular markers discussed previously, low expression of the brain and acute leukemia, cytoplasmic (*BAALC*) gene and ets-related gene (*ERG*) may also predict older patients who benefit from intensive chemotherapy.[92] In comparing the outcomes of older patients with AML in first remission who received two cycles of postremission therapy cytarabine (400 mg/m^2 for 5 days) with those who did not receive any postremission treatment in retrospective study, investigators from the Cleveland Clinic found no differences in DFS or OS.[93] Most randomized studies have compared the intensity or during of postremission therapy in older individuals. The NCRI found no difference in OS after one or four courses of moderate-intensity postremission therapy.[94] Both the AML Cooperative Group[69] and ALFA[95] groups found prolonged outpatient postre-mission therapy gave superior DFS and OS survival compared with one course of intensive consolidation. In contrast, the AMLSG found that one cycle of intensive consolidation was superior to 1 year of oral maintenance therapy.[96] Based on these data, it is reasonable to administer one or two courses of consolidation therapy to patients without adverse prognostic markers and comorbid conditions who have a good performance status. Conversely, patients with high-risk disease derive no clear benefit from consolidation chemotherapy and should be considered for novel postre-mission strategies.

Hematopoietic Stem Cell Transplantation

Despite the use of nonmyeloablative or reduced-intensity conditioning regimens to decrease TRM, allogeneic HCT remains an option for only a minority of older patients. In an intention-to-treat analysis, investigators at MDACC found that only 5% of older patients with AML underwent HCT because of such issues as age, comorbid condi-tions, patient choice, physician attitude, and lack of a suitable donor.[97] Most studies show HCT in older patients results in TRM in 20% to 30% with an OS rate of approx-imately 30%.[98–100] A retrospective study from the Cooperative German Transplant Study Group suggested that match unrelated and match sibling donor HCT results in comparable survival in older patients.[101] Current data are limited by small patient cohorts, heterogeneity of conditioning regimens, and patient selection. Ultimately, prospective randomized trials will be needed to determine if reduced-intensity condi-tioning HCT is superior to conventional consolidation chemotherapy in older patients.

Reduced-intensity Therapies

With the recognition that many older patients will not benefit from standard induction therapy, investigators have directed their efforts toward the development of less inten-sive therapeutic options (**Table 1**). As part of the NCRI AML14 trial, 217 patients deemed unfit for standard induction chemotherapy were randomized to receive low-dose cytarabine or hydroxyurea. Low-dose cytarabine produced a higher remis-sion rate (18% vs 1%) and OS than hydroxyurea; however, patients with adverse cyto-genetics did not benefit.[102] A variety of newer agents have also been studied in recent years with generally disappointing results. Tipifarnib, an oral farnesyl transferase

Table 1				
Reduced-intensity therapies for older adults with AML				
Agent	**Class**	**ORR/CR (%)**	**Median OS (mo)**	**30-Day mortality (%)**
Low-dose cytarabine[102]	Nucleoside analog	NR/18	5	NR
Tipifarnib[103]	Farnesyltransferase inhibitor	23/14	5.3	7
Laromustine[105]	Alkylating agent	32/20	3.2	14
Clofarabine[106,107]	Nucleoside analog	46–48/32-38	4.4–9.6	9.8–18
Azacitidine[a,110]	Hypomethylating agent	NR/18	24.5	NR
Decitabine (5-d)[111]	Hypomethylating agent	27/25	7.7	7
Decitabine (10-d)[112]	Hypomethylating agent	64/47	12.8	2
Lenalidomide[114]	Immunomodulator, antiangiogenic agent	30/9	4	24

Abbreviations: CR, complete remission; NR, not reported; ORR, overall response rate; OS, overall survival.
[a] Included only patients with <30% blasts.

inhibitor, produced remissions in 14% of elderly patients with previously untreated, poor-risk AML,[103] and a randomized Phase III trial comparing tipifarnib with supportive care failed to show a benefit in patients aged 70 years and older.[104] The novel alkylating agent laromustine produced responses in 32% of patients age 60 or older; however, the periinduction mortality rate was 14%, and 1-year OS was only 21%.[105]

The second-generation purine analog clofarabine, currently approved by the US Food and Drug Administration for children with relapsed and refractory acute lymphoblastic leukemia, has shown promise in the treatment of older patients with AML. A large Phase II study of clofarabine (30 mg/m^2 for 5 days) produced responses in 46% of patients, including those with poor-risk cytogenetics. The 30-day TRM was 9.8% and the median OS survival was approximately 10 months.[106] Similarly, in two sequential trials conducted in the United Kingdom, clofarabine produced responses in 48% of patients with a 30-day TRM of 18%.[107] These patients had a superior OS compared with the patients receiving low-dose cytarabine in the AML14 trial. In a small randomized study, the combination of clofarabine and low-dose cytarabine produced a higher response rate than clofarabine alone, but no difference in OS was seen.[108] When higher-doses of clofarabine and cytarabine were given in combination, responses were seen in 60% of patients aged 50 years of age or older but the regimen was associated with prolonged myelosuppression in more than 40% of patients.[109] Despite these encouraging results, no clear benefit to induction therapy with clofarabine has been demonstrated in older individuals with AML to date. A randomized study led by ECOG comparing clofarabine with standard induction with daunorubicin and cytarabine is now underway to address this question definitively.

Epigenetic approaches with hypomethylating agents, approved for use in myelodysplastic syndrome (MDS), have also been investigated in AML. In a Phase III randomized trial, azacitidine (75 mg/m^2/d for 7 days) significantly prolonged OS compared with conventional care regimens in patients with intermediate- and high-risk MDS. In a subset analysis of patients with AML as defined by the World Health Organization criteria with 20% blasts or more, the median survival for azacitidine-treated patients was 24.5 months, compared with 16 months for patients receiving conventional care regimens (**Fig. 4**). CR rates were 18% for patients receiving azacitidine, 15% for patients receiving low-dose cytarabine, and 55% for patients receiving intensive induction therapy.[110] Additional studies are required to determine if these results are applicable to older patients with higher blast counts and more rapidly proliferative disease. Decitabine (20 mg/m^2 for 5 days) produced remissions in 25% of patients, with a median OS of 7.7 months and a 30-day mortality rate of 7%.[111] With a 10-day schedule of decitabine, 47% of patients achieved CR without added toxicity.[112] Despite these encouraging results, in a randomized Phase III trial, decitabine produced CR in 18% of patients with AML aged 65 years and older but the improvement in OS was not statistically significant compared with patients receiving supportive care or low-dose cytarabine.[113] Novel approaches to exploit the activity of hypomethylating agents currently under investigation include a maintenance strategy in older patients and combination with standard chemotherapy in younger adults.

Lenalidomide, currently approved for the treatment of patients with lower-risk MDS associated with the del(5q) cytogenetic abnormality, has modest activity in older patients with AML. In a Phase II study conducted in patients 60 years of age or older with untreated AML, high-dose lenalidomide (50 mg/day for 28-day cycles for two courses followed by maintenance with 10 mg/day) produced responses in 30% of patients.[114] In a smaller Phase II study limited to patients with AML with del(5q), 14% of patients responded.[115] Although these low-intensity therapies can produce remissions in some patients, response rates observed to date have not been superior

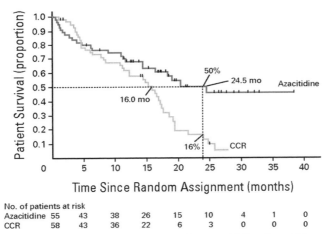

Fig. 4. Kaplan-Meier plot of OS in patients receiving azacitidine (n = 55) or conventional care regimens (CCR; n = 58). Significantly higher overall survival rate was seen in the azacitidine group versus the CCR group at month 20 (54.1% vs 19.1%; P = .0005); month 24 (50.2% vs 15.9%; P = .0007); and month 27 (45.6% vs 4.8%; P<.0001). (*From* Fenaux P, Mufti GJ, Hellström-Lindberg E, et al. Azacitidine prolongs overall survival compared with conventional care regimens in elderly patients with low bone marrow blast count acute myeloid leukemia. J Clin Oncol 2010;28:565; with permission.)

to standard induction regimens. Moreover, for some agents, it is unclear whether their toxicity profiles differ significantly from intensive chemotherapy in similar populations, because entry criteria in some studies allowed for discretion of individual treating physicians and patient choice. More effective, less toxic therapeutic options for older patients who cannot tolerate standard induction therapy are urgently needed. Combinations of these alternative agents with standard chemotherapy or other novel compounds are under active investigation.

INVESTIGATIONAL AGENTS AND FUTURE DIRECTIONS

AML results from multiple genetic and epigenetic lesions affecting differentiation, proliferation, and apoptosis. Consequently, targeting a single abnormality is unlikely to eradicate the leukemic clone. Nevertheless, increased understanding of the molecular pathogenesis of AML has provided novel therapeutic targets. Genetic alternations may result in activation of signal transduction pathways (eg, *FLT3*, *KIT*, and *RAS*); enhanced or repressed transcriptional activity (eg, *RML-RARA*, *RUNX1-RUNX1T1*, *CBFB-MYH11*, and *CEBPA*); or changes in function of nuclear cytoplasmic shuttling (eg, *NPM1*, *NUP98*, and *NUP214*).[116] With the exception of all-*trans* retinoic acid and arsenic trioxide in acute promyelocytic leukemia, which affect transcriptional regulation, most newer therapeutic strategies seek to inhibit constitutive tyrosine kinase activity. In this section, recently studied molecularly targeted approaches are highlighted, in addition to other novel chemotherapeutic strategies, which have now reached late Phase II and III development (**Table 2**).

FLT3 and Other Molecular Targets

Several *FLT3*-selective tyrosine kinase inhibitors, including midostaurin (PKC412),[117] lestaurtinib (CEP701),[118] tandutinib (MLN1518),[119] sunitinib,[120] and sorafenib,[121] have shown in vitro activity against AML cells. Most of these inhibitors have modest

Table 2
Investigational agents for AML in late-stage development

Agent	Mechanism of Action	Phase of Development	Comments
Midostaurin (PKC412)[125]	RTKI with *FLT3* inhibition	III	Phase III trial of daunorubicin + cytarabine induction and HiDAC consolidation ± midostaurin in newly diagnosed patients <60 years of age with *FLT3*+ AML is completed
AC220[126]	RTKI with *FLT3* inhibition	II	Phase III trial of AC220 versus salvage chemotherapy for relapsed/refractory *FLT3*-ITD+ AML and Phase I trial of AC220 + daunorubicin/cytarabine for newly diagnosed AML are planned
Tipifarnib[103]	Farnesyltransferase inhibition	II	Phase II trial for untreated older patients with specific *RASGRP1/APTX* ratio is ongoing
Sapacitabine[130]	Purine nucleoside analog	III	Phase III trial of sapacitabine + decitabine versus sapacitabine versus decitabine in untreated patients ≥70 years is ongoing
Elacytarabine[131]	Purine nucleoside analog	III	Phase III trial of elacytarabine versus investigator's choice for late-stage AML is ongoing
CPX-351[132–134]	Liposome encapsulated cytarabine and daunorubicin in a fixed molar ratio	II	Phase II trial for untreated patients aged 60–75 years is completed
Vosaroxin[135,136]	Quinoline with topoisomerase II inhibitory activity	III	Phase III trial of cytarabine ± vosaroxin for first relapsed or refractory AML is ongoing

Abbreviation: RTKI, receptor tyrosine kinase inhibitor.

single-agent activity in relapsed AML associated with transient reductions in peripheral blood blasts and, to a lesser extent, marrow blasts.[122,123] In a randomized study conducted with patients with AML in first relapse, the multitargeted kinase inhibitor lestaurtinib in combination with chemotherapy (HiDAC or mitoxantrone, etoposide, and cytarabine [MEC]) failed to improve responses compared with chemotherapy alone.[124] In a pilot study combining midostaurin with cytarabine and daunorubicin in previously untreated patients with AML, however, CRs were observed in 80% of all patients and in 92% of patients with an *FLT3* mutation.[125] Moreover, OS for patients with mutated and wild-type *FLT3* were similar. These data provide the rationale for an ongoing randomized trial comparing standard induction, postremission, and maintenance therapy with or without midostaurin in newly diagnosed patients with *FLT3* mutations. More recently, a novel agent, AC220, produced responses in 56% of patients with relapsed *FLT3*-ITD–positive relapsed AML; responses were also seen in some patients with wild-type *FLT3*.[126] Based on its activity as a single agent, trials investigating AC220 in combination with standard chemotherapy for patients with newly diagnosed AML are planned.

When studied in older patients with untreated poor-risk AML, tipifarnib, a farnesyl transferase inhibitor, produced CRs in only 14%.[103] By examining gene expression profiles for these patients, however, investigators found that a two-gene expression ratio (*RASGRP1/APTX*) was predictive of clinical response.[127] Overexpression of *RASGRP1*, a guanine nucleotide exchange factor that activates *RAS*, and downregulation of *APTX*, which is involved in DNA excision repair, were associated favorable responses. The predictive value of this two-gene classifier was confirmed retrospectively in a cohort of patients treated with the combination of tipifarnib and etoposide.[128] When a gene ratio cutoff of 5.2 was used, the overall response rate increased from 28% to 78%. There was no association between the two-gene ratio and clinical response in a cohort of patients with AML treated with other traditional chemotherapeutic regimens. A prospective trial evaluating tipifarnib in patients selected based on the *RASGRP1/APTX* expression ratio is planned. Such studies can provide a model of personalized treatment decisions based on molecular evaluation of an individual's tumor.

Chemosensitization Strategies

Results of priming with G-CSF have been equivocal, but other priming strategies seem promising. The CXCR4/SDF-1 axis is believed to function as a principal regulator of homing and retention of normal and malignant hematopoietic cells. Based on this observation, investigators from Washington University postulated that plerixafor, a small molecular inhibitor of CXCR4 currently licensed for stem cell mobilization, might increase the effects of chemotherapy. Patients with relapsed or refractory AML were treated with plerixafor followed by MEC in a Phase I and II trial.[129] CRs were seen in 50% of patients, which compares favorably to historical controls treated with MEC alone. These encouraging results provide the rationale for testing this strategy in larger, randomized trials in the setting of relapsed and refractory AML and in combination with standard induction therapy in untreated AML.

Novel Chemotherapeutic Agents

In addition to clofarabine, there are two other promising nucleoside analogs currently under investigation in AML. Sapacitabine is an oral agent that causes irreparable single-strand DNA breaks and induces G2 cell cycle arrest. A randomized Phase II study conducted in patients aged 70 years or older compared three dosing schedules. The overall response rates for the three schedules ranged from 25% to 45%, with a CR rate of 25% in the group receiving a 3-day per week regimen.[130] A randomized study comparing sapacitabine with decitabine in older patients with untreated AML is planned. Elacytarabine, another nucleoside analog, has mechanisms of action similar to cytarabine, but unlike cytarabine, its cellular uptake is independent of nucleoside transporters. Among patients with AML receiving elacytarabine as second salvage therapy, remissions were seen in 15%, a significantly higher rate than seen in historical controls. Moreover, treatment with elacytarabine provided an OS and TRM benefit compared with outcomes in the historical group.[131] A phase III trial is currently underway for patients with multiply relapsed or refractory AML. If successful, this compound may prove useful earlier in the treatment of AML.

CPX-351 is a liposomal formulation of cytarabine and daunorubicin at a 5:1 molar ratio that maximizes synergy.[132] In a randomized phase IIB study conducted in newly diagnosed patients aged 60 to 75 years, CPX-351 had a higher response rate compared with daunorubicin and cytarabine (66.7% vs 51.2%) with a trend toward decreased early mortality (4.7% vs 14.6%).[133] Higher response rates were seen in patients with adverse risk cytogenetics, those older than age 70 years, and those with secondary AML.[134] Vosaroxin (formerly voreloxin) is a first-in-class anticancer quinolone that induces site-selective DNA damage by intercalating DNA and inhibiting topoisomerase II. Antileukemic activity was seen in patients with relapsed and refractory AML in a Phase I trial.[135] Subsequently, vosaroxin as a single-agent produced remissions in 34% of untreated patients with AML 60 years of age or older.[136] A randomized Phase III study of intermediate-dose cytarabine with or without vosaroxin for patients with AML in first relapse is now underway.

SUMMARY

Although the past decade has brought improvements in the treatment of AML, particularly for younger individuals, most patients succumb to the disease. With current induction therapy, most patients achieve remission, but the optimal strategy for post-remission therapy is unclear. Refinements to risk classification systems that incorporate additional molecular markers may better guide physicians in recommendations for postremission therapy. The prognosis for older patients with AML remains uniformly poor, because only a minority can benefit from intensive chemotherapy and novel HCT strategies. Despite active investigation, no standard of care has emerged for patients who are not suitable candidates for standard induction therapy. The development of less toxic, more effective therapies for this population is sorely needed. Advances in molecular genetics, immunology, and the biology of normal and malignant hematopoiesis pathogenesis have led to an improved understanding of the pathogenesis of AML and to the discovery of potential therapeutic targets. Until a greater proportion of individuals with AML attain long-term survival, patients should routinely be referred to cancer centers and enrolled in investigational studies.

REFERENCES

1. Howlader N, Noone AM, Krapcho M, et al. SEER cancer statistics review, 1975-2008. Bethesda (MD): National Cancer Institute; 2010. Available at: http://seer.cancer.gov/csr/1975_2008/, based on November 2010 SEER data submission, posted to the SEER web site, 2011. Accessed September 29, 2011.
2. Estey E, Döhner H. Acute myeloid leukaemia. Lancet 2006;368:1894–907.
3. Bishop JF, Lowenthal RM, Joshua D, et al. Etoposide in acute nonlymphocytic leukemia: Australian Leukemia Study Group. Blood 1990;75:27–32.
4. Sekeres MA, Elson P, Kalaycio ME, et al. Time from diagnosis to treatment initiation predicts survival in younger, but not older, acute myeloid leukemia patients. Blood 2009;113:28–36.
5. Vogler WR, Velez-Garcia E, Weiner RS, et al. A phase III trial comparing idarubicin and daunorubicin in combination with cytarabine in acute myelogenous leukemia: a Southeastern Cancer Study Group study. J Clin Oncol 1992;10:1103–11.
6. Wiernik PH, Banks PLC, Case DC Jr, et al. Cytarabine plus idarubicin or daunorubicin as induction and consolidation therapy for previously untreated adult patients with acute myeloid leukemia. Blood 1992;79:313–9.
7. Berman E, Heller G, Santorsa J, et al. Results of a randomized trial comparing idarubicin and cytosine arabinoside with daunorubicin and cytosine arabinoside in adult patients with newly diagnosed acute myelogenous leukemia. Blood 1991;77:1666–74.
8. Arlin Z, Case DC Jr, Moore J, et al. Randomized multicenter trial of cytosine arabinoside with mitoxantrone or daunorubicin in previously untreated adult patients with acute nonlymphocytic leukemia (ANLL). Leukemia 1990;4:177–83.

9. Mandelli F, Vignetti M, Suciu S, et al. Daunorubicin versus mitoxantrone versus idarubicin as induction and consolidation chemotherapy for adults with acute myeloid Leukemia: the EORTC and Gimema groups study AML-10. J Clin Oncol 2009;27:5397–403.
10. Fernandez H, Sun Z, Yao X, et al. Anthracycline dose intensification in acute myeloid leukemia. N Engl J Med 2009;361:1249–59.
11. Pautas C, Merabet F, Thomas X, et al. Randomized study of intensified anthracycline doses for induction and recombinant interleukin-2 for maintenance in patients with acute myeloid leukemia age 50 to 70 years: results of the ALFA-9801 study. J Clin Oncol 2010;28:808–14.
12. Ohtake S, Miyawaki S, Fujita H, et al. Randomized study of induction therapy comparing standard-dose idarubicin with high-dose daunorubicin in adult patients with previously untreated acute leukemia: the JALSG AML201 study. Blood 2011;117:2358–65.
13. Weick JK, Kopecky KJ, Appelbaum FR, et al. A randomized investigation of high-dose versus standard-dose cytosine arabinoside with daunorubicin in patients with previously untreated acute myeloid leukemia: a Southwest Oncology Group study. Blood 1996;88:2841–51.
14. Bishop JF, Matthews JP, Young GA, et al. Randomized study of high-dose cytarabine in induction in acute myeloid leukemia. Blood 1996;87:1710–7.
15. Cassileth PA, Lee SJ, Litzow MR, et al. Intensified induction chemotherapy in adult acute myeloid leukemia followed by high-dose chemotherapy and autologous peripheral blood stem cell transplantation: an Eastern Cooperative Oncology Group trial (E4995). Leuk Lymphoma 2005;46:55–61.
16. Petersdorf SH, Rankin C, Head DR, et al. Phase II evaluation of an intensified induction therapy with standard daunomycin and cytarabine followed by high dose cytarabine for adults with previously untreated acute myeloid leukemia: a Southwest Oncology Group study (SWOG-9500). Am J Hematol 2007;82:1056–62.
17. Büchner T, Berdel WE, Schoch C, et al. Double induction containing either two courses or one course of high-dose cytarabine plus mitoxantrone and postremission therapy by either autologous stem-cell transplantation or by prolonged maintenance for acute myeloid leukemia. J Clin Oncol 2006;24:2480–9.
18. Löwenberg B, Pabst T, Vellenga E, et al. Cytarabine dose for acute myeloid leukemia. N Engl J Med 2011;364:1027–36.
19. Medeiros BC, Othus M, Fang M, et al. Prognostic impact of monosomal karyotype in young adult and elderly acute myeloid leukemia: the Southwest Oncology Group (SWOG) experience. Blood 2010;116:2224–8.
20. Hann IM, Stevens RF, Goldstone AH, et al. Randomized comparison of DAT versus ADE as induction chemotherapy in children and younger adults with acute myeloid leukemia. Results of the Medical Research Council's 10th AML trial (MRC AML10). Blood 1997;89:2311–8.
21. Estey EH, Thall PF, Cortes JE, et al. Comparison of idarubicin + ara-C, fludarabine + araC–, and Topotecan + ara-C–based regimens in treatment of newly diagnosed acute myeloid leukemia, refractory anemia with excess blasts in transformation, or refractory anemia with excess blasts. Blood 2001;98:3575–83.
22. Ossenkoppele GJ, Graveland WJ, Sonneveld P, et al. The value of fludarabine in addition to ARA-C and G-CSF in the treatment of patients with high-risk myelodysplastic syndromes and AML in elderly patients. Blood 2004;103:2908–13.
23. Milligan DW, Wheatley K, Littlewood T, et al. Fludarabine and cytosine are less effective than standard ADE chemotherapy in high-risk acute myeloid leukemia,

and addition of G-CSF and ATRA are not beneficial: results of the MRC AML-HR randomized trial. Blood 2006;107:4614–22.

24. List AF, Kopecky KJ, Willman CL, et al. Benefit of cyclosporine modulation of drug resistance in patients with poor-risk acute myeloid leukemia: a Southwest Oncology Group study. Blood 2001;98:3212–20.

25. Kolitz JE, George SL, Marcucci G, et al. P-glycoprotein inhibition using valspodar (PSC-833) does not improve outcomes for patients younger than age 60 years with newly diagnosed acute myeloid leukemia: Cancer and Leukemia Group B study 19808. Blood 2010;116:1413–21.

26. Rowe JM. Treatment of acute myeloid leukemia with cytokines: effect on duration of neutropenia and response to infections. Clin Infect Dis 1998;26:1290–4.

27. Amadori S, Suciu S, Jehn U, et al. Use of glycosylated recombinant human G-CSF (lenograstim) during and/or after induction chemotherapy in patients 61 years of age and older with acute myeloid leukemia: final results of AML13, a randomized phase 3 study of the European Organization for Research and Treatment of Cancer and Grippo Italiano Malattie Ematologiche dell Advito (EORTG/GIMEMA) Leukemia groups. Blood 2005;106:27–34.

28. Löwenberg B, van Putten W, Theobald M, et al. Effect of priming with granulocyte colony-stimulating factor on the outcome of chemotherapy for acute myeloid leukemia. N Engl J Med 2003;349:743–52.

29. Thomas X, Raffoux E, de Botton S, et al. Effect of priming with granulocyte-macrophage colony stimulating factor in younger adults with newly diagnosed acute myeloid leukemia: a trial by the Acute Leukemia French Association (ALFA) Group. Leukemia 2007;21:453–61.

30. Büchner T, Berdel WE, Hiddemann W. Priming with granulocyte colony stimulating factor – relation to high-dose cytarabine in acute myeloid leukemia [comment]. N Engl J Med 2004;350:2215–6.

31. Larson RA, Sievers EL, Stadtmauer EA, et al. Final report of the efficacy and safety of gemtuzumab ozogamicin (Mylotarg) in patients with CD33-positive acute myeloid leukemia in first recurrence. Cancer 2005;104:1442–52.

32. Petersdorf S, Kopecky K, Stuart RK, et al. Preliminary results of Southwest Oncology Group Study S0106: an international intergroup phase 3 randomized trial comparing the addition of gemtuzumab ozogamicin to standard induction therapy versus standard induction therapy followed by a second randomization to post-consolidation gemtuzumab ozogamicin versus no additional therapy for previously untreated acute myeloid leukemia. Blood (ASH Ann Meeting Abstracts) 2009;114:790.

33. Burnett AK, Hills RK, Milligan D, et al. Identification of patients with acute myeloblastic leukemia who benefit from the addition of gemtuzumab ozogamicin: results of the MRC AML15 trial. J Clin Oncol 2011;29:369–77.

34. Mayer RJ, Davis RB, Schiffer CA, et al. Intensive post-remission chemotherapy in adults with acute myeloid leukemia. N Engl J Med 1994;331:896–903.

35. Bloomfield CD, Lawrence D, Byrd JC, et al. Frequency of prolonged remission duration after high-dose cytarabine intensification in acute myeloid leukemia varies by cytogenetic subtype. Cancer Res 1998;58:4173–9.

36. Byrd JC, Dodge RK, Carroll A, et al. Patients with t(8;21)(q22;q22) and acute myeloid leukemia have superior failure-free and overall survival when repetitive cycles of high-dose cytarabine are administered. J Clin Oncol 1999;17:3767–75.

37. Byrd JC, Ruppert AS, Mrózek K, et al. Repetitive cycles of high-dose cytarabine benefit patients with acute myeloid leukemia and inv(16)(p13q22) or t(16;16)(p13;q22): results from CALGB 8461. J Clin Oncol 2004;22:1087–94.

38. Grimwade D, Walker H, Oliver F, et al. The importance of diagnostic cytogenetics on outcome in AML: analysis of 1,612 patients entered into the MRC AML 10 trial. Blood 1998;92:2322–33.
39. Cassileth PA, Harrington DP, Appelbaum FR, et al. Chemotherapy compared with autologous or allogeneic bone marrow transplantation in the management of acute myeloid leukemia in first remission. N Engl J Med 1998;339:1649–56.
40. Slovak ML, Kopecky KJ, Cassileth PA, et al. Karyotypic analysis predicts outcome of preremission and postremission therapy in adult acute myeloid leukemia: a Southwest Oncology Group/Eastern Cooperative Oncology Group study. Blood 2000;96:4075–83.
41. Schlenk RF, Benner A, Hartmann F, et al. Risk-adapted post-remission therapy in acute myeloid leukemia: results of the German Multicenter AML HD93 treatment trial. Leukemia 2003;17:1521–8.
42. Appelbaum FR, Kopecky KJ, Tallman MS, et al. The clinical spectrum of adult acute myeloid leukaemia associated with core binding factor translocations. Br J Haematol 2006;135:165–73.
43. Cornelissen JJ, van Putten WLJ, Verdonck LF, et al. Results of a HOVON/SAKK donor versus no-donor analysis of myeloablative HLA-identical sibling stem cell transplantation in first remission acute myeloid leukemia in young and middle aged adults: benefits for whom? Blood 2007;109:3658–66.
44. Yanada M, Matsuo K, Emi N, et al. Efficacy of allogeneic hematopoietic stem cell transplantation depends on cytogenetic risk for acute myeloid leukemia in first disease remission: a metaanalysis. Cancer 2005;103:1652–8.
45. Koreth J, Schlenk R, Kopecky KJ, et al. Allogeneic stem cell transplantation for acute myeloid leukemia in first complete remission: systematic review and meta-analysis of prospective clinical trials. JAMA 2009;301:2349–61.
46. Schlenk RF, Benner A, Krauter J, et al. Individual patient data-based meta-analysis of patients aged 16 to 60 years with core binding factor acute myeloid leukemia: a survey of the German Acute Myeloid Leukemia Intergroup. J Clin Oncol 2004;15:3741–50.
47. Nguyen S, Leblanc T, Fenaux P, et al. A white blood cell index as the main prognostic factor in t(8;21) acute myeloid leukemia (AML): a survey of 161 cases from the French AML Intergroup. Blood 2002;99:3517–23.
48. Delaunay J, Vey N, Leblanc T, et al. Prognosis of inv(16)/t(16;16) acute myeloid leukemia (AML): a survey of 110 cases from the French AML Intergroup. Blood 2003;102:462–9.
49. Paschka P, Marcucci G, Ruppert A, et al. Adverse prognostic significance of KIT mutations in adult acute myeloid leukemia with inv(16) and t(8;21): a Cancer and Leukemia Group B study. J Clin Oncol 2006;24:3904–11.
50. Schlenk R, Döhner K, Krauter J, et al. Mutations and treatment outcome in cytogenetically normal acute myeloid leukemia. N Engl J Med 2008;358:1909–18.
51. Paschka P, Schlenk RF, Gaidzik, et al. IDH1 and IDH2 mutations are frequent genetics alternations in acute myeloid leukemia and confer adverse prognosis in cytogenetically normal acute myeloid leukemia with NPM 1 mutation without FLT3 internal tandem duplication. J Clin Oncol 2010;28:3636–43.
52. Green CL, Evans CM, Zhao L, et al. The prognostic significance of IDH2 mutations in AML depends on the location of the mutation. Blood 2011;118:409–12.
53. Green CL, Koo KK, Hills RK, et al. Prognostic significance of CEBPA mutations in a large cohort of younger adult patients with acute myeloid leukemia: impact of double CEBPA mutations and the interaction with FLT3 and NPM1 mutations. J Clin Oncol 2010;28:2739–47.

54. Horowitz MM, Gale RP, Sondel PM, et al. Graft-versus- leukemia reactions after bone marrow transplantation. Blood 1990;75:555–62.

55. Zittoun RA, Mandelli F, Willemze R, et al. Autologous or allogeneic bone marrow transplantation compared with intensive chemotherapy in acute myelogenous leukemia. N Engl J Med 1995;332:217–23.

56. Burnett AK, Wheatley K, Goldstone AH, et al. The value of allogeneic bone marrow transplant in patients with acute myeloid leukaemia at different risk of relapse: results of the UK MRC 10 trial. Br J Haematol 2002;118:385–400.

57. Abdel-Wahab O, Mullally A, Hedvat C, et al. Genetic characterization of TET1, TET2, and TET3 alterations in myeloid malignancies. Blood 2009;114:144–7.

58. Breems DA, Van Putten LJ, De Greef GE, et al. Monosomal karyotype in acute myeloid leukemia: a better indicator of poor prognosis than a complex karyotype. J Clin Oncol 2008;26:4791–7.

59. Basara N, Schulze A, Wedding U, et al. Early related or unrelated haematopoietic cell transplantation results in higher overall survival and leukaemia-free survival compared with conventional chemotherapy in high-risk acute myeloid leukaemia patients in first complete remission. Leukemia 2009;23:635–40.

60. Krauter J, Heil G, Hoelzer D, et al. Role of consolidation therapy in the treatment of patients up to 60 years with high risk AML. Blood (Ann Meeting Abstracts) 2005;106:172.

61. Pagel J, Gooley T, Petersdorf E, et al. Outcome following hematopoietic cell transplantation for patients with AML-CR1: comparison between matched-sibling and unrelated allografts. Blood (Ann Meeting Abstracts) 2007;110:330.

62. Tallman MS, Dewald GW, Gandham S, et al. Impact of cytogenetics on outcome of matched unrelated donor hematopoietic stem cell transplantation for acute myeloid leukemia in first or second complete remission. Blood 2007;110:409–17.

63. Brunstein CG, Gutman JA, Weisdorf DJ, et al. Allogeneic hematopoietic cell transplantation for hematologic malignancy: relative risks and benefits of double umbilical cord blood. Blood 2010;116:4694–9.

64. Ciceri F, Labopin M, Aversa F, et al. A survey of fully haploidentical hematopoietic stem cell transplantation in adults with high-risk acute leukemia: a risk factor analysis of outcomes for patients in remission at transplantation. Blood 2008; 112:3574–81.

65. Burnett AK, Goldstone AH, Stevens RF, et al. Randomised comparison of addition of autologous bone-arrow transplantation to intensive chemotherapy for acute myeloid leukaemia in first remission: results of MRC AML 10 trial. Lancet 1998;351:700–8.

66. Harrousseau JL, Chan JY, Pignon B, et al. Comparison of autologous bone marrow transplantation and intensive chemotherapy as postremission therapy in adult acute myeloid leukemia. Blood 1997;90:2978–86.

67. Fernandez HF, Sun Z, Litzow MR, et al. Autologous transplantation gives encouraging results for young adults with favorable-risk acute myeloid leukemia, but is not improved with gemtuzumab ozogamicin. Blood 2011;177:5306–13.

68. Cassileth P, Lynch E, Hines J, et al. Varying intensity of post-remission therapy in acute myeloid leukemia. Blood 1992;79:1924–30.

69. Büchner T, Hiddemann W, Berdei W, et al. 6-thioguanine, cytarabine, and daunorubicin (TAD) and high-dose cytarabine and mitoxantrone (HAM) for induction, TAD for consolidation, and either prolonged maintenance by reduced monthly TAD or TAD-HAM-TAD and one course of intensive consolidation by sequential HAM in adult patients at all ages with de novo acute myeloid

leukemia (AML). A randomized trial of the German AML Cooperative Group. J Clin Oncol 2003;21:4496–504.

70. Hewlett J, Kopecky K, Head D, et al. A prospective evaluation of the roles of allogeneic marrow transplantation and low-dose monthly maintenance chemotherapy in the treatment of adult acute myelogenous leukemia (AML). A Southwest Oncology Group Study. Leukemia 1995;9:562–9.

71. Blaise D, Attal M, Reiffers J, et al. Randomized study of recombinant interleukin-2 after autologous bone marrow transplantation for acute leukemia in first complete remission. Eur Cytokine Netw 2000;11:91–8.

72. Lange BJ, Smith FO, Dinndorf PA, et al. Outcomes in CCG-2961, a Children's Cancer Group phase III trial for untreated acute myeloid leukemia (AML). Blood (ANN Meeting Abstracts) 2005;106:169.

73. Brune M, Castaigne S, Catalano J, et al. Improved leukemia-free survival after postconsolidation immunotherapy with histamine dihydrochloride and interleukin-2 in acute myeloid leukemia: results of a randomized phase 3 trial. Blood 2006;108:88–96.

74. Oka Y, Tsuboi A, Taguchi T, et al. Induction of WT1 (Wilms' tumor gene)-specific cytoxic T lymphocytes by WT1 peptide vaccine and the resultant cancer regression. Proc Natl Acad Sci U S A 2004;101:13885–90.

75. Keilholz U, Letsch A, Busse A, et al. A clinical and immunologic phase 2 trial of Wilms tumor gene product 1 (WT1) peptide vaccination in patients with AML and MDS. Blood 2009;113:6541–8.

76. Maslak PG, Dao T, Krug LM, et al. Vaccination with synthetic analog peptides derived from WT1 oncoprotein induces T-cell responses in patients with complete remission from acute myeloid leukemia. Blood 2010;(116):171–9.

77. Qazibash MH, Wieder E, Rios R, et al. Vaccination with the PR1 leukemia-associated antigen can induce complete remission in patients with myeloid leukemia. Blood (Ann Meeting Abstracts) 2004;104:259.

78. Van Tendeloo VF, Van de Velde A, Van Driessche A, et al. Induction of complete and molecular remissions in acute myeloid leukemia by Wilms' tumor 1 antigen-targeted dendritic cell vaccination. Proc Natl Acad Sci U S A 2010;107: 13824–9.

79. Appelbaum FR, Gundacker H, Head DR, et al. Age and acute myeloid leukemia. Blood 2005;107:3481–5.

80. Menzin J, Lang K, Earle CC, et al. The outcomes and costs of acute myeloid leukemia among the elderly. Arch Intern Med 2002;162:1597–603.

81. Juliusson G, Antunovic P, Derolf A, et al. Age and acute myeloid leukemia: real world data on decision to treat and outcomes from the Swedish Acute Leukemia Registry. Blood 2009;113:4179–87.

82. Wahlin A, Markevärn B, Golovleva I, et al. Prognostic significance of risk group stratification in elderly patients with acute myeloid leukaemia. Br J Haemat 2001; 115:25–33.

83. Valcárcel D, Montesinos P, Sánchenz-Ortega I, et al. A scoring system to predict the risk of death during induction with anthracycline plus cytarabine-based chemotherapy in patients with de novo acute myeloid leukemia. Cancer 2011. [Epub ahead of print].

84. Kantarjian H, O'Brien S, Cortes J, et al. Results of intensive chemotherapy in 998 patients age 65 years or older with acute myeloid leukemia or high-risk myelodysplastic syndrome: predictive prognostic models for outcome. Cancer 2006; 106:1090–8.

85. Kantarjian H, Ravandi F, O'Brien S, et al. Intensive chemotherapy does not benefit most older patients (age 70 years or older) with acute myeloid leukemia. Blood 2010;118:4422–9.

86. Rowe JM, Neuberg D, Friedenberg W, et al. A phase 3 study of three induction regimens and of priming with GM-CSF in older adults with acute myeloid leukemia: a trial by the Eastern Cooperative Oncology Group. Blood 2004; 103:479–85.

87. Löwenberg B, Ossenkoppele GJ, Van Putten W, et al. High-dose daunorubicin in older patients with acute myeloid leukemia. N Engl J Med 2009;361:1235–48.

88. Cripe LD, Uno H, Paietta EM, et al. Zosuquidar, a novel modulator of P-glycoprotein, does not improve the outcome of older patients with newly diagnosed acute myeloid leukemia: a randomized, placebo-controlled trial of the Eastern Cooperative Oncology Group 3999. Blood 2010;116:4077–85.

89. Stone RM, Berg DT, George SL, et al. Granulocyte-macrophage colony stimulating factor after initial chemotherapy for elderly patients with primary acute myelogenous leukemia. N Engl J Med 1995;332:1671–7.

90. Rowe JM, Andersen JW, Mazza JJ, et al. A randomized placebo-controlled phase III study of granulocyte-macrophage colony-stimulating factor in adult patients (>55 to 70 years of age) with acute myelogenous leukemia: a study of the Eastern Cooperative Oncology Group (E1490). Blood 1995;86:457–62.

91. Dombret H, Chastang C, Fenaux P, et al. A controlled study of recombinant human granulocyte colony-stimulating factor in elderly patients after treatment for acute myelogenous leukemia. N Engl J Med 1995;332:1678–783.

92. Schwind S, Marcucci G, Maharry K, et al. BAALC and ERG expression levels are associated with outcome and distinct gene- and microRNA-expression profiles in older patients with de novo cytogenetically normal acute myeloid leukemia: a Cancer and Leukemia Group B study. Blood 2010;116:5660–9.

93. Abou-Jawde RM, Sobecks R, Pohlman B, et al. The role of post-remission chemotherapy for older patients with acute myelogenous leukemia. Leuk Lymphoma 2006;47:689–95.

94. Goldstone AH, Burnett AK, Wheatley K, et al. Attempts to improve treatment outcomes in acute myeloid leukemia (AML) in older patients: the results of the United Kingdom Medical Research Council AML11 trial. Blood 2001;98:1302–11.

95. Gardin C, Turturee P, Fagot T, et al. Post-remission treatment of elderly patients with acute myeloid leukemia in first complete remission after intensive induction chemotherapy: results of the multi-center randomized Acute Leukemia French Associate (ALFA) 9803 trial. Blood 2007;109:5129–35.

96. Schlenk RF, Fröhling S, Martmann F, et al. Intensive consolidation versus oral maintenance therapy in patients 61 years or older with acute myeloid leukemia in first remission: results of second randomization of the AML HD98-B treatment trial [letter]. Leukemia 2006;20:748–50.

97. Estey E, de Lima M, Tibes R, et al. Prospective feasibility analysis of reduced-intensity conditioning (RIC) regimens for hematopoietic stem cell transplantation (HCT) in elderly patients with acute myeloid leukemia (AML and high-risk myelodysplastic syndrome (MDS). Blood 2007;109:1395–400.

98. Giralt S, Thall PF, Khouri I, et al. Melphalan and purine analog-containing preparative regimens: reduced-intensity conditioning for patients with hematologic malignancies undergoing allogeneic progenitor cell transplantation. Blood 2001;97:631–7.

99. Shimoni A, Kröger N, Zabelina T, et al. Hematopoietic stem-cell transplantation from unrelated donors in elderly patients (age >55 years) with hematologic

malignancies: older age is no longer a contraindication when using reduced intensity conditioning. Leukemia 2005;19:7–12.

100. Hegenbart U, Niederwieser D, Sandmaier BM, et al. Treatment for acute myelogenous leukemia by low-dose, total-body, irradiation-based conditioning and hematopoietic cell transplantation from related and unrelated donors. J Clin Oncol 2006;24:444–53.

101. Schetelig J, Bornhäuser M, Schmid C, et al. Matched unrelated or matched sibling donors result in comparable survival after allogeneic stem-cell transplantation in elderly patients with acute myeloid leukemia: a report from the Cooperative German Transplant Study Group. J Clin Oncol 2008; 26:5183–91.

102. Burnett AK, Milligan D, Prentice AG, et al. A comparison of low-dose cytarabine and hydroxyurea with or without all-trans retinoic acid for acute myeloid leukemia and high-risk myelodysplastic syndrome in patients not considered fit for intensive treatment. Cancer 2007;109:1114–24.

103. Lancet JE, Gojo I, Gotlib J, et al. A phase 2 study of farnesyltransferase inhibitor tipifarnib in poor-risk and elderly patients with previously untreated acute myelogenous leukemia. Blood 2007;109:1387–94.

104. Harousseau J-L, Martinelli G, Jedrzejczak WW, et al. A randomized phase 3 study of tipifarnib compared with best supportive care, including hydroxyurea, in the treatment of newly diagnosed acute myeloid leukemia in patients 70 years or older. Blood 2009;114:1166–73.

105. Schiller GJ, O'Brien SM, Pigneux A, et al. Single-agent laromustine, a novel alkylating agent, has significant activity in older patients with previously untreated poor-risk acute myeloid leukemia. J Clin Oncol 2009;28:815–21.

106. Kantarjian HM, Erba HP, Claxton D, et al. Phase II study of clofarabine monotherapy in previously untreated older adults with acute myeloid leukemia and unfavorable prognostic factors. J Clin Oncol 2010;28:549–55.

107. Burnett AK, Russell NH, Kell J, et al. European development of clofarabine as treatment for older patients with acute myeloid leukemia considered unsuitable for intensive chemotherapy. J Clin Oncol 2010;28:2389–95.

108. Faderl S, Ravandi F, Huang X, et al. A randomized study of clofarabine versus clofarabine plus low-dose cytarabine as front-line therapy for patients aged 60 years and older with acute myeloid leukemia and high-risk myelodysplastic syndrome. Blood 2008;112:1638–45.

109. Faderl S, Verstovsek S, Cortes J, et al. Clofarabine and cytarabine combination as induction therapy for acute myeloid leukemia (AML) in patients 50 years of age or older. Blood 2006;108:45–51.

110. Fenaux P, Mufti GJ, Hellström-Lindberg E, et al. Azacitidine prolongs overall survival compared with conventional care regimens in elderly patients with low bone marrow blast count acute myeloid leukemia. J Clin Oncol 2009;28:562–9.

111. Cashen AF, Schiller GJ, O'Donnell MR, et al. Multicenter, phase II study of decitabine for the first-line treatment of older patients with acute myeloid leukemia. J Clin Oncol 2009;28:556–61.

112. Blum W, Garzon R, Klisovic RB, et al. Clinical response and *miR-29b* predictive significance in older AML patients treated with a 10-day schedule of decitabine. Proc Natl Acad Sci U S A 2010;107:7475–8.

113. Thomas XG, Dmoszynska A, Wierzbowska A, et al. Results from a randomized phase III trial of decitabine versus supportive care or low-dose cytarabine for the treatment of older patients with newly diagnosed AML. J Clin Oncol ASCO Ann Meeting Proc 2011;29:6504.

114. Fehniger TA, Uy GL, Trinkaus K, et al. A phase 2 study of high-dose lenalido-mide as initial therapy for older patients with acute myeloid leukemia. Blood 2011;117:1828–33.
115. Sekeres MA, Gundacker H, Lancet J, et al. A phase 2 study of lenalidomide monotherapy in patients with deletion 5q acute myeloid leukemia: SWOG Study S0605. Blood 2011;118:523–8.
116. Krause DS, Van Etten RA. Tyrosine kinases as targets for cancer therapy. N Engl J Med 2005;353:172–87.
117. Weisberg E, Boulton C, Kelly LM, et al. Inhibition of mutant FLT3 receptors in leukemia cells by the small molecule tyrosine kinase inhibitor PKC412. Cancer Cell 2002;1:433–43.
118. Levis M, Allebach J, Tse KF, et al. A FLT3-targeted tyrosine kinase inhibitor is cytotoxic to leukemia cells in vitro and in vivo. Blood 2002;99:3885–91.
119. DeAngelo DJ, Stone RM, Heaney MA, et al. Phase 1 clinical results with tandu-tinib (MLN518), a novel FLT3 antagonist, in patients with acute myelogenous leukemia or high-risk myelodysplastic syndrome: safety, pharmacokinetics, and pharmacodynamics. Blood 2006;108:3674–81.
120. O'Farrell A-M, Abrams TJ, Yuen HA, et al. SU11248 is a novel FLT3 tyrosine kinase inhibitor with potent activity in vitro and in vivo. Blood 2003;101:3597–605.
121. Auclair D, Miller D, Yatsula V, et al. Antitumor activity of sorafenib in FLT3-driven leukemic cells. Leukemia 2007;21:439–45.
122. Stone RM, DeAngelo DJ, Klimek V, et al. Patients with acute myeloid leukemia and an activating mutation in FLT3 respond to a small-molecule FLT3 tyrosine kinase inhibitor, PKC412. Blood 2005;105:54–60.
123. Smith BD, Levis M, Beran M, et al. Single-agent CEP-701, a novel FLT3 inhibitor, shows biologic and clinical activity in patients with relapsed or refractory acute myeloid leukemia. Blood 2004;103:3669–76.
124. Levis M, Ravandi F, Wang ES, et al. Results from a randomized trial of salvage chemotherapy followed by lestaurtinib for patients with FLT3 mutant AML in first relapse. Blood 2011;117:3294–301.
125. Stone RM, Fischer T, Paquette R, et al. Phase Ib study of midostaurin (PKC412) in combination with daunorubicin and cytarabine induction and high-dose cytar-abine consolidation in patients under age 61 with newly diagnosed *de novo* acute myeloid leukemia: overall survival of patients whose blasts have FLT3 mutations is similar to those with wild-type FLT3. Blood (ASH Annual Meeting Abstracts) 2009;114:634.
126. Cortes J, Foran J, Ghirdaladze D, et al. AC220, a potent, selective, second generation FLT3 receptor tyrosine kinase (RTK) inhibitor, in a first-in-human (FIH) phase 1 AML study. Blood (ASH Annual Meeting Abstracts) 2009;114:636.
127. Raponi M, Lancet JE, Fan H, et al. A 2-gene classifier for predicting response to the farnesyltransferase inhibitor tipifarnib in acute myeloid leukemia. Blood 2008;111:2589–96.
128. Vener TI, Derecho C, Galkin S, et al. Correlation of RASVRP1:APTX expression assay with response to tipifarnib plus etoposide in elderly patients with newly diagnosed AML. J Clin Oncol ASCO Ann Meeting Proc 2011;29:6534.
129. Uy GL, Rettig MP, McFarland K, et al. A phase I/II study of chemosensitization with the CXCR4 antagonist plerixafor in relapsed or refractory AML. Blood (ASH Annual Meeting Abstracts) 2009;114:787.
130. Kantarjian HM, Garcia-Manero G, Luger S, et al. A randomized phase 2 study of sapacitabine, an oral nucleoside analogue, in elderly patients with AML

previously untreated or in first relapse. Blood (ASH Ann Meeting Abstracts) 2009;114:1061.

131. O'Brien S, Rizzieri DA, Vey N, et al. A phase II multicentre study with elacytarabine as second salvage therapy in patients with AML. Blood (ASH Ann Meeting Abstract) 2009;114:1042.

132. Feldman EJ, Lancet JE, Kolitz JE, et al. First-in-man study of CPX-351: a liposomal carrier containing cytarabine and daunorubicin in a fixed 5:1 molar ratio for the treatment of relapsed and refractory acute myeloid leukemia. J Clin Oncol 2011;29:979–85.

133. Lancet JE, Cortes JE, Hogge DE, et al. Phase 2B randomized study of CPX-351 vs. cytarabine and daunorubicin (7+3 regimen) in newly diagnosed AML patients aged 60-75. Blood (ASH Ann Meeting Abstracts) 2010;166:655.

134. Lancet JE, Cortes JE, Kovacosvics T, et al. CPX-351 versus cytarabine and daunorubicin therapy in newly diagnosed AML patients age 60-75: safety and efficacy in secondary AML. J Clin Oncol ASCO Ann Meeting Proc 2011;29:6519.

135. Lancet JE, Ravandi F, Ricklis RM, et al. A phase Ib study of vosaroxin, an anticancer quinolone derivative, in patients with relapsed or refractory acute leukemia. Leukemia 2011. [Epub ahead of print].

136. Stuart RK, Ravnadi Kashani F, Cripe LD, et al. Voreloxin singlxe-agent treatment of older patients (60 years or older) with previously untreated acute myeloid leukemia: final results from a phase II study with three schedules. J Clin Oncol ASCO Ann Meeting Proc 2010;28:6525.

Curing All Patients with Acute Promyelocytic Leukemia: Are We There Yet?

Muhamed Baljevic, MD[a], Jae H. Park, MD[b], Eytan Stein, MD[c],
Dan Douer, MD[c,d], Jessica K. Altman, MD[e],
Martin S. Tallman, MD[b,c,*]

KEYWORDS

- Acute promyelocytic leukemia • All-*trans* retinoic acid
- Arsenic trioxide • Targeted therapies • Cure

Acute promyelocytic leukemia (APL) is a distinct morphologic variant of acute myeloid leukemia (AML), accounting for approximately 10% to 15% of the adult cases of AML diagnosed in the United States annually.[1] The leukemia cells are usually easy to distinguish morphologically from others[2] and are characterized by a specific reciprocal translocation t(15;17),[3] which fuses the PML (promyelocyte) gene from chromosome 15 to the RAR-α (retinoic acid receptor-α) gene of chromosome 17.[4] Consistently found in all cases of t(15;17) APL, the resulting PML-RARα fusion gene on der(15) encodes a chimeric transcript of the 2 DNA-binding domains that shows altered transcriptional regulatory properties, eventually leading to the block of retinoic-acid–induced myeloid differentiation.[4]

The authors have nothing to disclose.
[a] Department of Medicine, New York-Presbyterian Hospital/Weill Cornell Medical Center, 525 East 68th Street, Box 130, New York, NY 10065, USA
[b] Leukemia Service, Department of Medicine, Memorial Sloan-Kettering Cancer Center, Weill Cornell Medical College, 1275 York Avenue, New York, NY 10065, USA
[c] Department of Medicine, Memorial Sloan-Kettering Cancer Center, Weill Cornell Medical College, 1275 York Avenue, New York, NY 10065, USA
[d] Acute Lymphoblastic Leukemia Program, Department of Medicine, Memorial Sloan-Kettering Cancer Center, Weill Cornell Medical College, 1275 York Avenue, New York, NY 10065, USA
[e] Department of Medicine, Robert H. Lurie Comprehensive Cancer Center, Northwestern University Feinberg School of Medicine, Chicago, IL, USA
* Corresponding author. Leukemia Service, Department of Medicine, Memorial Sloan-Kettering Cancer Center, Weill Cornell Medical College, 1275 York Avenue, New York, NY 10065.
E-mail address: TallmanM@mskcc.org

Ever since the seminal description by Hillestad in 1957,[5] APL has been well recognized as one of the most fatal forms of acute leukemia at presentation or during induction, primarily because of an associated complex and often catastrophic bleeding disorder.[1] However, the introduction of all-*trans* retinoic acid (ATRA) in 1985, combined with anthracycline-based chemotherapy, has revolutionized the prognosis of this disease, with unprecedented complete response (CR) rates in excess of 90%, and cure rates of approximately 80%. The pharmacologic concentrations of ATRA used in the treatment of APL lead to dissociation of N-CoR (nuclear corepressor) (a ubiquitous nuclear protein that mediates transcriptional repression) presumably permitting differentiation of the leukemic cells.[6] As a result, the long-term outcome in most patients with APL is favorable. Nevertheless, a small percentage of patients have a variant form of the disease with different fusion transcripts such as PLZF/RAR-α[7] or STAT5b/RAR-α[8] coding for fusion proteins that are almost invariably resistant to initial treatment with ATRA, necessitating the accurate baseline identification of candidates who can be expected to benefit from induction therapy with ATRA. FLT-3 mutations, particularly the internal tandem duplication (ITD) mutations, are also common in APL and seem to be present in approximately 40% of patients. These variants are often also characterized by the high white blood cell (WBC) count and the bcr3 PML breakpoint. Several retrospective studies have reported that the subgroup of patients with FLT-3 mutation have a higher death rate during induction chemotherapy without a significant difference in relapse rate or 5-year overall survival (OS).[9] Nevertheless, there have been reports that through univariate analysis showed higher relapse and lower survival rates in patients with an FLT3-ITD.[10]

The subsequent introduction of arsenic trioxide (ATO) further redefined the course of APL from a highly fatal to the most curable subtype of AML in adults. After several studies reported that the combination of ATRA and ATO is a highly effective and potentially curative treatment, an exciting new treatment strategy has emerged, which aims to eliminate exposure to conventional cytotoxic chemotherapy in treatment of many, if not most, patients with APL. Despite the advances in molecular biology and treatment approaches that have led to substantially decreased relapse rates, even among high-risk patients, the persistent challenge of the complex and life-threatening coagulopathy[11] before and during induction therapy has remained the principal cause of early death and has emerged as the major cause of treatment failure among patients with APL. Other questions of importance in APL are centered on defining the best treatment of patients with high-risk disease, the role of ATO in initial therapy, and the roles of maintenance therapy and molecular monitoring. Nevertheless, implementing rapid, aggressive, and comprehensive strategies that mitigate early death has become one of the most important goals in APL treatment and is sure to further increase the cure rate of APL.

In this review, the therapeutic approaches that have led to the current frontline treatment in APL are summarized, focusing on development of new and rationally targeted therapeutic approaches that aim to eliminate toxicities of conventional chemotherapy without compromising cure rates; the importance of strategies to further increase the cure rate of APL by addressing early hemorrhagic deaths is also highlighted.

INDUCTION THERAPY

In the age preceding the therapeutic use of ATRA, APL was treated much like other subtypes of AML, with the standard induction regimens based on an anthracycline and cytarabine (Ara-C) yielding 70% CR rates among newly diagnosed patients.[12–14]

However, even among those patients who initially achieved CR, between 50% and 65% subsequently relapsed, whereas only 30% to 50% remain alive at 2 years.[12,15]

Initial Studies of ATRA in APL

The evolution of creative treatment approaches for APL was spurred by an initial report, which documented CR rates of 85% with ATRA as a single induction agent.[16] Among the first large studies to explore the role of ATRA either as a single agent or in combination with chemotherapy,[16–19] the first North American Intergroup study I0129/E2491 reported an equivalent remission rate of 70% with single-agent ATRA compared with induction with Ara-C and daunorubicin.[17] These encouraging results were tempered by studies of ATRA as a single agent that reported relapse of these patients from CR without further chemotherapy. As a result, subsequent trials such as that conducted by the European APL (EAPL) group focused on improving the clinical outcome through a combination of ATRA and chemotherapy. These investigators reported equal remission rates of 92% among the groups randomized to induction with concurrent therapy with ATRA plus chemotherapy with Ara-C and daunorubicin, versus sequential ATRA followed by chemotherapy.[20] However, a reduced relapse rate at 2 years (6% vs 16%) was observed in the arm with concurrent versus sequential therapy. After validation in multiple large multicenter trials[21–24] (**Table 1**), these results led to the simultaneous administration of ATRA and anthracycline-based chemotherapy as the current standard induction approach in newly diagnosed patients with APL, with outstanding disease-free survival (DFS) rates (**Fig. 1**).

Choice of Anthracyclines

There is no clear evidence that one anthracycline is superior to another when combined with ATRA because no prospective randomized trials have directly compared daunorubicin and idarubicin in the ATRA era. The best available evidence stems from the pre-ATRA era. Even though it seems to suggest that idarubicin is associated with an improved outcome compared with daunorubicin or amsacrine,[25] there is no distinct superiority between the two because both seem equally effective in APL.

Role of Ara-C in Initial Therapy

The question of the importance of the addition of Ara-C to anthracyclines in the induction regimen has been addressed with disparate results. The cooperative groups Gruppo Italiano Malattie Ematologiche dell'Adulto (GIMEMA) and the Programa

Table 1
Outcome of major contemporary trials in APL

Groups (References)	Year	N	CR (%)	D(E)FS (%)	Therapy
EAPL group[29]	1999	99	92%	84	ATRA + DA
GIMEMA[22]	1997	240	95	79	ATRA + IDA
North American study[17]	1997	172	72	75	ATRA-based induction/maintenance
PETHEMA[24]	1999	123	89	92	ATRA + IDA (Ara-C, etoposide in consolidation)
GAMLCG[21]	2000	51	92	88	HiDAC + ATRA

Abbreviations: DA, daunorubicin; D(E)FS, disease (event)-free survival; GAMLCG, The German Acute Myeloid Leukemia Cooperative Group; HiDAC, high dose Ara-C; IDA, idarubicin; N, number.

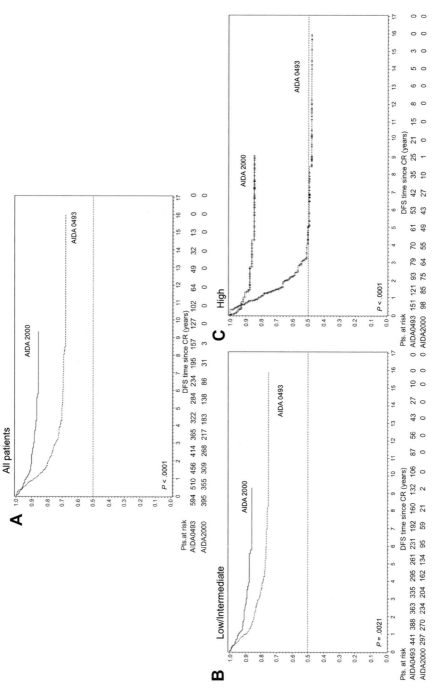

Fig. 1. (A-C) Current DFS after initial treatment of APL.

Español de Tratamientos en Hematología (PETHEMA) omitted Ara-C during induction in nonrandomized prospective clinical trials, showing that ATRA plus idarubicin (AIDA) is as effective in inducing CR as a regimen containing Ara-C, with CR rates of 89% to 95% that were not influenced by the presenting WBC count.[24,26] The National Cancer Research Institute (NCRI) in the United Kingdom (UK) reported no overall difference in response, relapse, or survival rates between the arms randomized to AIDA and ATRA plus daunorubicin and Ara-C. However, they did observe less myelosuppression without the use of cytarabine.[27] In a contrasting report, the EAPL group (APL 2000) in a randomized study observed a statistically significant increase in relapse risk (13.4% vs 29%) and OS (92.9% vs 83.3%) without the addition of Ara-C in both induction and consolidation regimens.[28,29] Despite the discrepancy of these reports, which can be attributed possibly to the choice and cumulative doses of anthracyclines, as well as differences in the consolidation regimens and the number of total consolidation courses, the choice of induction therapy is defined by the ability to tolerate anthracyclines and by whether the patient had high-risk or low-risk disease based on the WBC count at diagnosis.[30] It seems that Ara-C can be omitted from ATRA plus anthracycline-based induction regimen in most patients, even those considered high-risk (WBC count >10,000/µL). The optimal anthracycline has not been determined. However, idarubicin seems to be sufficient to induce CR in almost all patients who survive the initial risk of early death during induction.[31]

CONSOLIDATION THERAPY

Unlike the aim of induction therapy, which focuses on reduction of the total disease burden to less than the cytologically detectable level of approximately 10^9 cells, the goal of consolidation therapy in APL is to eliminate the remaining malignant leukemic stem cells that through replicative resilience lead to eventual relapse. Induction failure of any subgroup of patients with APL is generally related to bleeding, the APL differentiation syndrome, or infection and not disease progression.[31] There is essentially no primary resistance in APL. Although ATRA-based induction therapy has a greater than 90% CR rate in APL,[22] patients are invariably destined to relapse, necessitating effective consolidation therapy that provides durable remission. The benefit of adding ATRA in induction in improving DFS and OS by reducing relapse has been amply reported. Although not shown in any randomized trial, consecutive trials by the GIMEMA[32] and PETHEMA groups[33] have shown improvement in outcome by the addition of ATRA in consolidation. The optimal choice and intensity of consolidation regimens remain controversial, because many of the investigative efforts of the past decade have promoted the development of risk-adapted approaches that guide the treatment intensity as defined by the risk factors predictive of relapse.

Risk-adapted Approach to Consolidation Therapy

The necessity for a risk-adapted approach is reflected in the higher mortality of 19% in patients in CR older than 70 years, compared with mortality of 1% in those younger than 60 years.[34] The currently used risk model stems from the 2 PETHEMA trials,[33,35] which have identified 3 different groups of patients at risk for relapse: high-risk defined by presenting WBC counts 10,000/µL or greater and platelet count less than 40,000/µL; intermediate-risk with WBC count less than 10,000/µL and platelet count less than 40,000/µL and a low-risk with WBC count less than 10,000/µL and platelet count greater than 40,000/µL.

The results of the LPA99 trial of significantly improved outcome with the inclusion of ATRA in consolidation treatment were confirmed by the new AIDA-2000 trial of the Italian GIMEMA group.[32] The PETHEMA group study (LPA2005) randomized high-risk patients younger than 60 years to receive Ara-C combined with ATRA and idarubicin in the first and third consolidation courses, reporting significantly lower relapse rate of 11% at 3 years (this is compared with 26% relapse rate in the historical cohort in the LPA99 trial, $P = .03$).[31] More importantly, the study also investigated reducing the overall toxicity in low-risk and intermediate-risk patients by lowering the dose of mitoxantrone for the second consolidation course and eliminating Ara-C during the 3 consolidation courses. This treatment resulted in a comparable clinical outcome but with a significant reduction of toxicity (as reflected in the duration of neutropenia and thrombocytopenia) and a shorter overall hospital stay (17 days vs 22 days in the LPA99 trial; $P<.001$).[31] The GIMEMA group (AIDA2000), which also included ATRA as a part of the consolidation regimen, similarly reported no difference in OS and a significant reduction of infections (40% vs 80%) and prolonged neutropenia with improved DFS at 6 years (85.9% vs 76.6% in the AIDA0493) for the low-risk and intermediate-risk patients who had Ara-C omitted from their consolidation courses.[32] An additional study conducted by the UK NCRI failed to show any benefit of Ara-C regardless of risk stratification.[27] With the goal of further reduction in toxicity, the North American Intergroup Trial C9710 randomized patients after CR to receive either 2 courses of 25 days of ATO (5 days a week for a total of 5 weeks) followed by a standard postremission regimen with 2 courses of ATRA plus daunorubicin, or postremission therapy alone. Treatment with ATO, particularly in the high-risk subgroup, showed significantly better event-free survival (EFS) and OS.[36] This finding represents an attractive alternative among those patients with a high-risk disease who may be in particular need of a less cardiotoxic consolidation regimen.

Given the overall body of evidence, it seems that high-risk patients benefit from either the addition of intermediate-dose Ara-C to consolidation or ATO as an early consolidation course with synergistic antileukemic effect of combination therapy.[37]

MAINTENANCE (POSTCONSOLIDATION) THERAPY

The response to completed consolidation therapy is routinely assessed using reverse transcriptase-polymerase chain reaction (RT-PCR) in the bone marrow, the goal being complete molecular remission (MR). The best therapeutic approach to maintenance therapy was controversial even in the pre-ATRA era, and despite the 2 randomized controlled trials that have reported a substantial benefit with ATRA-based maintenance therapy,[20,38] its systematic use remains controversial. This situation is particularly true for those patients considered nonhigh risk, or those who achieve MR after consolidation treatment. Moreover, parallel to evolution of not only induction but also consolidation regimens that have incorporated ATO into first-line treatment of APL, the significance of maintenance therapy may have been reduced even further.

The North American Intergroup study I0129/E2491 reported a superior 5-year DFS (61% vs 36%), with a reduction in relapse rate (22% vs 39%), proving clinical benefit with ATRA-based maintenance therapy.[17,38] The APL93 trial similarly confirmed the beneficial effect of adding ATRA to maintenance therapy in a randomized study in which the regimen consisting of continuous low-dose 6-mercaptopurine (6-MP), methotrexate (MTX), and intermittent ATRA showed the lowest relapse rate (8%) at 2 years, compared with relapse for 6-MP plus MTX (13%), ATRA alone (21%) versus no maintenance (35%).[20] More importantly, this group recently updated the results of their previous study to indicate that the clinical benefit of maintenance therapy was mainly evident in high-risk patients whereas the low-risk and intermediate-risk patients experienced only marginal benefit.[39] With contrasting results, randomized trials by the GIMEMA[40] and Japanese Adult Leukemia Study Group (JALSG)[41] have reported no difference in DFS with postconsolidation therapy, with follow-up of up to 12 years. However, the observations of the JALSG group trial may not entirely be applicable, because ATRA was not included in maintenance therapy. Furthermore, data from the AIDA study appeared to suggest that patients who test molecularly negative after the consolidation therapy experience no real benefit from maintenance therapy.[42]

These studies differed significantly in the treatment approach. Both the JALSG[41] and the GIMEMA[40] groups administered a higher number of consolidation cycles with idarubicin as a choice of anthracycline therapy for induction and consolidation chemotherapy; in contrast, the EAPL[20,39] and North American Intergroup[17,38] trials administered only 2 consolidation courses with daunorubicin. Moreover, whereas studies by the GIMEMA and JALSG groups may have been confounded because all study patients tested negative for PML/RARα at the end of consolidation, the North American Intergroup and EAPL studies did not examine the MR status at the end of consolidation, raising a question whether the benefit that was observed by the maintenance therapy in their study largely reflected the response of patients with residual disease after consolidation treatment.

Overall, the sum of reported studies points to discrepancies that suggest that the benefit of maintenance treatment may be dependent on preceding induction and consolidation therapy, as well as PML/RARα molecular status after consolidation, which has clearly been shown to correlate with the relapse risk.[43,44] Together with RT-PCR, which should be completed to document postconsolidation MR, subsequent molecular monitoring of patients can be performed based on the perceived risk of relapse. Furthermore, studies suggest that low-risk and intermediate-risk patients and those who achieve complete MR after consolidation may not benefit from the combination maintenance therapy. However, for high-risk patients, maintenance therapy for 1 to 2 years with intermittent ATRA and low-dose chemotherapy with 6-MP and MTX is recommended. Furthermore, molecular monitoring every 3 months for 2 years during maintenance for high-risk subgroups is also recommended, with the aim of monitoring and identifying potential molecular relapse. Because there are no prospective trial data in comparing 1 versus 2 years of maintenance therapy, we recommend continuation of maintenance therapy for 2 years unless toxicity develops. In those patients who develop cytopenias and have a negative molecular test with RT-PCR, a marrow analysis is recommended for evaluation of new cytogenetic anomalies that may represent therapy-related myelodysplastic syndrome (MDS) or AML.

MINIMAL RESIDUAL DISEASE MONITORING

Minimal residual disease (MRD) monitoring entails identification of the molecular product of the chimeric PML-RARα transcript. The development of the real-time quantitative PCR (RQ-PCR) allowed more precise assessment of the kinetics of treatment response and relapse, setting foundation to MRD-directed therapy. Taking into account that frank relapse in APL can be complicated by a major risk of death because of hemorrhagic complications, and evidence that impending relapses can be reliably predicted by MRD monitoring with RT-PCR,[45,46] there has been a growing interest inadopting MRD monitoring as a tool to guide and deliver preemptive therapy. Nevertheless, the optimal use of sequential MRD monitoring in treatment of APL remains controversial because of limited prospective data.

A prospective study by the PETHEMA group reported improved survival in patients salvaged with ATRA and anthracycline-based chemotherapy in molecular relapse compared with those who were treated only at frank hematologic relapse (historical control population).[46] However, OS of 44% at 2 years for the historical cohort patients was considerably lower than what is currently achieved with ATO-based regimens.[47] The UK NCRI prospective study[48] has similarly reported a benefit from MRD-directed preemptive therapy using ATO, showing the evidence for MRD monitoring being far superior to presenting WBC count as a therapy guide and the strongest predictor of relapse-free survival (RFS) with less toxicity and reduced rates of frank relapses. However, there remain many unanswered questions from the trial. Given that half of the trial patients (MRC AML15) received maintenance after consolidation treatment, the difference in kinetics of PML-RARα transcripts and time from molecular to hematologic relapse among the group that did and did not receive maintenance therapy is unclear; furthermore, although the key aim of monitoring was to trigger preemptive therapy, more than half of the patients failed to have the salvage therapy initiated because of various technical reasons, questioning the large-scale practicality of this approach; the clinical outcome of patients in this trial reported in the 5-year RFS of 35% and OS of 41% remains less than optimal, implying that primary focus should be placed on improving the initial therapy in high-risk patients to prevent against, rather than detect, disease relapse.[49]

The limited prospective data and the improved antileukemic efficacy of currently available standard treatments together question the true benefit of systematic molecular monitoring after consolidation therapy. As a result, the role of MRD monitoring as part of currently standard practice is changing, particularly for low-risk and intermediate-risk patients. The main reasons are the unanswered questions that pertain to the cumulative cost of serial testing, the implications of positive MRD screen, the chance of successful treatment at the time of MRD versus at the time of hematologic relapse as well as persistent anxiety potentially conferred by frequent testing.

Rigorous sequential RQ-PCR monitoring has been found to be the strongest predictor of RFS in APL and, when coupled with preemptive therapy, represents a valid strategy toward reducing rates of clinical relapse.[48] Low-risk and intermediate-risk patients have a more favorable outcome with extremely low risk of relapse with currently available treatment protocols. Consequently, serious doubts can be raised about the usefulness of molecular monitoring in this group of patients if they are treated with contemporary strategies and followed with routine complete blood counts.[50] On the other hand, the high-risk patients carry a relapse risk of approximately 10%, which seems to suggest there may be a greater benefit for sequential MRD monitoring in this patient population[48,51]; the optimal schedule for monitoring is still the subject for future research. Molecular monitoring may guide an appropriate salvage therapy for these patients based on the available evidence that suggests a higher relapse rate after a PCR-positive autologous hematopoietic stem cell transplantation (HSCT).[52] In addition, a small subset of the high-risk patients may have the propensity for a central nervous system relapse. After achieving second morphologic remission, these patients are strongly recommended to receive intrathecal chemotherapy.[53] Allogeneic transplantation should be reserved for those patients who have evidence of persistent disease despite salvage therapy.

Keeping in mind the pace at which new effective therapeutic strategies are evolving with less residual disease to detect, MRD monitoring in APL may soon become less important for most patients.[48] Nevertheless, although still advised in the high-risk patients with APL, it is highly recommended that it be performed in reference laboratories with extensive expertise.

Role of HSCT

Those patients who experience persistence of disease after appropriate initial therapy or fail to achieve second molecular CR after salvage ATO at first relapse should be considered for allogeneic HSCT. Patients who relapse after initial therapy and achieve a second molecular CR after ATO salvage therapy do well with autologous HSCT. The choice between autologous versus allogeneic HSCT in second molecular CR was initially answered in a study that showed that for those patients with APL in second CR, autologous bone marrow transplantation (ABMT) with PML/RAR-α–negative marrow cells is likely to result in prolonged clinical and MRs. Conversely, patients who tested PCR-positive after reinduction required the use of alternative aggressive approaches, including unrelated allogeneic HSCT.[51] This finding was also further investigated by the EAPL group, who showed an OS rate of 75% for patients with PCR-negative autologous HSCT, versus 52% for those who underwent allogeneic HSCT.[54] Differences in the survival were likely reflective of cumulatively higher treatment-related mortality for the allogeneic HSCT arm. Allogeneic and autologous stem cell transplantations (SCTs) were directly compared in the same retrospective study, which concluded that if performed in MR, ABMT is effective in patients who relapse after initial treatment with ATRA. At the same time, allogeneic SCT was found to be associated with high treatment-related mortality when performed after salvage with intensive chemotherapy.[54] Salvage with ATO instead, which has lower toxicity, promises to further improve the outcome of relapsing patients with APL.

INCREASING APL CURE RATES WITH EARLY DEATH REDUCTION

Since the first report of APL 50 years ago, rapid and unprecedented progress has been made in our understanding of the biology and therapeutic options available for APL, making its story epical in the chronicles of modern medicine. More recently, several studies have contributed to the optimization of the antileukemic efficacy of the current regimens for APL. Despite this and in the face of highly effective therapy, early death rates remain high,[55] and more efforts are need to reduce the early deaths in this highly curable disease.

Although infection is the principal cause of death in AML, hemorrhagic complications of the induction therapy are still often the primary cause of early death in APL.[56] Other associating factors significantly related to the severe bleeding and early death also include late diagnosis and delayed treatment initiation, in addition to increased WBC count.[56] Even although earlier multicenter cooperative studies report an approximate 5% to 10% early death rate within 1 month after the initiation of treatment,[17,20,22–24] several population-based observational studies recently reported higher early death rates in unselected patients with APL,[57,58] the largest of which involved a cohort of 1400 patients and reported a 17.3% early death rate despite use of ATRA (**Fig. 2**).[59] These results indicate that the availability and routine use of ATRA per se are not sufficient to eliminate the major cause of treatment failure in APL. They also further highlight the essence of educating a range of health care providers across a wide spectrum of medical fields who may be the first to evaluate patients suspected of having APL with the knowledge necessary to approach them as a medical emergency that requires swift initiation of ATRA, aggressive supportive care to correct the coagulopathy, and transfer to experienced medical centers.

ATRA has been shown to rapidly improve biochemical parameters of the coagulopathy associated with APL, thereby reducing the severity of bleeding and the amount of blood products needed to maintain hemostatic stability.[60] ATRA should be started immediately on the first suspicion of the diagnosis. Although the real impact of ATRA

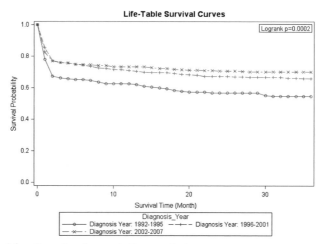

Fig. 2. Survival functions by diagnosis time periods.

in reducing the early death rate remains to be determined,[17,20,61] it is the correct approach to presume a favorable risk/benefit ratio of its initiation, because the agent is unlikely to have any deleterious systemic effects should the final diagnostic assessment fail to confirm the diagnosis of APL. Much like with ATRA, supportive measures to reverse life-threatening coagulopathy including fresh frozen plasma, cryoprecipitate, fibrinogen and platelet transfusions to keep the fibrinogen concentration more than 100 to 150 mg/dL and platelet count more than 50,000/μL need to be instituted instantly. Posttransfusion values must be followed with the same vigilance, ensuring adequate repletion of all coagulation factors.[62] Intense monitoring and aggressive correction of the same should be maintained during induction therapy for all patients suspected of having APL, irrespective of whether they may potentially be variant subtypes virtually resistant to the ATRA induction, until the disappearance of any clinical or laboratory signs of coagulopathy.

Whereas genetic verification of the specific PML-RARα fusion transcript is a prerequisite to definitive diagnosis of APL, fluorescence in situ hybridization and reverse RT-PCR (the turnaround time of which is 1 to 2 days) may not even be available at more decentralized health care centers. Immunostaining with anti-PML monoclonal antibodies performed on dry smears of bone marrow or even peripheral blood samples has been shown to have the sufficiently high sensitivity and specificity to establish a rapid diagnosis, which in this way is made in less than 4 hours.[63] This test may be of particular value in smaller centers lacking immediate access to sophisticated molecular diagnostics laboratories, and has further been shown in a large South American trial[64] to reduce early mortality by facilitating the rapid confirmation of the diagnosis. Nevertheless, even in the setting in which these tests are readily available, there should be no delay in initiation of ATRA if a sufficiently high index of suspicion is present. The immediate transfer of patients when stable to more experienced centers with a capacity to administer ATRA and provide aggressive repletion of the blood products may be beneficial.

IN SEARCH OF A CHEMOTHERAPY-FREE CURE FOR APL

Contemporary investigative efforts have influenced the therapeutic approach to the treatment of neoplastic processes, particularly hematologic malignancies in the direction of molecularly targeted therapies. In APL, it is in this spirit and on the weight of the breakthrough discoveries of agents such as ATRA and ATO that the adoption of novel treatment approaches devoid of conventional chemotherapy has begun. Although treatment of newly diagnosed APL with anthracycline-based regimens augmented with ATRA has been proved to be highly effective, eliminating the exposure of patients to cytotoxicity of conventional DNA-disrupting chemotherapy has been the primary focus of recent studies. Reducing the potential for treatment-associated cardiomyopathy of anthracyclines, as well as infection risk associated with prolonged neutropenia, may further improve the overall outcome of patients with APL. Furthermore, although the risk of therapy-related MDS and AML is low in published series,[65–67] removing this risk of therapy-related secondary malignancy may improve the outcome profile of patients with APL being treated with curative intent.

THE ROLE OF ATO

As a cytostatic agent, ATRA effectively induces complete differentiation of the promyelocyte clones, but it rarely gives rise to durable remissions when used as a single agent.[68] As a potent promoter of apoptosis[69,70] ATO is not a direct activator of transcription or terminal differentiation, and, unlike ATRA, has been shown to be curative in APL, even as a single agent.

Recent insights into the molecular nature and the in vivo and in vitro dynamics of leukemic cells in APL have challenged the historical dogma that assumes the disappearance of the disease with the differentiation of APL leukemic clones. Current understanding suggests that the degradation of the chimeric product of translocation (PML-RARα), initially considered to be a mere aftermath of differentiation therapy, plays a pivotal role in not only the loss of self-renewal capacity of APL clones but also the eradication of leukemic cancer stem cells (termed leukemia initiating cells) and ultimately stable disease remission.[71–73]

ATRA functions by inducing proteasome-dependent degradation of RAR alpha moiety,[74] whereas ATO acts on the PML part of the fusion protein, resulting in rapid degradation of the PML-RARα transcript.[75,76] Given specific and divergent mechanisms of action of ATRA and ATO on the PML-RARα protein, it is possible to hypothesize that combination of the 2 agents would degrade the fusion protein in synergy, leading to cooperative cure in APL. This hypothesis is what has been shown in murine models in which degradation of the fusion product leads to the disease clearance.[52,77,78] Although data from clinical trials suggest that ATO does not seem to be sufficient for many patients as a single frontline therapy,[79,80] the combination of ATRA and ATO leads to cure of many patients despite the absence of conventional chemotherapy.[36,81–85]

In the clinical arena, ATO as a single agent has been shown to be equivalent to ATRA-based regimens with induction CRs of 85% to 86% in previously untreated patients with APL (**Table 2**).[79,80] Nevertheless, the outcome of high-risk patients defined in this study with WBC count greater than 5000/μL at diagnosis (what would otherwise not be defined as high risk) in which patients were randomized to receive sequential ATO induction, 28-day consolidation, and a 6-month postconsolidation therapy was found to be inferior, with an EFS of 60% at 5 years, when compared with a similar subset of patients treated with ATRA-based chemotherapy.[79] The same outcome is evident when risk-stratifying patients by the conventional relapse risk grouping[35] with an EFS of less than 60% in high-risk patients.[79] In contrast, a study that followed shortly thereafter reported no difference in clinical outcome with the same ATO induction and consolidation therapy, irrespective of the presenting WBC

Table 2
ATO-based treatment and outcomes in APL

Groups (References)	N	Median Age, Years (Ranges)	Follow-up (mo)	Outcomes (%)
Mathews et al[79]	72	28 (3–75)	60	ED: 13.9 CR: 86.1 5-y DFS: 80 5-y OS: 74.2
Ghavamzadeh et al[80]	197	29 (11–71)	38	ED: 14.7 CR: 85.8 5-y DFS: 66.7 5-y OS: 64.4
Shanghai Institute of Hematology[81]	61	30.5 (14–74)	18	ED: 5 CR: 95 Median DFS: 13 mo
		39.5 (15–69)		ED: 10 CR: 90 Median DFS: 16 mo
		34 (14–62)		ED: 4.8 CR: 95.2 Median DFS: 20 mo
Shanghai Institute of Hematology[82]	85	N/A	70	ED: 5.9 CR: 94.1 5-y EFS: 89.2 5-y OS: 91.7
MDACC[84]	82	47 (14–81)	25	ED: 8.5 CR: 92 3-yr OS: 85
ALLG[85]	124	44 (3–78)	20	ED: 3 CR: 97 3-y EFS: 87 3-y OS: 93
North American Intergroup C9710[36]	481	N/A (15–79)	54	ED: 8 CR: 90 3-y DFS: 70–90 3-y OS: 81–86
Gore et al[86]	45	50 (19–70)	32	ED: 8.9 CR: 91.1 3-y DFS: 88.7 3-y EFS: 76 3-y OS: 88

Abbreviations: ALLG, Australasian Leukemia and Lymphoma Group; CR, complete remission; ED, early death; MDACC, MD Anderson Cancer Center; N, number of patients; N/A, not available.

count.[80] For patients who presented with a WBC count greater than 50×10^9/L (the value used to define hyperleukocytosis) and despite allowing the use of hydroxyurea, which was given to 73.6% of patients, and anthracyclines administered to 11% of patients, there was a higher early death rate of 13.9% to 14.7% because of hemorrhagic complications, suggesting that ATO as a single-agent frontline therapy may not be sufficient or appropriate for some patients with APL.

Building on the preclinical evidence of the synergistic effect of ATRA and ATO combination therapy,[52,77,78] several rationally targeted studies have been launched for newly diagnosed patients with APL, with the aim to investigate the effect of this approach in the absence of significant exposure to conventional DNA-targeting chemotherapy. A randomized clinical trial from Shanghai in which patients were randomized to receive induction therapy with either ATRA, ATO, or the combination of the two,[81] with subsequent consolidation and maintenance courses, resulted in the lowest rates of relapse, a faster CR rate, and a greater reduction in the number of PML-RARα transcripts, without apparent greater toxicity compared with ATRA or ATO alone. The 7-year follow-up update on this report[82] confirms the high efficacy and minimal toxicity of the combination treatment, with no difference in early death rates among the different treatment arms, and an overall early death rate of 6.5%. In a similar fashion, the study from the MD Anderson Cancer Center reported the combination ATRA and ATO treatment to be an effective regimen in previously untreated patients with APL with presenting WBC count less than $10 \times 10^9/L$, with a CR rate of 96% and few relapses even when eliminating conventional chemotherapy from consolidation course.[84] These investigators also reported, unlike investigators of a comparable study,[81] that chemotherapy can be eliminated in consolidation, resulting in durable responses with few late relapses. Nevertheless, high-risk patients in this study who presented with WBC count $10 \times 10^9/L$ or greater achieved an inferior CR rate of 79% to 81% and a lower EFS (65% vs 90% at 2 years) because of early treatment failure from fatal hemorrhage and APL differentiation syndrome despite the addition of gemtuzumab ozogamicin (GO) or idarubicin during induction.[84]

More recently, 124 patients with newly diagnosed APL were studied in the Australasian Leukemia and Lymphoma Group. These patients were treated with ATRA, ATO, and idarubicin during induction, followed by 2 courses of consolidation therapy with ATRA and ATO and 2-year postconsolidation therapy with ATRA, MTX, and 6-MP. After a median follow-up of 20 months, the 3-year OS and EFS rates were 93% and 87%, respectively.[85] The North American Intergroup randomized patients during induction to receive 2 cycles of consolidation of ATRA plus daunorubicin, either immediately after induction therapy or preceded by 2 25-day cycles of ATO plus ATRA.[36] Adding the ATO as an initial consolidation therapy significantly improved the 3-year DFS (90% vs 70%) and OS (86% vs 81%) irrespective of the risk stratification by presenting WBC count. With considerably reduced amount of anthracyclines coupled with a single cycle of ATO, a similar phase II study reported comparable outcomes with DFS 90% and OS 88% at a 2.7-year median follow-up (see **Table 2**).[86]

Overall, although limited by the nonrandomized trial design, the body of evidence points toward a potential cooperative mechanism of disease suppression and elimination with combination therapy with ATRA and ATO, raising the possibility of minimizing or perhaps even eliminating the use of conventional chemotherapy in the treatment of APL, particularly as it pertains to low-risk and intermediate-risk disease (commonly defined as those patients who present with WBC count $<10 \times 10^9/L$). Furthermore, according to the National Comprehensive Cancer Network Guidelines, ATRA and ATO represent an attractive alternative for older patients or patients otherwise unfit for conventional anthracycline therapy because of severe comorbidities of cardiovascular or other organ systems, secondary anthracycline-related APL, or women with previous breast cancer. Nevertheless, evidence suggests that in high-risk patients who present with increased WBC count, concomitant use of conventional chemotherapy such as anthracyclines remains critical to prevent rapid progression of leukocytosis and consequent APL differentiation syndrome. Ongoing randomized trials by several cooperative groups who will compare ATRA plus ATO with ATRA plus chemotherapy will shed further light into the safety of additional deintensification of APL therapy in high-risk patients without the compromise of cure rates.

TOWARD CURATIVE STRATEGIES IN APL

The introduction of the cytostatic, differentiating agent ATRA has transformed APL into one of the most curable subtypes of adult AML. Further institution of ATO to the therapeutic arsenal has brought forth the development of several frontline rationally targeted treatment protocols with the aim of limiting or eliminating exposure to traditional cytotoxic chemotherapy, reducing the treatment-associated complications and toxicities in most patients. Through risk-adapted approaches without the use of the cytotoxic chemotherapy, these questions are being tested in several multi-center trials.

In efforts to optimize the front-line therapies, colleagues in the GIMEMA group will compare ATRA plus ATO with minimal chemotherapy to control the WBC count during the induction to AIDA for intermediate-risk and high-risk patients (presenting WBC count 10×10^9/L or less). The British NCRI (AML17 trial) with investigators from France will use the same randomization in all patients irrespective of the presenting WBC count. The role of maintenance therapy in high-risk patients who are induced and consolidated with ATO-containing regimens is to be answered through future prospective clinical trials.

An essential part of the strategy to further increase the cure rate and improve overall outcome of patients with APL are efforts focusing on successful implementation of strategies that will reduce early hemorrhagic deaths. This goal can be achieved through the education of a wide range of health care providers, who may be the first to encounter patients with APL in a variety of clinical settings that will prompt swift initiation of ATRA followed by aggressive blood product support and transfer to more equipped and specialized medical centers.

The ensuing decade will bring exciting answers and perhaps significant changes in the way we approach frontline treatment of patients with newly diagnosed APL. Soon, APL might be better individually tailored and rationally targeted with reduced exposure to conventional cytotoxic chemotherapy in most, if not all, patients as we learn more from data on the short-term and long-term safety and efficacy of ATRA and ATO-based nonchemotherapy treatment protocols being investigated in ongoing clinical trials. Furthermore, novel formulations of the same targeted agents such as the oral formulation of ATO and an oral synthetic retinoid (Tamibarotene) designed to overcome ATRA resistance[87] may be promising new therapeutic options for patients with relapsed disease.

REFERENCES

1. Tallman MS, Altman JK. Curative strategies in acute promyelocytic leukemia. Hematology Am Soc Hematol Educ Program 2008;391–9.
2. Bennett JM, Catovsky D, Daniel MT, et al. Proposals for the classification of the acute leukaemias. French-American-British (FAB) co-operative group. Br J Haematol 1976;33(4):451–8.
3. Rowley JD, Golomb HM, Dougherty C. 15/17 translocation, a consistent chromosomal change in acute promyelocytic leukaemia. Lancet 1977;1(8010):549–50.
4. Grignani F, Ferrucci PF, Testa U, et al. The acute promyelocytic leukemia-specific PML-RAR alpha fusion protein inhibits differentiation and promotes survival of myeloid precursor cells. Cell 1993;74(3):423–31.
5. Hillestad LK. Acute promyelocytic leukemia. Acta Med Scand 1957;159:189–94.
6. Guidez F, Ivins S, Zhu J, et al. Reduced retinoic acid-sensitivities of nuclear receptor corepressor binding to PML- and PLZF-RARalpha underlie molecular

pathogenesis and treatment of acute promyelocytic leukemia. Blood 1998;91: 2634.

7. Melnick A, Licht JD. Deconstructing a disease: RARalpha, its fusion partners, and their roles in the pathogenesis of acute promyelocytic leukemia. Blood 1999;93: 3167.

8. Dong S, Tweardy DJ. Interactions of STAT5b-RARalpha, a novel acute promyelocytic leukemia fusion protein, with retinoic acid receptor and STAT3 signaling pathways. Blood 2002;99:2637.

9. Gale RE, Hills R, Pizzey AR, et al. Relationship between FLT3 mutation status, biologic characteristics, and response to targeted therapy in acute promyelocytic leukemia. Blood 2005;106:3768–76.

10. Barragán E, Montesinos P, Camos M, et al. Prognostic value of FLT3 mutations in patients with acute promyelocytic leukemia treated with all-trans retinoic acid and anthracycline monochemotherapy. Haematologica 2011;96(10):1470–7.

11. Tallman MS, Kwaan HC. Reassessing the hemostatic disorder associated with acute promyelocytic leukemia. Blood 1992;79(3):543–53.

12. Cunningham I, Gee TS, Reich LM, et al. Acute promyelocytic leukemia: treatment results during a decade at Memorial Hospital. Blood 1989;73(5):1116–22.

13. Fenaux P, Degos L. Treatment of acute promyelocytic leukemia with all-trans retinoic acid. Leuk Res 1991;15(8):655–7.

14. Head DR, Kopecky KJ, Willman C, et al. Treatment outcome with chemotherapy in acute promyelocytic leukemia: the Southwest Oncology Group (SWOG) experience. Leukemia 1994;8(Suppl 2):S38–41.

15. Degos L, Dombret H, Chomienne C, et al. All-trans-retinoic acid as a differentiating agent in the treatment of acute promyelocytic leukemia. Blood 1995; 85(10):2643–53.

16. Huang ME, Ye YC, Chen SR, et al. Use of all-trans retinoic acid in the treatment of acute promyelocytic leukemia. Blood 1988;72(2):567–72.

17. Tallman MS, Andersen JW, Schiffer CA, et al. All-trans-retinoic acid in acute promyelocytic leukemia. N Engl J Med 1997;337(15):1021–8.

18. Chen ZX, Xue YQ, Zhang R, et al. A clinical and experimental study on all-trans retinoic acid-treated acute promyelocytic leukemia patients. Blood 1991;78(6): 1413–9.

19. Castaigne S, Chomienne C, Daniel MT, et al. All-trans retinoic acid as a differentiation therapy for acute promyelocytic leukemia. I. Clinical results. Blood 1990; 76(9):1704–9.

20. Fenaux P, Chastang C, Chevret S, et al. A randomized comparison of all transretinoic acid (ATRA) followed by chemotherapy and ATRA plus chemotherapy and the role of maintenance therapy in newly diagnosed acute promyelocytic leukemia. The European APL Group. Blood 1999;94(4):1192–200.

21. Lengfelder E, Reichert A, Schoch C, et al. Double induction strategy including high dose cytarabine in combination with all-trans retinoic acid: effects in patients with newly diagnosed acute promyelocytic leukemia. German AML Cooperative Group. Leukemia 2000;14(8):1362–70.

22. Mandelli F, Diverio D, Avvisati G, et al. Molecular remission in PML/RAR alpha-positive acute promyelocytic leukemia by combined all-trans retinoic acid and idarubicin (AIDA) therapy. Gruppo Italiano-Malattie Ematologiche Maligne dell'Adulto and Associazione Italiana di Ematologia ed Oncologia Pediatrica Cooperative Groups. Blood 1997;90(3):1014–21.

23. Asou N, Adachi K, Tamura J, et al. Analysis of prognostic factors in newly diagnosed acute promyelocytic leukemia treated with all-trans retinoic acid and

chemotherapy. Japan Adult Leukemia Study Group. J Clin Oncol 1998;16(1): 78–85.

24. Sanz MA, Martin G, Rayon C, et al. A modified AIDA protocol with anthracycline-based consolidation results in high antileukemic efficacy and reduced toxicity in newly diagnosed PML/RARalpha-positive acute promyelocytic leukemia. PETHEMA group. Blood 1999;94(9):3015–21.

25. Berman E, Little C, Kher U, et al. Prognostic analysis of patients with acute promyelocytic leukemia [abstract]. Blood 1991;78:43a.

26. Avvisati G, Lo Coco F, Diverio D, et al. AIDA (all-trans retinoic acid + idarubicin) in newly diagnosed acute promyelocytic leukemia: a Gruppo Italiano Malattie Ematologiche Maligne dell'Adulto (GIMEMA) pilot study. Blood 1996;88(4): 1390–8.

27. Burnett AK, Hills RK, Grimwade D, et al. Idarubicin and ATRA is as effective as MRC chemotherapy in patients with acute promyelocytic leukaemia with lower toxicity and resource usage: preliminary results of the MRC AML15 Trial. ASH Annual Meeting Abstracts. 2007;110(11):589.

28. Ades L, Chevret S, Raffoux E, et al. Is cytarabine useful in the treatment of acute promyelocytic leukemia? Results of a randomized trial from the European Acute Promyelocytic Leukemia Group. J Clin Oncol 2006;24(36):5703–10.

29. Ades L, Raffoux E, Chevret S, et al. Is AraC required in the treatment of standard risk APL? Long term results of a randomized trial (APL 2000) from the French Belgian Swiss APL Group. ASH Annual Meeting Abstracts. 2010;116(21):13.

30. O'Donnell MR, Abboud CN, Altman J, et al. Acute myeloid leukemia. J Natl Compr Canc Netw 2011;9(3):280–317.

31. Sanz MA, Montesinos P, Rayon C, et al. Risk-adapted treatment of acute promyelocytic leukemia based on all-trans retinoic acid and anthracycline with addition of cytarabine in consolidation therapy for high-risk patients: further improvements in treatment outcome. Blood 2010;115(25):5137–46.

32. Lo-Coco F, Avvisati G, Vignetti M, et al. Front-line treatment of acute promyelocytic leukemia with AIDA induction followed by risk-adapted consolidation for adults younger than 61 years: results of the AIDA-2000 trial of the GIMEMA Group. Blood 2010;116(17):3171–9.

33. Sanz MA, Martin G, Gonzalez M, et al. Risk-adapted treatment of acute promyelocytic leukemia with all-trans-retinoic acid and anthracycline monochemotherapy: a multicenter study by the PETHEMA group. Blood 2004;103(4):1237–43.

34. Sanz MA, Vellenga E, Rayon C, et al. All-trans retinoic acid and anthracycline monochemotherapy for the treatment of elderly patients with acute promyelocytic leukemia. Blood 2004;104(12):3490–3.

35. Sanz MA, Lo Coco F, Martin G, et al. Definition of relapse risk and role of nonanthracycline drugs for consolidation in patients with acute promyelocytic leukemia: a joint study of the PETHEMA and GIMEMA cooperative groups. Blood 2000; 96(4):1247–53.

36. Powell BL, Moser B, Stock W, et al. Arsenic trioxide improves event-free and overall survival for adults with acute promyelocytic leukemia: North American Leukemia Intergroup Study C9710. Blood 2010;116(19):3751–7.

37. Flanagan SA, Meckling KA. All- trans-retinoic acid increases cytotoxicity of 1-beta-D-arabinofuranosylcytosine in NB4 cells. Cancer Chemother Pharmacol 2003;51(5):363–75.

38. Tallman MS, Andersen JW, Schiffer CA, et al. All-trans retinoic acid in acute promyelocytic leukemia: long-term outcome and prognostic factor analysis from the North American Intergroup protocol. Blood 2002;100(13):4298–302.

39. Ades L, Guerci A, Raffoux E, et al. Very long-term outcome of acute promyelocytic leukemia after treatment with all-trans retinoic acid and chemotherapy: the European APL Group experience. Blood 2010;115(9):1690–6.
40. Avvisati G, Lo-Coco F, Paoloni FP, et al. AIDA 0493 protocol for newly diagnosed acute promyelocytic leukemia: very long-term results and role of maintenance. Blood 2011;117(18):4716–25.
41. Asou N, Kishimoto Y, Kiyoi H, et al. A randomized study with or without intensified maintenance chemotherapy in patients with acute promyelocytic leukemia who have become negative for PML-RARalpha transcript after consolidation therapy: the Japan Adult Leukemia Study Group (JALSG) APL97 study. Blood 2007;110(1): 59–66.
42. Avvisati G, Petti MC, Lo Coco F, et al. AIDA: the Italian way of treating acute promyelocytic leukemia (APL), final act. Blood 2003;102(Suppl 1): [abstract 487].
43. Lo Coco F, Diverio D, Falini B, et al. Genetic diagnosis and molecular monitoring in the management of acute promyelocytic leukemia. Blood 1999;94(1):12–22.
44. Grimwade D, Lo Coco F. Acute promyelocytic leukemia: a model for the role of molecular diagnosis and residual disease monitoring in directing treatment approach in acute myeloid leukemia. Leukemia 2002;16(10):1959–73.
45. Lo Coco F, Diverio D, Avvisati G, et al. Therapy of molecular relapse in acute promyelocytic leukemia. Blood 1999;94(7):2225–9.
46. Esteve J, Escoda L, Martin G, et al. Outcome of patients with acute promyelocytic leukemia failing to front-line treatment with all-trans retinoic acid and anthracycline-based chemotherapy (PETHEMA protocols LPA96 and LPA99): benefit of an early intervention. Leukemia 2007;21(3):446–52.
47. Thirugnanam R, George B, Chendamarai E, et al. Comparison of clinical outcomes of patients with relapsed acute promyelocytic leukemia induced with arsenic trioxide and consolidated with either an autologous stem cell transplant or an arsenic trioxide-based regimen. Biol Blood Marrow Transplant 2009; 15(11):1479–84.
48. Grimwade D, Jovanovic JV, Hills RK, et al. Prospective minimal residual disease monitoring to predict relapse of acute promyelocytic leukemia and to direct pre-emptive arsenic trioxide therapy. J Clin Oncol 2009;27(22):3650–8.
49. Park JH, Tallman MS. Managing acute promyelocytic leukemia without conventional chemotherapy: is it possible? Expert Rev Hematol 2011;4(4):427–36.
50. Grimwade D, Tallman MS. Should minimal residual disease monitoring be the standard of care for all patients with acute promyelocytic leukemia? Leuk Res 2011;35(1):3–7.
51. Meloni G, Diverio D, Vignetti M, et al. Autologous bone marrow transplantation for acute promyelocytic leukemia in second remission: prognostic relevance of pre-transplant minimal residual disease assessment by reverse-transcription polymerase chain reaction of the PML/RAR alpha fusion gene. Blood 1997;90(3):1321–5.
52. Lallemand-Breitenbach V, Guillemin MC, Janin A, et al. Retinoic acid and arsenic synergize to eradicate leukemic cells in a mouse model of acute promyelocytic leukemia. J Exp Med 1999;189(7):1043–52.
53. de Botton S, Sanz MA, Chevret S, et al. Extramedullary relapse in acute promyelocytic leukemia treated with all-trans retinoic acid and chemotherapy. Leukemia 2006;20:35–41.
54. de Botton S, Fawaz A, Chevret S, et al. Autologous and allogeneic stem-cell transplantation as salvage treatment of acute promyelocytic leukemia initially treated with all-trans-retinoic acid: a retrospective analysis of the European acute promyelocytic leukemia group. J Clin Oncol 2005;23:120–6.

55. de la Serna J, Montesinos P, Vellenga E, et al. Causes and prognostic factors of remission induction failure in patients with acute promyelocytic leukemia treated with all-trans retinoic acid and idarubicin. Blood 2008;111(7):3395–402.
56. Breccia M, Latagliata R, Cannella L, et al. Early hemorrhagic death before starting therapy in acute promyelocytic leukemia: association with high WBC count, late diagnosis and delayed treatment initiation. Haematologica 2010;95(5):853–4.
57. Alizadeh AA, McClellan JS, Gotlib JR, et al. Early mortality in acute promyelocytic leukemia may be higher than previously reported. Blood 2009;114:1015.
58. Micol J, Raffoux E, Boissel N, et al. Do early events excluding patients with acute promyelocytic leukemia (APL) from trial enrollment modify treatment result evaluation? Real-life management of 100 patients referred to the University Hospital Saint-Louis between 2000 and 2010. Blood (ASH Annual Meeting Abstracts), 116, Abstract 1083 (2010).
59. Park JH, Qiao B, Panageas KS, et al. Early death rate in acute promyelocytic leukemia remains high despite all-trans retinoic acid. Blood 2011;118(5):1248–54.
60. Di Bona E, Avvisati G, Castaman G, et al. Early haemorrhagic morbidity and mortality during remission induction with or without all-trans retinoic acid in acute promyelocytic leukaemia. Br J Haematol 2000;108(4):689–95.
61. Visani G, Gugliotta L, Tosi P, et al. All-trans retinoic acid significantly reduces the incidence of early hemorrhagic death during induction therapy of acute promyelocytic leukemia. Eur J Haematol 2000;64(3):139–44.
62. Sanz MA, Grimwade D, Tallman MS, et al. Management of acute promyelocytic leukemia: recommendations from an expert panel on behalf of the European LeukemiaNet. Blood 2009;113(9):1875–91.
63. Dimov ND, Medeiros LJ, Kantarjian HM, et al. Rapid and reliable confirmation of acute promyelocytic leukemia by immunofluorescence staining with an antipromyelocytic leukemia antibody. Cancer 2010;116(2):369–76.
64. Rego EM, Kim H, Ruiz-Arguelles GJ, et al. Improving the treatment outcome of acute promyelocytic leukemia in developing countries through international cooperative network. Report on the International Consortium on Acute Promyelocytic Leukemia Study Group. ASH Annual Meeting Abstracts. 2009;114(6).
65. Andersen MK, Pedersen-Bjergaard J. Therapy-related MDS and AML in acute promyelocytic leukemia. Blood 2002;100(5):1928–9 [author reply: 1929].
66. Garcia-Manero G, Kantarjian HM, Kornblau S, et al. Therapy-related myelodysplastic syndrome or acute myelogenous leukemia in patients with acute promyelocytic leukemia (APL). Leukemia 2002;16(9):1888.
67. Latagliata R, Petti MC, Fenu S, et al. Therapy-related myelodysplastic syndrome-acute myelogenous leukemia in patients treated for acute promyelocytic leukemia: an emerging problem. Blood 2002;99(3):822–4.
68. Hu J, Shen ZX, Sun GL, et al. Long-term survival and prognostic study in acute promyelocytic leukemia treated with all-trans-retinoic acid, chemotherapy, and As2O3: an experience of 120 patients at a single institution. Int J Hematol 1999;70(4):248–60.
69. Shen ZX, Chen GQ, Ni JH, et al. Use of arsenic trioxide (As2O3) in the treatment of acute promyelocytic leukemia (APL): II. Clinical efficacy and pharmacokinetics in relapsed patients. Blood 1997;89:3354–60.
70. Soignet SL, Maslak P, Wang ZG, et al. Complete remission after treatment of acute promyelocytic leukemia with arsenic trioxide. N Engl J Med 1998;339:1341–8.
71. Nasr R, Guillemin MC, Ferhi O, et al. Eradication of acute promyelocytic leukemia-initiating cells through PML-RARA degradation. Nat Med 2008;14(12):1333–42.

72. Licht JD. Acute promyelocytic leukemia–weapons of mass differentiation. N Engl J Med 2009;360(9):928–30.
73. Ablain J, de The H. Revisiting the differentiation paradigm in acute promyelocytic leukemia. Blood 2011;117(22):5795–802.
74. Zhu J, Gianni M, Kopf E, et al. Retinoic acid induces proteasome-dependent degradation of retinoic acid receptor alpha (RARalpha) and oncogenic RARalpha fusion proteins. Proc Natl Acad Sci U S A 1999;96(26):14807–12.
75. Shao W, Fanelli M, Ferrara FF, et al. Arsenic trioxide as an inducer of apoptosis and loss of PML/RAR alpha protein in acute promyelocytic leukemia cells. J Natl Cancer Inst 1998;90(2):124–33.
76. Chen GQ, Shi XG, Tang W, et al. Use of arsenic trioxide (As2O3) in the treatment of acute promyelocytic leukemia (APL): I. As2O3 exerts dose-dependent dual effects on APL cells. Blood 1997;89(9):3345–53.
77. Zheng PZ, Wang KK, Zhang QY, et al. Systems analysis of transcriptome and proteome in retinoic acid/arsenic trioxide-induced cell differentiation/apoptosis of promyelocytic leukemia. Proc Natl Acad Sci U S A 2005;102(21):7653–8.
78. Gianni M, Koken MH, Chelbi-Alix MK, et al. Combined arsenic and retinoic acid treatment enhances differentiation and apoptosis in arsenic-resistant NB4 cells. Blood 1998;91(11):4300–10.
79. Mathews V, George B, Chendamarai E, et al. Single-agent arsenic trioxide in the treatment of newly diagnosed acute promyelocytic leukemia: long-term follow-up data. J Clin Oncol 2010;28(24):3866–71.
80. Ghavamzadeh A, Alimoghaddam K, Rostami S, et al. Phase II study of single-agent arsenic trioxide for the front-line therapy of acute promyelocytic leukemia. J Clin Oncol 2011;29(20):2753–7.
81. Shen ZX, Shi ZZ, Fang J, et al. All-trans retinoic acid/As2O3 combination yields a high quality remission and survival in newly diagnosed acute promyelocytic leukemia. Proc Natl Acad Sci U S A 2004;101(15):5328–35.
82. Hu J, Liu YF, Wu CF, et al. Long-term efficacy and safety of all-trans retinoic acid/ arsenic trioxide-based therapy in newly diagnosed acute promyelocytic leukemia. Proc Natl Acad Sci U S A 2009;106(9):3342–7.
83. Estey E, Garcia-Manero G, Ferrajoli A, et al. Use of all-trans retinoic acid plus arsenic trioxide as an alternative to chemotherapy in untreated acute promyelocytic leukemia. Blood 2006;107(9):3469–73.
84. Ravandi F, Estey EH, Cortes JE, et al. Phase II study of all-trans retinoic acid (ATRA), arsenic trioxide (ATO), with or without gemtuzumab ozogamicin (GO) for the frontline therapy of patients with acute promyelocytic leukemia (APL). Blood (ASH Annual Meeting Abstracts). 116, Abstract 1080 (2010).
85. Iland H, Frank F, Supple S. et al. Interim analysis of the APML4 trial incorporating all-trans retinoic acid (ATRA), idarubicin, and intravenous arsenic trioxide (ATO) as initial therapy in acute promyelocytic leukaemia (APL): an Australasian Leukaemia and Lymphoma Group (ALLG) study. International Oral Arsenic Union & 38th Annual Scientific Meeting Hong Kong Society of Haematology 2010;16 [abstract 6].
86. Gore SD, Gojo I, Sekeres MA, et al. Single cycle of arsenic trioxide-based consolidation chemotherapy spares anthracycline exposure in the primary management of acute promyelocytic leukemia. J Clin Oncol 2010;28(6):1047–53.
87. Di Veroli A, Ramadan SM, Divona M, et al. Molecular remission in advanced acute promyelocytic leukaemia after treatment with the oral synthetic retinoid Tamibarotene. Br J Haematol 2010;151(1):99–101.

Oddballs: Acute Leukemias of Mixed Phenotype and Ambiguous Origin

David P. Steensma, MD

KEYWORDS

- Acute leukemia • Leukemia pathology • Immunophenotype
- Leukemias of ambiguous lineage • Bilineage • Biphenotypic
- Mixed phenotype acute leukemia
- Acute undifferentiated leukemia

Using currently available diagnostic tools, skilled hematopathologists can assign most pediatric and adult acute leukemias to myeloid, B-lymphoid, or T-lymphoid lineages without much difficulty.[1] However, a subset of more challenging cases (depending on the particular criteria used for lineage assignment, this subset may represent as many as 5% of all acute leukemias) cannot be easily classified, despite integration of data from flow cytometric, immunohistochemical, cytochemical, cytogenetic, and molecular genetic investigations.[2,3]

This uncommon and heterogeneous group of acute leukemias has received a degree of attention disproportionate to its prevalence, and has been described using a variety of terms: *bilineage, biphenotypic, hybrid, polyphenotypic, mixed lineage, mixed phenotype, ambiguous lineage, uncertain origin.*[4] The most recent (2008, fourth edition) World Health Organization (WHO) *Classification of Tumours of Haematopoietic and Lymphoid Tissues*[5] includes 7 categories of varying specificity within an "acute leukemias of ambiguous origin" diagnostic group, including bilineage and biphenotypic leukemias, which are classified together as "mixed phenotype acute leukemias" (MPAL) (**Table 1**). The WHO ambiguous-origin leukemias also include an "other ambiguous lineage leukemias" category, which contains a provisional entity, "natural killer cell lymphoblastic leukemia/lymphoma,"[6] as well as 2 categories defined by both immunophenotype and by one of a pair of specific molecular genetic findings, *BCR-ABL* fusion and *MLL* rearrangement. With the exception of *BCR-ABL1* fusion,

Conflicts of Interest/Disclosures: The author has no relevant disclosures or conflicts of interest.
Funding source: None reported.
Adult Leukemia Program, Department of Medical Oncology, Dana-Farber Cancer Institute, 450 Brookline Avenue, Suite D1B30 (Mayer 1B21), Boston, MA 02215, USA
E-mail address: david_steensma@dfci.harvard.edu

Hematol Oncol Clin N Am 25 (2011) 1235–1253
doi:10.1016/j.hoc.2011.09.014
0889-8588/11/$ – see front matter © 2011 Elsevier Inc. All rights reserved.

Table 1
World Health Organization (WHO) 2008 (4th edition) classification of "acute leukemias of ambiguous lineage"

Category	Definition and Comments
Acute undifferentiated leukemia	*An acute leukemia that does not express any marker that is considered specific for either lymphoid or myeloid lineage.*[a] Nonhematopoietic tumors (eg, germ cell tumors) and acute leukemias of unusual lineage (eg, those derived from myeloid or plasmacytoid dendritic cell precursors, NK-cell precursors, basophils) must be excluded. Blasts may express HLA-DR, CD34, or CD38 and may be positive for TdT.
Mixed phenotype acute leukemia with t(9;22)(q34;q11.2); *BCR-ABL1*	*An acute leukemia that meets diagnostic criteria[b] for MPAL, in which the blasts also have the t(9;22) chromosome translocation or the BCR-ABL1 rearrangement.* Patients known to have had chronic myeloid leukemia before developing blast phase should not be assigned to this category, even if they meet diagnostic criteria for MPAL.
Mixed phenotype acute leukemia with t(v;11q23); *MLL* rearranged	*An acute leukemia that meets diagnostic criteria[b] for MPAL, in which the blasts also have a translocation involving the MLL gene at 11q23.* Cases of ALL that express myeloid antigens but do not meet criteria for MPAL should not be assigned to this category.
Mixed phenotype acute leukemia, B/myeloid, NOS	*An acute leukemia that meets diagnostic criteria for assignment to both B and myeloid lineage*, in which the blasts lack genetic abnormalities involving *BCR-ABL1* or *MLL*
Mixed phenotype acute leukemia, T/myeloid, NOS	*An acute leukemia that meets diagnostic criteria for assignment to both T and myeloid lineage*, in which the blasts lack genetic abnormalities involving *BCR-ABL1* or *MLL*
Mixed phenotype acute leukemia, NOS – rare types	*An acute leukemia with a mixed phenotype that is not listed above.* Examples would include a lymphoid leukemia with both B and T lineage commitment, or a leukemia with evidence of trilineage (ie, B/T/myeloid) markers. Erythroleukemias and megakaryocytic leukemias are clearly of myeloid origin, but do not typically express MPO, so B/ or T/erythroleukemia, or B/ or T/megakaryocytic leukemia, if they exist (they had not yet been described at the time of the 2008 WHO classification, but a case report of B/erythroleukemia appeared shortly thereafter[87]), would fit in this category.

(continued on next page)

Table 1 (*continued*)	
Category	**Definition and Comments**
Other ambiguous lineage leukemias	*An acute leukemia that expresses an unusual combination of markers that does not allow classification as either AUL, MPAL, or a single lineage leukemia (eg, a form of AML or ALL) using WHO diagnostic criteria[c] for lineage assignment.* This category includes a rare provisional entity: (Precursor) natural killer cell lymphoblastic leukemia/lymphoma, which expresses CD56 along with immature T-associated markers, and lacks B-cell and myeloid markers as well as T-cell clonal gene rearrangement. CD94 1A and CD161 might be expressed, but currently are rarely tested in clinical practice.

Abbreviations: ABL1, Abelson tyrosine kinase 1; ALL, acute lymphoblastic leukemia; BCR, break-point cluster region; CD, cluster of differentiation/designation; MLL, mixed lineage leukemia; MPAL, mixed phenotype acute leukemia; MPO, myeloperoxidase; NK, natural killer; NOS, not otherwise specified; TdT, terminal deoxynucleotidyl transferase.

[a] By definition, acute undifferentiated leukemias lack cytoplasmic CD3 (T lineage defining), lack MPO (myeloid lineage defining), do not express B-cell–specific markers (eg, cytoplasmic CD22, cyto-plasmic CD79a, or strong expression of CD19), and lack specific features of other lineages, such as plasmacytoid dendritic cells, erythroblasts, or megakaryocytes. For further discussion of lineage-specific markers, see **Tables 2** and **3** and relevant text.

[b] Diagnostic criteria for "mixed phenotype acute leukemia" require assignment of blast cells to 2 or 3 lineages, using lineage-defining criteria in **Table 3**. Mixed phenotype may result from either 2 distinct blast cell populations or 2 or more lineage-associated markers on the same blast cells.

[c] These cases must be distinguished from blastic plasmacytoid dendritic cell neoplasm (BPDCN), which was not clearly part of the 2001 WHO classification but is included as a distinct entity in the 2008 WHO classification.[88] BPDCN tumor cells express CD4, CD56, CD43, CD45RA, and the plasma-cytoid dendritic cell neoplasm markers CD123, CD303 (BDCA2), TCL1, CLA, and MxA; 50% of cases express CD68, whereas CD7, TdT, and CD33 expression are common. Names used in the past for this neoplastic entity (BPDCN) include the following: blastic NK cell lymphoma, agranular CD4+ NK cell leukemia, blastic NK leukemia/lymphoma, or agranular CD4+ CD56+ hematodermic neoplasm/tumor.[54,88] These cases also must be distinguished from myeloid/NK cell acute leukemia, which is a form of AML with minimal differentiation, possibly of precursor NK cell origin (but early NK cells express no specific markers).

Data from Borowitz MJ, Béné MC, Harris NL, et al. Acute leukaemias of ambiguous lineage. In: Swerdlow SH, Campo E, Harris NL, et al, editors. World Health Organization (WHO) Classification of Tumours of Haematopoietic and Lymphoid Tissues, 4th edition. Lyon (France): International Agency for Research on Cancer (IARC) Press; 2008. p. 150–5.

the oncogenic protein product of which can be inhibited using targeted tyrosine kinase inhibitors,[7,8] the clinical relevance of the other WHO-defined ambiguous leukemia distinctions remains unclear.

The general perception among clinicians is that whether they appear in adults or children, leukemias of ambiguous origin are as difficult to treat successfully as they are to classify definitively (**Fig. 1**).[1,9–12] Indeed, in most published series, outcomes are poorer for leukemias of ambiguous origin than for more typical cases of acute myeloid leukemia (AML) or acute lymphoblastic leukemia (ALL), and allogeneic hema-topoietic stem cell transplantation is commonly offered to transplant-eligible patients,[10] albeit more as an act of desperation in the face of extremely high relapse risk than as a data-driven care choice. Improved treatment approaches will almost

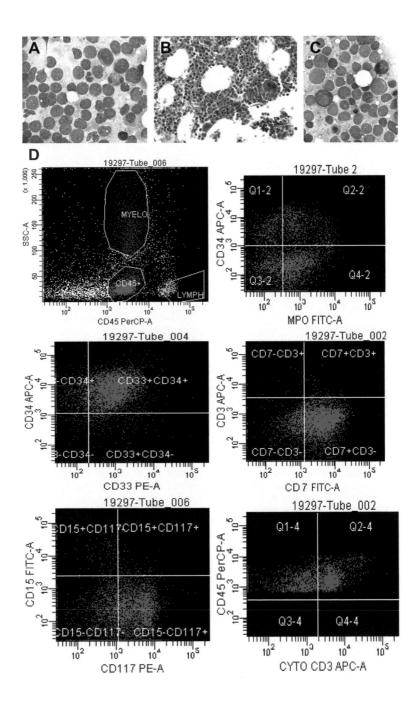

certainly require moving beyond immunophenotyping and cytochemistry, and toward better understanding of the molecular pathobiology of these uncommon disorders. The evolution of diagnostic criteria, current understanding, and potential approaches to therapy for leukemias of ambiguous lineage are reviewed in this article.

HISTORICAL DEVELOPMENTS AND DIAGNOSTIC CRITERIA
Developments Before 1991

Because lineage infidelity in leukemic blasts could not be described until lineage-associated markers became widely available, recognition of the more peculiar varieties of leukemia is, in the history of hematological oncology, a relatively recent development. This development is closely tied to the advent of routine cytochemical evaluation of marrow specimens in the 1970s, introduction of monoclonal antibodies in the early 1980s, and increasing use of multiparameter flow cytometry in leukemia phenotyping during the late 1980s and early 1990s.[4]

Before 1980, clinicians and morphologists assigned leukemia diagnoses on the basis of clinical presentation and cell morphologic features, such as the cytoplasmic appearance and presence or absence of Auer rods, supplemented by basic cytochemical stains, such as Sudan Black B, chloroacetate esterase, and the periodic acid-Schiff reaction.[13] The lineage and corresponding cytologic appearance and immunophenotype of blast cells in acute leukemia was believed to cleanly reflect malignant transformation and maturation arrest at a particular stage of hematopoietic

◀ ───

Fig. 1. Photomicrographs of (A) Wright-Giemsa–stained bone marrow aspirate (original magnification ×400), (B) hematoxylin and eosin–stained bone marrow core biopsy (original magnification ×100), and (C) myeloperoxidase (original magnification ×400) (MPO) immunohistochemistry with Wright-Giemsa counterstaining of a marrow aspirate from a 34-year-old man who presented with a hemoglobin of 4.6 g/dL, platelet count of 82×10^9/L, and a white blood cell count of 11×10^9/L with 20% circulating undifferentiated blasts. The aspirate (A) and core biopsy (B) samples indicated a 60% cellular marrow with 71% blasts; the blasts exhibited scant cytoplasm, prominent nucleoli, and occasional cytoplasmic granules. MPO staining (C) highlighted normal neutrophils and MPO-positive blasts (brown cytoplasm), which comprised more than 3% of the total blast population; numerous MPO-negative blasts were also visible. Blasts were negative for both specific and nonspecific esterase by cytochemistry, and negative for periodic acid-Schiff (PAS) staining. Flow cytometry of the marrow aspirate (D; 6 representative scattergrams) revealed a population of immature cells positive for CD45 (dim), CD34, terminal deoxynucleotidyl transferase (TdT, small subset), and both myeloid lineage-associated markers (ie, MPO, CD33, and CD117) and T-cell markers (ie, cytoplasmic CD3 and CD7). The cells were negative for HLA-DR, CD13, CD15, and other monocytic, B and T lymphoid markers. Karyotyping failed at the time of diagnosis; fluorescent in situ hybridization (FISH) tests were negative for BCR-ABL fusion and MLL gene rearrangement, and subsequent karyotypes were normal. The final diagnosis using the WHO classification was "Acute leukemia of ambiguous origin, mixed phenotype acute leukemia, T/myeloid, not otherwise specified." The patient was treated with 2 cycles of an acute myeloid leukemia chemotherapy regimen, daunorubicin and cytarabine, because of the MPO positivity, to which he did not respond, but he achieved remission with high-dose cytarabine. He was then referred to our center for consideration of allogeneic stem cell transplantation and underwent transplantation from an unrelated donor with busulfan and cyclophosphamide conditioning, which resulted in a brief remission. After relapse (similar immunophenotype), the patient received clofarabine without response, then combination chemotherapy with mitoxantrone and etoposide and high-dose cytarabine, a donor lymphocyte infusion, and a second full transplant with a different donor, all without achieving durable remission. (*Courtesy of* Olga Pozdnyakova, MD, PhD, Department of Pathology, Brigham & Women's Hospital, Boston, MA.)

differentiation, with acute lymphoid malignancies originating in lymphoid progenitors and acute myeloid malignancies originating in early myeloid series cells.[14,15]

Several observations in the 1980s challenged this assumption, however. Expression of the terminal deoxynucleotidyl transferase (TdT) enzyme, thought to be an exclusive marker of lymphoid lineage for several years following its discovery by McCaffrey and colleagues in blasts from children with ALL in 1973,[16–19] was found by 1981 to occur in 10% to 20% of cases of AML.[20] (In fact, if more sensitive techniques are used, TdT activity is detectable in blasts in as many as 55% of AML cases, albeit usually at a much lower level of expression than is typically seen in TdT-positive ALL.[21]) Similarly, in the 1980s morphologists also learned that myeloperoxidase (MPO) expression, considered to be a myeloid lineage-defining marker after its initial description in the 1940s, is detectable by either cytochemistry or immunohistochemistry in more than 20% of B-ALL cases.[22–24]

Additionally, in the late 1970s and early 1980s, a series of case reports and small series appeared in which investigators described detecting either 2 distinct populations of blasts of differing putative origin simultaneously in the same patient ("bilineage" leukemias), or a homogeneous population of blasts expressing markers of more than one lineage ("biphenotypic" leukemias).[14,22,25] The relationship between bilineage and biphenotypic leukemias remained unclear, and in some instances leukemic blasts that expressed markers most suggestive of one cell differentiation program at the time of initial diagnosis would subsequently exhibit a different immunophenotype consistent with another lineage at relapse (eg, B-cell ALL at diagnosis, but AML without lymphoid lineage markers at relapse following ALL-directed chemotherapy).

In 1985, Mirro and colleagues[26] assessed 123 consecutive pediatric leukemia cases diagnosed at St Jude Children's Research Hospital in Memphis, Tennessee, or in Calgary, Alberta, Canada, using a panel of myeloid and lymphoid-associated antibodies, and found that ALL blasts coexpressed at least one myeloid marker in 19% of cases, whereas the leukemic blasts in 25% of AML cases expressed at least one lymphoid-associated marker. Although this landmark study highlighted the frequency of lineage infidelity in leukemia, the antibodies used to assign lineage in the study by Mirro and colleagues[26] (ie, CD2 [T-11 antibody], CD3e [T-3], CD5 [T-101], and CD10 [J5 CALLA] for lymphoid; CD11b [Mo1 antibody], CD13 [MCS.2 and SJ-D1], CD15 [My-1], and CD36 [5F1] for myeloid) would, with the exception of CD3e, no longer be considered lineage-defining markers.[4,5]

Investigators compiling adult leukemia series soon noted that a large proportion of patients with AML or ALL express at least one lineage infidelity marker, but that the presence of only a single such antigen does not alter clinical behavior or response to treatment.[27–29] Further complicating matters, some markers initially thought to be tightly lineage-associated later proved to be so commonly expressed in malignancies of other lineages as to no longer even be considered aberrant. One such example is the CD15 carbohydrate adhesion molecule, which is expressed on normal neutrophils and on blast cells in most AML cases so was once considered myeloid-associated, but is also very commonly detected in B-cell ALL lacking CD10 expression and in other non-myeloid neoplasms (eg, Hodgkin lymphoma).[30]

Development of European Group for the Immunologic Characterization of Leukemias Criteria

A growing number of case reports and small series in the 1980s highlighted increasing diagnostic confusion related to mixed lineage acute leukemias, and the need for more formal definitions of these somewhat puzzling disorders became increasingly clear. Catovsky and a group of European colleagues[31] proposed the first scoring system for defining biphenotypic acute leukemia (BAL) in 1991, which weighed various cyto-chemical/immunohistochemical and immunophenotypic markers according to their perceived lineage specificity.

In 1995, the European Group for the Immunologic Characterization of Leukemias (EGIL) refined this 1991 system (**Table 2**) to make it somewhat more stringent, requiring a lineage-associated marker score of more than 2 points in each of 2 lineages to define BAL, as well as demoting several markers that Catovsky and colleagues[31] had proposed as supporting lineage assignment (ie, immunoglobulin heavy chain gene rearrangement for B lineage; CD11b/c and CD12 for myeloid lineage) while adding or refining several others (ie, CD20 and CD79a for B lineage; TdT, CD1a, CD7, CD8, and CD10 for T lineage; CD13, CD64, and CD65 for myeloid lineage).[32] The EGIL system was modified in 1998[33] to add CD117 as a putative myeloid-specific marker,[34] but soon a few ALL cases were found that expressed CD117.[35]

Clinicians and investigators quickly raised concerns about the EGIL criteria, such as the lack of specificity of certain EGIL-proposed markers, especially CD79a expression for defining B lineage and MPO positivity for defining myeloid lineage.[4] In addition, the EGIL system used varying and arbitrary thresholds of cellular antigen expression required to qualify as "positive" (eg, 20% for most markers, but 10% for MPO, CD3, TdT, and CD79a), did not distinguish between biphenotypic and bilineage leukemia, did not assess intensity of antigen expression,[36] and also failed to incorporate cytoge-netic data. The latter proved to be a particularly troublesome limitation, because leukemia subtypes that were already well defined by routine G-banded karyotyping by the time the EGIL system was introduced (and, later, were further clarified using molecular genetic techniques) often express a degree of lineage infidelity, yet have other uniform features or may respond similarly to therapy regardless of immunophe-notype. For example, t(8;21) AML often expresses a subset of B-cell antigens, whereas acute promyelocytic leukemia (APL), especially the hypogranular variant, frequently expresses T-cell markers, particularly CD2, and T-cell marker expression in APL has no effect on response to all-trans retinoic acid therapy.[37–39] In addition,

Table 2
European Group for the Immunologic Characterization of Leukemias (EGIL) scoring system for biphenotypic acute leukemias, 1998 version

Score	B Lineage	T Lineage	Myeloid Lineage
2 points	• Cytoplasmic CD79a • Cytoplasmic IgM • Cytoplasmic CD22	• CD3 (cytoplasmic or membrane) • T cell receptor (α/β or γ/δ)	• Myeloperoxidase • Lysozyme
1 point	• CD19 • CD10 • CD20	• CD2 • CD5 • CD8 • CD10	• CD13 • CD33 • CD65 • CD117
0.5 point	• TdT • CD24	• TdT • CD7 • CD1a	• CD14 • CD15 • CD64

More than 2 points from 2 different lineages defines biphenotypic acute leukemia.
Abbreviations: CD, cluster of differentiation/designation; IgM, immunoglobulin M; TdT, terminal deoxynucleotidyl transferase.
Data from Béné MC, Castoldi G, Knapp W, et al. Proposals for the immunologic classification of acute leukemias. European Group for the Immunologic Characterization of Leukemias (EGIL). Leukemia 1995;9(10):1783–6; and Bene MC, Bernier M, Casasnovas RO, et al. The reliability and spec-ificity of c-kit for the diagnosis of acute myeloid leukemias and undifferentiated leukemias. The European Group for the Immunologic Classification of Leukemias (EGIL). Blood 1998;92(2):596–9.

CD79a can be found in both T-ALL and myeloid leukemia, so lacks the B-cell specificity accorded to it by the EGIL system.[40–43]

World Health Organization Criteria: Third and Fourth Editions

In the third edition of the WHO Classification of Tumours of Haematopoietic and Lymphoid Tissues proposed in 1999 and published in 2001, the WHO working group included a 2-page description of a classification of "acute leukemias of ambiguous lineage," composed of 3 categories: bilineage, biphenotypic, and undifferentiated acute leukemias.[44] Although the third edition WHO classification referenced the 1995 EGIL system (with the 1998 CD117 addition), the WHO third edition text unfortunately included a typographical error in its Table 4.03, stating that only 2 points, rather than more than 2 points, were necessary to assign a leukemia case to a given lineage. In one series, these slightly less stringent criteria tripled the number of cases defined as biphenotypic compared with EGIL criteria, and the reassignment was of dubious clinical value.[45]

Perhaps because of this debacle, the 2008 fourth edition of the WHO classification did away with lineage scoring entirely in favor of descriptive but relatively specific requirements for assigning more than one lineage to a single blast population (**Table 3**). Although the WHO fourth edition classification retained the category of acute leukemias of ambiguous lineage, the updated system also incorporated 5 major changes with respect to the third edition classification.

First, because of frequent ambiguity about whether mixed lineage markers are truly coexpressed by the same blasts or by 2 distinct populations of leukemic cells, WHO did away with the terms "bilineal" and "biphenotypic" in favor of the collective term "mixed phenotype acute leukemia" (MPAL). Second, the criteria that define the myeloid, T-lymphoid, and B-lymphoid components of MPAL were altered and simplified (see **Table 3**), although the same criticisms persisted about lineage specificity of proposed markers. Third, cases that are clearly acute leukemia with recurrent genetic abnormalities were excluded from MPAL, even if they express a mixed lineage

Table 3 2008 World Health Organization criteria for defining lineage assignment in acute leukemia		
Lineage	Criterion #1	Criterion #2
B lineage	Strong CD19, plus at least 1 of CD79a (cytoplasmic or membrane), cytoplasmic CD22, or surface CD10 also strongly expressed	Weak CD19, plus at least 2 of CD79a, cytoplasmic CD22, CD10
T lineage	Cytoplasmic expression of CD3 (detected by flow cytometry with antibodies against the epsilon chain of CD3[a])	Surface CD3 (rare)
Myeloid	Myeloperoxidase positivity in >3% of blasts (detected by flow cytometry, immunohistochemistry, or cytochemistry)	At least 2 of the following monocytic differentiation markers: CD11c, CD14, CD64, lysozyme, nonspecific (butyrate) esterase

[a] Immunohistochemistry using polyclonal anti-CD3 antibodies is not adequate, as this assay may detect CD3 zeta chain, which is not T-cell specific.

Data from Borowitz MJ, Béné MC, Harris NL, et al. Acute leukaemias of ambiguous lineage. In: Swerdlow SH, Campo E, Harris NL, et al, editors. World Health Organization (WHO) Classification of Tumours of Haematopoietic and Lymphoid Tissues, 4th edition. Lyon (France): International Agency for Research on Cancer (IARC) Press; 2008. p. 150–5.

phenotype that would otherwise qualify. Such entities include cases classified as AML with recurrent genetic abnormalities (eg, t[15;17], t[8;21], and inv[16]), but the WHO committee did not feel comfortable extending this "trumping" of immunophenotype by genetic and molecular markers to provisional entities, such as AML with mutated NPM1 or CEBPA. Similarly excluded regardless of lineage expression are cases known to represent chronic myeloid leukemia (CML) in blast phase, therapy-related AML, or AML arising from a myelodysplastic syndrome.

The fourth change between third and fourth editions of the WHO classification was inclusion of 2 molecularly defined diagnostic categories in the acute leukemia of ambiguous lineage group: BCR-ABL1–positive and MLL-rearranged acute leukemias. In many series of EGIL-defined BAL, t(9;22) and t(11q23) translocations have been overrepresented, probably because loss of ABL tyrosine kinase activity or MLL fusions with associated HOX dysregulation severely disrupts normal differentiation programs.[46] Indeed, the MLL gene took its name from its association with "mixed lineage leukemia" or "myeloid-lymphoid leukemia."[47]

Unfortunately, although well intentioned, these molecularly defined acute leukemia of ambiguous origin categories quickly caused confusion. MLL-rearranged acute leukemias without a mixed lineage phenotype are elsewhere classified by WHO both as "AML with t(9;11)(p22;q23); MLLT3-MLL" and variants, and as "B lymphoblastic leukemia/lymphoma with t(v;11q23); MLL rearranged." These entities may be seen with a much greater frequency to MPAL with MLL rearrangement, and the prognosis and treatment are determined by the genotype rather than the immunophenotype.

In addition, patients who previously had unrecognized chronic myeloid leukemia (CML) and first present to medical attention at a late stage (ie, in blast crisis), are not easy to distinguish from those with BCR-ABL1–positive de novo ALL or AML, as p190 and p210 transcripts can be detected in either setting.[48] Although the WHO classification states, "this diagnosis (ie, MPAL with t[9;22][q34;q11.2; BCR-ABL1]) should not be made in patients known to have had CML," the stage at which the patient presents for medical attention is a poor criterion on which to base a disease classification, as delay in diagnosis does not reflect a genuine biologic difference and may be because of socioeconomic or other personal factors.

A fifth change between the 2001 and 2008 classifications is that in the 2008 edition, the WHO committee also included an "other ambiguous lineage leukemias" category for truly bizarre cells. For instance, leukemia cases that express T-cell lineage markers but not cytoplasmic CD3, or cases that express several myeloid markers but not MPO, do not fit into any of the other MPAL categories.

These cases are considered distinct from cases with no lineage-specific markers at all, which WHO designates as acute undifferentiated leukemia (AUL) and should be diagnosed only after a cautious, thorough evaluation.[49] AUL cases should express CD34, HLA-DR, or CD38—something to exclude the possibility of a nonhematopoietic neoplasm—but, by definition, lack specific myeloid or lymphoid antigens. Some AUL cases have a t(9;9) translocation that results in fusion of SET, a nuclear phosphoprotein that inhibits activity of protein phosphatase 2A (PP2A), to the oncoprotein CAN/NUP214 involved in the more common t(6;9) in AML.[50–52]

Finally, the difficult-to-define entity of natural killer cell lymphoblastic leukemia/lymphoma[6] was included as a provisional category within the miscellaneous "other ambiguous lineage leukemias" category in the fourth WHO classification, whereas those cases more clearly designated as originating from plasmacytoid dendritic cells (also CD56 positive, like natural killer cells) were reclassified as a new entity, blastic plasmacytoid dendritic cell neoplasms (BPDCNs). By definition, BPDCNs coexpress

CD4 and CD56, and usually also express CD123 or CD303 (BDCA2) (see **Table 1** footnotes).[53,54]

Limitations of Current Criteria

In addition to the concerns raised about lineage specificity of particular markers and variable intensity of marker expression, clinicians have expressed concerns that to some extent trying to pigeonhole leukemias of ambiguous origin is an exercise in futility. It is not clear whether, for example, T/myeloid leukemia and B/myeloid leukemia are genuinely distinct conditions requiring a different therapeutic approach, and whether the WHO 2008 criteria are really defining "real" entities in the sense of clinically actionable unique disorders.

There are also technical concerns. Currently, pathologists primarily perform immunophenotyping of new leukemia cases by flow cytometry, and flow is to some extent operator-dependent, with results varying depending on such parameters as gating and reagent quality.[3] In addition, most clinical laboratories, even those at major academic centers, normally do not use all the flow markers in the EGIL panel or even all of the major WHO markers, so biphenotypic/bilineage expression may be missed.[46] A conference convened in 2006 in Bethesda, Maryland, defined a consensus set of reagents suitable for general use in the diagnosis and monitoring of hematopoietic neoplasms, but did not recommend the full panel necessary for defining biphenotypic leukemia according to EGIL criteria.[55] For example, many laboratories do not routinely perform cytoplasmic CD79a as part of a standard new leukemia diagnostic flow panel, in part because as stated, this "B-lineage–specific" marker also is regularly found in cases of AML (especially t[8;21] or APL[42,56]) and T-ALL.[57,58]

PREVALENCE AND PROGNOSIS

Although it is common for acute leukemia cells to aberrantly express a lineage infidelity marker, as discussed previously, cases meeting EGIL diagnostic criteria for BAL represent no more than 5% of all cases of acute leukemia.[59] Furthermore, acute leukemias of ambiguous lineage defined using WHO 2008 criteria are even less common than EGIL-defined BAL, likely less than 3% of acute leukemia cases overall.[4]

Hematopathologists Weinberg and Arber of Stanford University retrospectively applied WHO 2008 criteria to 8 case series published between 1998 and 2009 in which EGIL criteria had been used to define BAL: 2 pediatric series, 2 adult series, and 4 series including all age groups, cumulatively comprising 7627 patients with acute leukemia.[4] Although 213 patients (2.8% overall, range 0.1%–8.0%) in these 8 series met EGIL criteria for BAL, only 119 (1.6%) met WHO 2008 criteria for MPAL, and in individual series, the frequency of WHO 2008–defined MPAL ranged between 0.1% and 2.6%. (The series with the lowest incidence rate included only bilineage leukemias, not biphenotypic.[1]) In one published series, clinical outcomes were better for pediatric patients with the more strictly defined WHO 2008 MPAL compared with EGIL-qualifying BAL.[10]

Since the Stanford review, at least one additional series comparing EGIL bilineage and WHO MPAL criteria has appeared.[29] In 2010, van den Ancker and colleagues[29] from Amsterdam described a series of 517 acute leukemia cases diagnosed at their hospital between 2000 and 2008, which they characterized with a battery of B-lineage, T-lineage, and myeloid-lineage associated markers. Altogether, 31 (5.8%) of the 517 Dutch cases could be characterized as BAL using EGIL criteria, whereas only 8 cases (1.5%) met WHO 2008 criteria for MPAL and only 6 cases (1.1%) would have met both

BAL and MPAL criteria. van den Ancker and colleagues[29] pointed out that because most published series of acute leukemias of ambiguous origin have used EGIL criteria for BAL, the finding of a relatively low degree of overlap between EGIL and the new WHO criteria means that the clinical behavior of MPAL cases defined using WHO 2008 criteria may be different from published series, and this needs to be defined in prospective clinical studies.

The relative frequency of the different combinations and subtypes of BAL and MPAL varies between series, and may also differ between children and adults. Xu and colleagues, from Shanghai, China, reported 21 new cases (4.6%) of EGIL-defined BAL among 452 new leukemia diagnoses over 7 years, and also summarized 9 other series[1,9,45,59–64] published between 1996 and 2007 and ranging in size between 19 and 63 patients.[65] The Chinese investigators confirmed the poor prognosis of the biphenotypic cases compared with more typical AML or ALL, and found that the most common BAL subtype overall is B/myeloid leukemia (excluding one outlier series,[1] the frequency of B/myeloid among BAL cases was 59%–72% in different series), followed by T/myeloid (21%–32%). B/T lymphoid and triple B/T/myeloid were the rarest types, with only one example of each seen in the Xu series (and the B/T lymphoid case engendered some skepticism from an editorialist[46]). Other clinical features of the BAL cases in the Xu series included a higher incidence of CD34 antigen expression on BAL blasts, higher frequency of complex karyotype, more frequent extramedullary disease, and more rapid relapse with resistance to therapy after relapse, compared with AML or ALL.[65]

In contrast, in a pediatric series from St Jude Children's Research Hospital, T/myeloid cases were more common than B/myeloid, and biphenotypic blasts were much more frequent (91%) than bilineal.[66] A large Johns Hopkins series that emphasized the rarity of bilineal leukemias found a relatively even split between T/myeloid and B/myeloid cases.[1]

MOLECULAR AND CYTOGENETIC FINDINGS

Most patients with leukemias of ambiguous origin have an abnormal karyotype.[62] In one report, 83% of cases (ie, 19 of 23 EGIL biphenotypic cases, among 676 acute leukemia cases) had a gene rearrangement detectable by either conventional G-banded karyotyping (68% of cases), fluorescent in situ hybridization, or polymerase chain reaction.[59] In almost all published series, the most common (cyto)genetic findings have been *BCR-ABL1* and *MLL* gene rearrangement, with *BCR-ABL1* dominating in adults and *MLL* more frequent in pediatric patients.[61,62,66] Cases without these rearrangements have unique gene expression patterns and may represent distinct biologic entities, even if their distinct clinical behavior is not apparent.[66]

The frequency of MLL involvement is estimated to be about 20% of ALL and 5% of AML, a much higher frequency than the reported incidence of WHO-defined MPAL.[67] As mentioned previously, although the WHO 2008 classification specified that MLL-rearranged cases must meet the other criteria for MPAL to be considered acute leukemias of ambiguous origin, it is not clear that MLL cases meeting WHO criteria (**Fig. 2**) differ in any consequential way from other *MLL* rearranged leukemias. Other common chromosomal abnormalities in MPAL include deletion (6q), rearrangements of chromosome 12p11.2, and abnormalities of chromosomes 5 and 7.[59] A German pediatric series found a high incidence of trisomy 8 and of ETV6/RUNX1 fusion.[11] Although numerical chromosomal abnormalities have provided relatively little insight into disease pathobiology in leukemia to date, cloning rare translocations may yield new discoveries.[68]

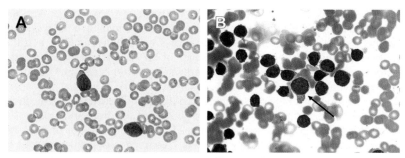

Fig. 2. Photomicrographs of (A) hematoxylin-eosin–stained peripheral blood smear (original magnification ×400) and (B) Wright-Giemsa–stained bone marrow aspirate from a 43-year-old woman who presented with anemia (hemoglobin 8.8 g/dL)(original magnification ×400), thrombocytopenia (platelet count 36 × 10⁹/L), leukocytosis (white blood count 101 × 10⁹/L) and 93% circulating immature blasts. Although most of the neoplastic cells resembled lymphoblasts morphologically, and the presence of numerous "hand-mirror" cells (B, arrow) initially suggested T-cell ALL, another subset of cells resembled monoblasts. Immunophenotype was initially suggestive of a B precursor (pro-B) cell origin, as flow cytometry demonstrated only HLA-DR, CD19, and TdT positivity; a subset of CD45-positive cells were also CD34 positive. CD15 is frequently expressed in CD10-negative ALL, but was only weakly expressed in this case. A small population of blasts was MPO-positive. All other tested markers were negative, including other B-cell markers (CD10, CD11c, CD20, cytoplasmic CD22, CD23, CD24, CD25, CD38, CD52, CD79a, CD103, surface immunoglobulins), T-cell markers (CD2, CD3, CD4, CD5, CD7, CD8), NK cell markers (CD16, CD56, CD57, CD94), and stem cell and myeloid markers (CD11b, CD13, CD14, CD33, CD64, glycophorin). In a more typical leukemia case, not all of these markers would have been assayed. Immunohistochemistry and cytochemical stains did not reveal any additional lineage-specific markers. Metaphase cytogenetics demonstrated t(4;11)(q21;q23) representing an *AF4-MLL* gene rearrangement, as well as del(20q) as a secondary clonal anomaly. After cytoreduction with hydroxyurea and methylprednisolone, the patient was treated on a clinical trial for younger adults with acute lymphoblastic leukemia using a pediatriclike regimen, and was referred for allogeneic stem cell transplantation once remission was achieved. By WHO criteria, because of expression of both MPO and CD19 on blast cells (albeit without other B cell markers), this case could have been termed "Mixed phenotype acute leukemia with t(v;11q23); MLL rearranged." (*Courtesy of* Elizabeth A. Morgan, MD, Department of Pathology, Brigham & Women's Hospital, Boston, MA.)

Whole genome sequencing (WGS) has not yet been performed on cases of MPAL or other leukemias of ambiguous origin without *BCR-ABL1* or *MLL* rearrangements, and such ambiguous lineage cases are not included in the ongoing 500-patient AML genome sequencing project that is part of The Cancer Genome Atlas (http://cancergenome.nih.gov/cancersselected/acutemyeloidleukemia) funded by the National Cancer Institute and the National Human Genome Research Institute (personal communication, Timothy Graubert, Washington University in St Louis, September 2011). It is possible that unique molecular aberrations characterizing the different subtypes of leukemia of ambiguous lineage and specifying specific differentiation programs might be discovered, just as WGS identified recurrent *IDH1* and *DNMT3A* mutations in AML.[69,70]

Alternatively, because acute leukemia cases explored to date with WGS approaches have exhibited at least 10 to 12 nonsynonymous or nonsense somatic mutations in conserved coding regions of the genome,[71] it is possible that biphenotypic cases may result from coexistence of multiple mutations or others specifying more than one differentiation program. A parallel example is the peculiar mixed myelo-proliferative neoplasm/myelodysplastic syndrome (MPN/MDS) subtype refractory anemia with ring sideroblasts and thrombocytosis (RARS-T), in which *JAK2* mutations drive thrombocytosis, whereas coexisting mutations in *SF3B1* encoding an RNA splicing factor underlie the sideroblastic anemia,[72,73] or del(5q) MDS, in which RPS14 haploinsufficiency accounts for anemia, whereas underexpression of micro-RNAs miR145A and miR146 may contribute to thrombocytosis.[74,75] The alternative explanation, however, is that, just as MLL rearrangements disrupt homeobox (HOX) expression and cause affected leukemic stem cells to follow a disordered differentia-tion program, other mutations might also force abnormal progenitor differentiation with confused lineage specification.[76,77]

TREATMENT

Because no specific treatment programs exist for acute leukemias of ambiguous origin, the key decision that clinicians face when encountering patients with these conditions is whether to use a combination chemotherapy regimen designed for ALL therapy, an AML regimen, or some type of hybrid regimen. In a British series in which both AML-active and ALL-active treatments were combined, the induction mortality was unexpectedly high (25%), leading the investigators to recommend that either one or the other be chosen.[9] Patients with BAL commonly have unfavorable cytogenetics with p-glycoprotein (multidrug resistance) expression, which may contribute to poor therapeutic outcomes.[60]

ALL regimens incorporate numerous drugs that are active in AML. AML regimens, in contrast, are simpler, with the most common induction regimens consisting of only 2 or 3 cytotoxic drugs, and AML regimens also incorporate a considerably shorter consolidation phase than for ALL therapy. Given the high rate of relapse described in BAL and MPAL series, a longer-duration ALL-like regimen may make more sense, especially for patients who do not go on to allogeneic stem cell transplantation. In pediatric cases, response rates seem to be higher with ALL-like therapy, such as the higher-risk St Jude "Total Therapy" protocols, and many patients refractory to AML therapy can be "salvaged" with an ALL regimen.[66]

In a Croatian series of 21 patients with BAL according to EGIL criteria, the complete response rate was 100% with an ALL regimen but only 60% with an AML regimen.[78] In an M. D. Anderson series of 31 adult patients, the complete response rate was 78% for the 24 patients treated with an ALL regimen, compared with 57% for the 7 patients who received AML therapy first; 2-year survival was 60%.[45] Because these data were not derived from prospective randomized trials, some selection bias may have played a role in which patients received which regimens, however. At many institutions, patients with MPAL or BAL are treated as ALL, unless they express MPO strongly.

As for other forms of high-risk leukemia, allogeneic stem cell transplantation is commonly offered to patients with BAL and MPAL in first remission[11]; however, the efficacy is unclear. At least one series found that most pediatric patients do not require transplantation if treated with an AML regimen, with an ALL regimen available as backup for poor responders.[66] Korean investigators observed that transplantation did not improve outcomes compared with chemotherapy, albeit based on only 25 cases.[79] Among 16 patients with acute bilineage leukemia at Johns Hopkins, only 2 were alive 2.5 years after stem cell transplantation.[1] A German (Berlin-Frankfurt-Münster) series of 92 pediatric patients suggested that cases with lymphoid morphology, ETV6/RUNX1 expression, or CD22/CD79a expression benefited from ALL therapy without transplant, whereas stem cell transplantation is appropriate for other cases.[11] Allogeneic transplantation may be particularly important in infantile leukemia (<1 year old), which is almost always associated with MLL rearrangement.[80]

In BCR-ABL1–positive ALL, clinical outcomes may be improved by combining conventional chemotherapy regimens with molecularly targeted therapy (eg, imatinib[7] or dasatinib[81]). Although no controlled trials have been done, outcomes with chemotherapy plus a tyrosine kinase inhibitor seem superior to historical controls with chemotherapy alone.[82–84] The same is likely to be true of MPAL with BCR-ABL1. Whether MLL-rearranged leukemias will also be targetable by small-molecule approaches, for example, DOT1L inhibitors (DOT1L is a key mediator of MLL fusion-induced aberrant H3K79 methylation across the genome, with consequent alteration in leukemia cell gene expression patterns[85,86]), is a promising area for future investigation.

SUMMARY

From the standpoint of the hematopathologist, attempts to dissect the immunophenotype and other lineage-defining characteristics of the puzzling group of acute leukemias of ambiguous origin have prompted considerable discussion and debate. For clinicians, however, such definitions, although academically interesting, as yet give relatively little insight into the most appropriate therapy, and patients with MPAL continue to do poorly compared with more typical AML or ALL cases. The most recent WHO 2008 MPAL definitions are provocative, but represent a major change from the previous EGIL BAL classification, and the clinical relevance of this change has yet to be established. Only further insight from the molecular biology laboratory can help define the true cell of origin and molecular drivers of ambiguous leukemias. New molecular information will allow clinicians and pathologists to refine classification of these challenging entities, and most importantly, should permit improved treatment for patients.

REFERENCES

1. Weir EG, Ali Ansari-Lari M, Batista DA, et al. Acute bilineal leukemia: a rare disease with poor outcome. Leukemia 2007;21(11):2264–70.
2. Weir EG, Borowitz MJ. Flow cytometry in the diagnosis of acute leukemia. Semin Hematol 2001;38(2):124–38.
3. Peters JM, Ansari MQ. Multiparameter flow cytometry in the diagnosis and management of acute leukemia. Arch Pathol Lab Med 2011;135(1):44–54.
4. Weinberg OK, Arber DA. Mixed-phenotype acute leukemia: historical overview and a new definition. Leukemia 2010;24(11):1844–51.
5. Borowitz MJ, Béné MC, Harris NL, et al. Acute leukaemias of ambiguous lineage. In: Swerdlow SH, Campo E, Harris NL, et al, editors. World Health Organization (WHO) Classification of Tumours of Haematopoietic and Lymphoid Tissues, 4th edition. Lyon (France): International Agency for Research on Cancer (IARC) Press; 2008. p. 150–5.
6. Ham MF, Ko YH. Natural killer cell neoplasm: biology and pathology. Int J Hematol 2010;92(5):681–9.
7. Druker BJ, Sawyers CL, Kantarjian H, et al. Activity of a specific inhibitor of the BCR-ABL tyrosine kinase in the blast crisis of chronic myeloid leukemia and acute lymphoblastic leukemia with the Philadelphia chromosome. N Engl J Med 2001;344(14):1038–42.
8. Druker BJ, Tamura S, Buchdunger E, et al. Effects of a selective inhibitor of the Abl tyrosine kinase on the growth of Bcr-Abl positive cells. Nat Med 1996;2(5):561–6.

9. Killick S, Matutes E, Powles RL, et al. Outcome of biphenotypic acute leukemia. Haematologica 1999;84(8):699–706.
10. Al-Seraihy AS, Owaidah TM, Ayas M, et al. Clinical characteristics and outcome of children with biphenotypic acute leukemia. Haematologica 2009;94(12):1682–90.
11. Gerr H, Zimmermann M, Schrappe M, et al. Acute leukaemias of ambiguous lineage in children: characterization, prognosis and therapy recommendations. Br J Haematol 2010;149(1):84–92.
12. Matutes E, Morilla R, Farahat N, et al. Definition of acute biphenotypic leukemia. Haematologica 1997;82(1):64–6.
13. Beard ME. Classification of acute leukaemias using Romanowsky, sudan black and periodic acid Schiff stains. Recent Results Cancer Res 1973;43:21–2.
14. Scamurra DO, Davey FR, Nelson DA, et al. Acute leukemia presenting with myeloid and lymphoid cell markers. Ann Clin Lab Sci 1983;13(6):496–502.
15. Greaves MF, Delia D, Robinson J, et al. Exploitation of monoclonal antibodies: a "who's who" of haemopoietic malignancy. Blood Cells 1981;7(2):257–80.
16. McCaffrey R, Smoler DF, Baltimore D. Terminal deoxynucleotidyl transferase in a case of childhood acute lymphoblastic leukemia. Proc Natl Acad Sci U S A 1973;70(2):521–5.
17. Bollum FJ. Terminal deoxynucleotidyl transferase as a hematopoietic cell marker. Blood 1979;54(6):1203–15.
18. Coleman MS, Greenwood MF, Hutton JJ, et al. Serial observations on terminal deoxynucleotidyl transferase activity and lymphoblast surface markers in acute lymphoblastic leukemia. Cancer Res 1976;36(1):120–7.
19. Gordon DS, Hutton JJ, Smalley RV, et al. Terminal deoxynucleotidyl transferase (TdT), cytochemistry, and membrane receptors in adult acute leukemia. Blood 1978;52(6):1079–88.
20. McGraw TP, Folds JD, Bollum FJ, et al. Terminal deoxynucleotidyl transferase-positive acute myeloblastic leukemia. Am J Hematol 1981;10(3):251–8.
21. Drexler HG, Sperling C, Ludwig WD. Terminal deoxynucleotidyl transferase (TdT) expression in acute myeloid leukemia. Leukemia 1993;7(8):1142–50.
22. Lanham GR, Bollum FJ, Williams DL, et al. Simultaneous occurrence of terminal deoxynucleotidyl transferase and myeloperoxidase in individual leukemia blasts. Blood 1984;64(1):318–20.
23. Arber DA, Snyder DS, Fine M, et al. Myeloperoxidase immunoreactivity in adult acute lymphoblastic leukemia. Am J Clin Pathol 2001;116(1):25–33.
24. Ferrari S, Mariano MT, Tagliafico E, et al. Myeloperoxidase gene expression in blast cells with a lymphoid phenotype in cases of acute lymphoblastic leukemia. Blood 1988;72(3):873–6.
25. Biphenotypic leukaemia. Lancet 1983;2(8360):1178–9.
26. Mirro J, Zipf TF, Pui CH, et al. Acute mixed lineage leukemia: clinicopathologic correlations and prognostic significance. Blood 1985;66(5):1115–23.
27. Khalidi HS, Medeiros LJ, Chang KL, et al. The immunophenotype of adult acute myeloid leukemia: high frequency of lymphoid antigen expression and comparison of immunophenotype, French-American-British classification, and karyotypic abnormalities. Am J Clin Pathol 1998;109(2):211–20.
28. Ossenkoppele GJ, van de Loosdrecht AA, Schuurhuis GJ. Review of the relevance of aberrant antigen expression by flow cytometry in myeloid neoplasms. Br J Haematol 2011;153(4):421–36.
29. van den Ancker W, Terwijn M, Westers TM, et al. Acute leukemias of ambiguous lineage: diagnostic consequences of the WHO2008 classification. Leukemia 2010;24(7):1392–6.

30. Maynadie M, Campos L, Moskovtchenko P, et al. Heterogenous expression of CD15 in acute lymphoblastic leukemia: a study of ten anti-CD15 monoclonal antibodies in 158 patients. Leuk Lymphoma 1997;25(1–2):135–43.
31. Catovsky D, Matutes E, Buccheri V, et al. A classification of acute leukaemia for the 1990s. Ann Hematol 1991;62(1):16–21.
32. Béné MC, Castoldi G, Knapp W, et al. Proposals for the immunological classification of acute leukemias. European Group for the Immunological Characterization of Leukemias (EGIL). Leukemia 1995;9(10):1783–6.
33. Béné MC, Bernier M, Casasnovas RO, et al. The reliability and specificity of c-kit for the diagnosis of acute myeloid leukemias and undifferentiated leukemias. The European Group for the Immunological Classification of Leukemias (EGIL). Blood 1998;92(2):596–9.
34. Hans CP, Finn WG, Singleton TP, et al. Usefulness of anti-CD117 in the flow cytometric analysis of acute leukemia. Am J Clin Pathol 2002;117(2):301–5.
35. Suggs JL, Cruse JM, Lewis RE. Aberrant myeloid marker expression in precursor B-cell and T-cell leukemias. Exp Mol Pathol 2007;83(3):471–3.
36. Paietta E, Racevskis J, Bennett JM, et al. Differential expression of terminal transferase (TdT) in acute lymphocytic leukaemia expressing myeloid antigens and TdT positive acute myeloid leukaemia as compared to myeloid antigen negative acute lymphocytic leukaemia. Br J Haematol 1993;84(3):416–22.
37. Albano F, Mestice A, Pannunzio A, et al. The biological characteristics of CD34+ CD2+ adult acute promyelocytic leukemia and the CD34 CD2 hypergranular (M3) and microgranular (M3v) phenotypes. Haematologica 2006;91(3):311–6.
38. Chapiro E, Delabesse E, Asnafi V, et al. Expression of T-lineage-affiliated transcripts and TCR rearrangements in acute promyelocytic leukemia: implications for the cellular target of t(15;17). Blood 2006;108(10):3484–93.
39. Valbuena JR, Medeiros LJ, Rassidakis GZ, et al. Expression of B cell-specific activator protein/PAX5 in acute myeloid leukemia with t(8;21)(q22;q22). Am J Clin Pathol 2006;126(2):235–40.
40. Hashimoto M, Yamashita Y, Mori N. Immunohistochemical detection of CD79a expression in precursor T cell lymphoblastic lymphoma/leukaemias. J Pathol 2002;197(3):341–7.
41. Pilozzi E, Pulford K, Jones M, et al. Co-expression of CD79a (JCB117) and CD3 by lymphoblastic lymphoma. J Pathol 1998;186(2):140–3.
42. Arber DA, Jenkins KA, Slovak ML. CD79 alpha expression in acute myeloid leukemia. High frequency of expression in acute promyelocytic leukemia. Am J Pathol 1996;149(4):1105–10.
43. Bhargava P, Kallakury BV, Ross JS, et al. CD79a is heterogeneously expressed in neoplastic and normal myeloid precursors and megakaryocytes in an antibody clone-dependent manner. Am J Clin Pathol 2007;128(2):306–13.
44. Brunning RD, Matutes E, Borowitz M, et al. Acute leukemias of ambiguous lineage. In: Jaffe ES, Harris NL, Stein H, et al, editors. World Health Organization Classification of Tumours. Tumours of Haematopoietic and Lymphoid Tissues. 3rd edition. Lyon (France): International Agency for Research on Cancer (IARC); 2001. p. 106–7.
45. Aribi A, Bueso-Ramos C, Estey E, et al. Biphenotypic acute leukaemia: a case series. Br J Haematol 2007;138(2):213–6.
46. Béné MC. Biphenotypic, bilineal, ambiguous or mixed lineage: strange leukemias! Haematologica 2009;94(7):891–3.
47. Ziemin-van der Poel S, McCabe NR, Gill HJ, et al. Identification of a gene, MLL, that spans the breakpoint in 11q23 translocations associated with human leukemias. Proc Natl Acad Sci U S A 1991;88(23):10735–9.

48. van Rhee F, Hochhaus A, Lin F, et al. p190 BCR-ABL mRNA is expressed at low levels in p210-positive chronic myeloid and acute lymphoblastic leukemias. Blood 1996;87(12):5213–7.
49. Bernier M, Massy M, Deleeuw N, et al. Immunological definition of acute minimally differentiated myeloid leukemia (MO) and acute undifferentiated leukemia (AUL). Leuk Lymphoma 1995;18(Suppl 1):13–7.
50. Minakuchi M, Kakazu N, Gorrin-Rivas MJ, et al. Identification and characterization of SEB, a novel protein that binds to the acute undifferentiated leukemia-associated protein SET. Eur J Biochem 2001;268(5):1340–51.
51. Ozbek U, Kandilci A, van Baal S, et al. SET-CAN, the product of the t(9;9) in acute undifferentiated leukemia, causes expansion of early hematopoietic progenitors and hyperproliferation of stomach mucosa in transgenic mice. Am J Pathol 2007;171(2):654–66.
52. von Lindern M, Fornerod M, van Baal S, et al. The translocation (6;9), associated with a specific subtype of acute myeloid leukemia, results in the fusion of two genes, dek and can, and the expression of a chimeric, leukemia-specific dek-can mRNA. Mol Cell Biol 1992;12(4):1687–97.
53. Feuillard J, Jacob MC, Valensi F, et al. Clinical and biologic features of CD4(+) CD56(+) malignancies. Blood 2002;99(5):1556–63.
54. Chen J, Zhou J, Qin D, et al. Blastic plasmacytoid dendritic cell neoplasm. J Clin Oncol 2011;29(2):e27–9.
55. Wood BL, Arroz M, Barnett D, et al. 2006 Bethesda International Consensus recommendations on the immunophenotypic analysis of hematolymphoid neoplasia by flow cytometry: optimal reagents and reporting for the flow cytometric diagnosis of hematopoietic neoplasia. Cytometry B Clin Cytom 2007; 72(Suppl 1):S14–22.
56. Kozlov I, Beason K, Yu C, et al. CD79a expression in acute myeloid leukemia t(8;21) and the importance of cytogenetics in the diagnosis of leukemias with immunophenotypic ambiguity. Cancer Genet Cytogenet 2005;163(1):62–7.
57. Thalhammer-Scherrer R, Mitterbauer G, Simonitsch I, et al. The immunophenotype of 325 adult acute leukemias: relationship to morphologic and molecular classification and proposal for a minimal screening program highly predictive for lineage discrimination. Am J Clin Pathol 2002;117(3):380–9.
58. Lai R, Juco J, Lee SF, et al. Flow cytometric detection of CD79a expression in T-cell acute lymphoblastic leukemias. Am J Clin Pathol 2000;113(6):823–30.
59. Owaidah TM, Al Beihany A, Iqbal MA, et al. Cytogenetics, molecular and ultrastructural characteristics of biphenotypic acute leukemia identified by the EGIL scoring system. Leukemia 2006;20(4):620–6.
60. Legrand O, Perrot JY, Simonin G, et al. Adult biphenotypic acute leukaemia: an entity with poor prognosis which is related to unfavourable cytogenetics and P-glycoprotein over-expression. Br J Haematol 1998;100(1):147–55.
61. Lee JH, Min YH, Chung CW, et al. Prognostic implications of the immunophenotype in biphenotypic acute leukemia. Leuk Lymphoma 2008;49(4):700–9.
62. Carbonell F, Swansbury J, Min T, et al. Cytogenetic findings in acute biphenotypic leukaemia. Leukemia 1996;10(8):1283–7.
63. Mi Y, Bian S, Meng Q, et al. Study on the clinical characteristics of biphenotypic acute leukemia. Zhonghua Xue Ye Xue Za Zhi 2000;21(7):352–4 [in Chinese].
64. Shen Y, Li J, Xue Y, et al. Acute biphenotypic leukemia in the adults. Zhonghua Zhong Liu Za Zhi 2002;24(4):375–7.
65. Xu XQ, Wang JM, Lu SQ, et al. Clinical and biological characteristics of adult biphenotypic acute leukemia in comparison with that of acute myeloid leukemia

and acute lymphoblastic leukemia: a case series of a Chinese population. Haematologica 2009;94(7):919–27.

66. Rubnitz JE, Onciu M, Pounds S, et al. Acute mixed lineage leukemia in children: the experience of St Jude Children's Research Hospital. Blood 2009;113(21):5083–9.

67. Meyer C, Kowarz E, Hofmann J, et al. New insights to the MLL recombinome of acute leukemias. Leukemia 2009;23(8):1490–9.

68. Steensma DP, Neiger JD, Porcher JC, et al. Rearrangements and amplification of IER3 (IEX-1) represent a novel and recurrent molecular abnormality in myelodysplastic syndromes. Cancer Res 2009;69(19):7518–23.

69. Mardis ER, Ding L, Dooling DJ, et al. Recurring mutations found by sequencing an acute myeloid leukemia genome. N Engl J Med 2009;361(11):1058–66.

70. Ley TJ, Ding L, Walter MJ, et al. DNMT3A mutations in acute myeloid leukemia. N Engl J Med 2010;363(25):2424–33.

71. Ley TJ, Mardis ER, Ding L, et al. DNA sequencing of a cytogenetically normal acute myeloid leukaemia genome. Nature 2008;456(7218):66–72.

72. Visconte V, Makishima H, Jankowska A, et al. SF3B1, a splicing factor is frequently mutated in refractory anemia with ring sideroblasts. Leukemia Sep 2 2011. [Epub ahead of print].

73. Steensma DP, Tefferi A. JAK2 V617F and ringed sideroblasts: not necessarily RARS-T. Blood 2008;111(3):1748.

74. Ebert BL, Pretz J, Bosco J, et al. Identification of RPS14 as a 5q- syndrome gene by RNA interference screen. Nature 2008;451(7176):335–9.

75. Starczynowski DT, Kuchenbauer F, Argiropoulos B, et al. Identification of miR-145 and miR-146a as mediators of the 5q- syndrome phenotype. Nat Med 2010;16(1): 49–58.

76. Argiropoulos B, Humphries RK. Hox genes in hematopoiesis and leukemogenesis. Oncogene 2007;26(47):6766–76.

77. Ernst P, Mabon M, Davidson AJ, et al. An MLL-dependent Hox program drives hematopoietic progenitor expansion. Curr Biol 2004;14(22):2063–9.

78. Mikulic M, Batinic D, Sucic M, et al. Biological features and outcome of biphenotypic acute leukemia: a case series. Hematol Oncol Stem Cell Ther 2008;1(4):225–30.

79. Park JA, Ghim TT, Bae K, et al. Stem cell transplant in the treatment of childhood biphenotypic acute leukemia. Pediatr Blood Cancer 2009;53(3):444–52.

80. Jacobsohn DA, Hewlett B, Morgan E, et al. Favorable outcome for infant acute lymphoblastic leukemia after hematopoietic stem cell transplantation. Biol Blood Marrow Transplant 2005;11(12):999–1005.

81. Ravandi F, O'Brien S, Thomas D, et al. First report of phase 2 study of dasatinib with hyper-CVAD for the frontline treatment of patients with Philadelphia chromosome-positive (Ph+) acute lymphoblastic leukemia. Blood 2010;116(12):2070–7.

82. Fielding AK, Rowe JM, Richards SM, et al. Prospective outcome data on 267 unselected adult patients with Philadelphia chromosome-positive acute lymphoblastic leukemia confirms superiority of allogeneic transplantation over chemotherapy in the pre-imatinib era: results from the International ALL Trial MRC UKALLXII/ECOG2993. Blood 2009;113(19):4489–96.

83. Schultz KR, Bowman WP, Aledo A, et al. Improved early event-free survival with imatinib in Philadelphia chromosome-positive acute lymphoblastic leukemia: a Children's Oncology Group study. J Clin Oncol 2009;27(31):5175–81.

84. Yanada M, Takeuchi J, Sugiura I, et al. High complete remission rate and promising outcome by combination of imatinib and chemotherapy for newly diagnosed BCR-ABL-positive acute lymphoblastic leukemia: a phase II study by the Japan Adult Leukemia Study Group. J Clin Oncol 2006;24(3):460–6.

85. Bernt KM, Zhu N, Sinha AU, et al. MLL-rearranged leukemia is dependent on aberrant H3K79 methylation by DOT1L. Cancer Cell 2011;20(1):66–78.
86. Daigle SR, Olhava EJ, Therkelsen CA, et al. Selective killing of mixed lineage leukemia cells by a potent small-molecule DOT1L inhibitor. Cancer Cell 2011; 20(1):53–65.
87. Lee JC, Yang S, Zou Y, et al. Erythroid/B-cell biphenotypic acute leukemia: first case report. Leukemia 2009;23(10):1920–3.
88. Lucioni M, Novara F, Fiandrino G, et al. Twenty-one cases of blastic plasmacytoid dendritic cell neoplasm: focus on biallelic locus 9p21.3 deletion. Blood Sep 7 2011. [Epub ahead of print].

Current Therapeutic Strategies in Adult Acute Lymphoblastic Leukemia

Adele K. Fielding, MB BS, PhD, FRCP, FRCPath

KEYWORDS

• Acute lymphoblastic leukaemia • Adult • Therapy
• Combination chemotherapy

OVERVIEW

Approximately half of all adults with acute lymphoblastic leukemia (ALL) now survive long term. An elegant study of unselected registry data, in which point estimates of survival were made for two 5-year time periods, 20 years apart, demonstrated highly significant 14% to 20% survival improvements for each age group except the over-60 group, in which no significant improvement in outcome had occurred.[1] This article summarizes the current approaches to treating ALL in adults, with a focus on a pragmatic approach to decision making, based on available data. A major problem in treating adults with ALL is that few physicians or institutions have a large personal practice, because the disease is rare. Coupled with a particularly punishing and often complex combination chemotherapy treatment regimen, treatment-related morbidity (TRM) and mortality are frequent and individual patient decisions on how to best balance efficacy with toxicity can be difficult. This article focuses on such situations. As examples, dealing with the toxicity of induction regimens and treating older people with ALL are both scenarios that vex clinicians and areas in which there are few conclusive answers in the literature. In many situations, it can be concluded that there is still "no right answer." Thankfully, there is a vibrant academic interest in ALL, both scientifically and clinically. The field will change significantly over the next few years as many ongoing clinical studies report and molecular insights are translated into providing prognostic information and novel therapeutic targets. Monoclonal antibodies are likely to make a considerable contribution to the treatment of ALL and are discussed in a separate article.

The author has received laboratory research funding from MEDAC GmBH.
UK National Cancer Research Institute (NCRI) Adult ALL Subgroup, University College London, Royal Free Campus, Rowland Hill Street, London NW3 2PF, UK
E-mail address: a.fielding@ucl.ac.uk

Hematol Oncol Clin N Am 25 (2011) 1255–1279
doi:10.1016/j.hoc.2011.09.008

DIAGNOSIS

ALL is a medical emergency. It should be diagnosed and treated without delay. A bone marrow aspirate should be examined morphologically by an expert hematopathologist. Bone marrow—or peripheral blood, if the blast count is high—should be examined using a panel of monoclonal antibodies to T-cell–associated and B-cell–associated antigens, which identify almost all cases of ALL. Aberrant expression of myeloid antigens is not uncommon and should not deflect from the correct diagnosis.[2] In the differential diagnosis, blastic transformation of chronic myeloid leukemia should be specifically ruled out by morphologic examination. Trephine biopsy examination is sometimes helpful, but the result is not required before starting treatment. Cytogenetic examination of the blast cells is mandatory and should comprise both examination of metaphases and fluorescence in situ hybridization with specific probes (eg, for BCR-ABL and MLL-AF4L). Screening by polymerase chain reaction (PCR) for the potential BCR-ABL transcripts, p190 and p210, should be performed. MLL-AF4 translocations can also be sought by PCR. Standardized primer sets are specified.[3] It is important that a specimen also be examined by molecular methods for the detection of patient-specific immunoglobulin and T-cell receptor (Ig/TCR) rearrangements[4–8] or by flow cytometry[9,10] to detect a specific immunophenotype, both tests can be used for minimal residual disease (MRD) quantification. If this is not performed at diagnosis, the opportunity to quantify MRD after therapy is lost unless a patient has a specific marker, such as BCR-ABL. At present, quantification of Ig/TCR rearrangements is the only standardized method for detection of MRD.[6] If bone marrow transplant is a possible part of a patient's future therapy, tissue typing of any patient siblings who are willing to be typed should also be performed at diagnosis. If there are no HLA-matched siblings, consideration should be given to prompt initiation of an unrelated donor search.

PROGNOSTIC FACTORS

Many factors that can be identified at—or soon after—diagnosis have a bearing on outcome (**Table 1**). These prognostic factors often form the basis for treatment decisions in ALL, although there is little convincing evidence that currently available therapeutic strategies other than allogeneic haematopoietic stem cell transplantation (alloHSCT) are able to overcome the adverse factors. When planning matching a potentially effective—but toxic—therapy, however, such as alloHSCT, a high risk of death as a result of ALL can be balanced against a more risky treatment strategy. Decisions of this nature are used in clinical practice and as tools to stratify patients within clinical trials. In contrast to pediatric practice, examination of prognostic factors cannot yet define a set of adults who have a particularly good prognosis. Hence, there is currently no strategy with which to limit therapy for adults on the basis of an expectation of particularly good outcome.

Minimal Residual Disease

The measurement of MRD deserves a specific discussion due to its pivotal role in the management of ALL. Long accepted as vital for management in pediatric practice, it has been conclusively demonstrated as carrying the same important prognostic information in adult ALL. Its adoption into standard practice, however, has been less quick.

MRD can be quantified by both molecular quantification of patient-specific Ig/TCR rearrangements[6]: by quantification of specific molecular abnormalities, such as BCR-ABL or MLL-AF4, or by flow cytometry,[10,31] where leukemia-specific immunophenotypes can be identified and quantified after initial treatment.

Table 1
Prognostic factors for adult acute lymphoblastic leukemia

Factor	Detail	Selected References
At diagnosis		
Age	Worse outcome with advancing age—no clear age cutoff in adults	11–14
Presenting white blood cell count	>30 × 10^9/L (B), >100 × 10^9/L (T)	11,13
Immunophenotype	In adults, T ALL can have a better outcome than B ALL CD20 expression has been associated with a less good outcome	11,13,15,16
Cytogenetics	Poor: t(9;22), t(4;11), complex (>5 abnormalities), low hypodiploidy near triplody	17,18
Specific molecular abnormalities	JAK2 IKFZ1 PAX5	4,19–23
Response to therapy		
Steroid responsiveness	Response to steroids has clear relationship with outcome in childhood ALL. Less well defined and tested in adult ALL.	24
Speed of initial response	Rapid initial response—CR within 4 weeks predicts better outcome. Not uniformly demonstrated.	25
Minimal residual disease	Clear relationship between MRD at protocol-specific time points and outcome in several studies.	9,26–30

The molecular techniques are sensitive and specific and have a sensitive range of approximately 1 in 100,000 cells. They can be accurately quantitative at the level of 1 in 10,000 cells. Molecular and flow cytometric techniques are patient specific and require a good-quality diagnostic sample. Both techniques, when performed properly, are labor intensive and expensive to carry out. Both techniques should be performed in reference laboratories according to standardized protocols. All techniques require a diagnostic sample. For treating clinicians, their clinical meaning is protocol dependent. MRD in adult ALL is an excellent example of what can be achieved by interlaboratory cooperation; the European Study Group overseen by VanDongen is a successful and thriving association of more than 30 laboratories from different countries that run standardized protocols for molecular MRD determination and are also working on joint strategies for standardized flow cytometric techniques.

A particular attraction of determination of MRD in adult ALL is that it can give information on patients d otherwise classified as "standard risk." An impressive illustration of this concept was provided by the German Multicenter Study Group for Adult Acute Lymphoblastic Leukemia (GMALL). Bruggeman and colleagues[28] demonstrated that quantification of MRD separates those who will have a poor outcome from those who will do better at several time points along the standard treatment protocol. It is a protocol-specific choice, however, as to which time point should be chosen for an intervention or intensification of therapy, such as bone marrow transplantation. At 1 year into treatment, for example, MRD-positive patients fare poorly but it is likely too late to intervene.

Another potential use of MRD is in post-therapy monitoring. The concept of molecular relapse is a realistic one in ALL, as shown by a recent study from Raff and colleagues,[32] also on behalf of the GMALL. Because the median time from MRD reappearance to clinical relapse was 9.5 months, an opportunity for intervention was offered. It remains to be seen what interventions would be appropriate in this situation.

STRATEGIES DURING INDUCTION TREATMENT
Induction Therapy—General Points

The aim of initial treatment is to achieve complete remission (CR), which is currently defined on a morphologic basis as less than 5% blasts in the bone marrow in the presence of overall hematopoietic recovery. Because treatments of ALL have evolved, an increasing intensity of therapy has been applied to achieve CR.[33,34] As a result, serious adverse effects are commonplace and treatment-related mortality is a significant risk. Hence, the highest standard of supportive care is imperative.

Supportive care

Before starting any treatment, patients should be well hydrated and receive appropriate medication to prevent urate nephropathy. ALL can be exquisitely sensitive to small doses of treatment and tumor lysis syndrome is not uncommon, especially in patients with bulky extramedullary disease. Allopurinol should be started 24 hours before induction chemotherapy and should be continued for a minimum of 5 days. Rasburicase should be considered an alternative to allopurinol if the white blood cell count is high (ie, >100×10^9/L) if a patient has bulky disease (eg, large mediastinal mass or elevated urate at diagnosis). Adults with ALL receive high doses of myelosuppressive chemotherapy along with steroids. They are, therefore, at high risk of infectious complications particularly during the induction phase of treatment. Adherence to strict anti-infective strategies is important. All patients should receive prophylaxis against herpes simplex virus and varicella-zoster virus reactivation.[35] Generally, patients are given acyclovir throughout therapy, although local policies may be followed.

All patients need prophylaxis against *Pneumocystis jeroveci* from the start of therapy. The recommended prophylaxis is co-trimoxazole (twice a day for 2 or 3 days each week), avoiding any day on which methotrexate (MTX) is given. In the event of the allergy to co-trimoxazole, alternative prophylactic agents include nebulized pentamidine or dapsone.

Antifungal prophylaxis is strongly recommended for all patients on ALL therapy from the time of induction. Azoles must be avoided when a patient is on vincristine due to potentiation of neurotoxicity.[36,37] There is no clear evidence to suggest which antifungal prophylaxis regimen should be used in this situation. An international randomized controlled trial comparing liposomal amphotericin with placebo is under way. Antifungal prophylaxis is not generally required when a patient is on maintenance therapy unless that patient is deemed at high risk for fungal disease.

The use of granulocyte colony-stimulating factor is strongly recommended for all patients to hasten neutrophil recovery, particularly after induction.[38–40]

Steroid prephase

Corticosteroids are among the most important drugs in the treatment of ALL, and recent trials in pediatric ALL patients have suggested that the use of dexamethasone, as opposed to prednisolone, may improve outcome. This is based on data suggesting that dexamethasone has greater in vitro antileukemia activity than prednisolone, has better penetration of the central nervous system (CNS), and causes fewer thromboembolic events.[41] Randomized trials have demonstrated improved survival in children receiving dexamethasone as opposed to prednisolone, although this has not been shown in every study.[42] Based on these data, many adult regimens substitute a discontinuous schedule of dexamethasone for prednisolone during induction.

Induction therapy

The primary goal of induction therapy is a complete eradication of ALL cells from blood, bone marrow, and CNS or other extramedullary sites (when initially involved). This should be achieved as early as possible and with as few toxic side effects as possible to start rapidly the postremission therapy. Most regimens use phases of induction, often called phases 1 and 2 or parts a and b, with the second part applied regardless of CR after induction 1. Many examples of highly effective induction protocols have been reported,[1,39,43–47] all of which result in CR rates of 90% or more. Due to the complexity of existing induction regimens and the fact that it is already possible to obtain a CR in 90% to 95% or more of unselected adult patients, evaluation of any new treatment elements during induction requires either the documentation of an improvement in event-free survival (EFS) or in overall survival (OS) or evaluation of an alternative, precisely quantitative, endpoint such as MRD.

Induction regimens in adult ALL are composed of steroid, vincristine, anthracycline (often daunorubicin or doxorubicin) and L-asparaginase (L-asp). Cyclophosphamide and cytarabine may also be included. Because more anthracycline is used in adult practice than in pediatric practice, prolonged myelosuppression is common. The intensity of anthracycline for maximal benefit during induction has already been reached and studies attempting to improve outcome by further intensification have not shown enhanced outcomes.[48]

Dealing with Problems and Delays During Induction Therapy

L-asparaginase and coagulation problems

Induction treatment is frequently complicated by problems that relate to a particular drug used. The most common reported cause of severe side effects of therapy relate to the bacterial enzyme L-asp. L-asp is regarded as one of the most important drugs in the treatment of ALL but is also one of the most difficult drugs to dose and manage. Expert panel guidance has recently been made,[49] although the evidence base for the management of L-asp toxicity in adults is scant.

A major problem with L-asp is the occurrence of abnormalities of coagulation. The management of the coagulation issues during treatment with L-asp varies widely worldwide and there is little clear evidence base particularly in the management of adult ALL. Although L-asp is associated with deranged coagulation as measured in the laboratory, thrombosis is the most commonly encountered clinical problem. Data indicate that thrombosis occurs in 10% to 20% of adults who are receiving L-asp therapy. There is little or no evidence that infusion of fresh frozen plasma can appropriately correct regulation abnormalities nor can it prevent thrombosis or bleeding events. In the French CAPELAL study, the mean antithrombin and fibrinogen levels increased from 61% to 88% and from 1 g/L to 1.4 g/L after infusion of antithrombin or fibrinogen, respectively, whereas both levels remained unchanged after the infusion of fresh frozen plasma. Additionally, there is some evidence that infusion of fresh frozen plasma can contribute to the replenishment of the asparginase pool that the drug is used to deplete.[50] Hence, using fresh frozen plasma to replenish coagulation factors does not seem a sensible option. Fibrinogen concentrates can be used to elevate fibrinogen levels more successfully. A median dose of 0.03 g/kg was required in the CAPELAL study to increase levels from 1.0 ± 0.3 g/L to 1.4 ± 0.45 g/L. Infusion of fibrinogen, however, was not associated with a lower incidence of bleeding complications and—unlike thrombotic events—hemorrhagic events were not associated with any difference in patients' survival.[51] There is some evidence that antithrombin concentrate can reduce the number of thromboses that occur during L-asp therapy. In a clinical study of adults undergoing ALL treatment, the occurrence of thrombosis was associated with a less good outcome, even though none of the thrombotic events, in and of themselves, was fatal. One explanation for this may be that thrombosis resulted in delay to or reduction in dose of therapy.[51] When patients treated for ALL experience a thrombosis, it can be difficult to decide whether to continue with L-asp treatment. Because the greatest risk of thrombosis is during induction therapy, cessation of one of the major components of the treatment strategy at that stage is likely to have an adverse impact on outcome. Strategies to reduce the risk of thrombosis are important. The presence of a central venous catheter considerably increases the risk of thrombosis and many treating centers delay placing indwelling central venous catheter until patients have reached CR at the end of the first phase of induction therapy. When catheter-associated thrombosis occurs, low-molecular-weight heparin is the treatment of choice. When a patient experiences a central nervous system thrombosis, the use of low-molecular-weight heparin is more contentious—patients treated with heparin should receive appropriate monitoring, because a proportion of patients have heparin resistance due to the depletion of antithrombin. When patients experience thrombosis, replacement of antithrombin is likely valuable. In the French CAPELAL study, patients who received antithrombin concentrates less frequently had delays or omissions to L-asp and a lower rate of thrombosis.[51]

There are several preparations of L-asp, which are variously licensed and marketed in different countries.[52] In pediatric practice, a pegylated version of the *Escherichia coli* enzyme is commonly used[53] and there is increasing evidence of its usefulness.[54] The advantage of this agent is that it has a long half-life; thus, administration results in prolonged asparagine depletion. A phase 2 study demonstrated that this drug can be given successfully to adult patients and was able to adequately deplete asparagine.[55] Increasing age, however, was associated with a less successful asparagine depletion as a result of fewer doses and more side effects. The role of pegylated L-asp and the optimal dose are not established in adults and are the subject of more than one clinical trial.

Liver function abnormalities and pancreatitis

It common for patients to develop transaminitis and hyperbilirubinemia during induction therapy. Again, L-asp is often implicated in the pathogenesis.[56] Experiencing severe sepsis exacerbates the problem. Most patients recover from this liver insult given time, but severe delays to therapy often result, compromising overall efficacy.

Pancreatitis is a life-threatening complication of L-asp treatment, seen more often in children than adults. It is a contradindication to further use of the drug.[57]

POSTREMISSION TREATMENT
CNS-Directed Prophylaxis

The presence of leukemic blasts in the CNS is a more frequent occurrence in patients with ALL than acute myeloid leukemia and the importance of prophylactic treatment to prevent the development of progression to the CNS has long been recognized.[2] The role of prophylactic cranial irradiation in the era of combined intrathecal and high-dose systemic therapy has been questioned in recent studies, with the intent of reducing the risk of late sequelae. This is of particular interest to pediatricians because the late effects of cranial irradiation in children are well documented. Trials in children have already demonstrated that CNS irradiation can be eliminated without worsening overall outcome.[58] In adults, several trials have reported CNS recurrence rates of less than 10% with the combined use of high-dose systemic and intrathecal chemotherapy without the use of cranial irradiation; thus, it is not considered an essential component of therapy.[44,47,59]

MTX is the most common chemotherapy drug used for CNS-directed prophylaxis. It is by no means without specific toxicity, however, even when delivered at low doses via the intrathecal route. MTX-related encephalopathy is a particular problem, although less common in adults than in children.[60] It presents with fits, focal neurologic deficit, or impaired consciousness and typically occurs within 1 day to approximately 3 weeks of exposure to intrathecal MTX. Full recovery is usual but the clinical presentation is dramatic and can be terrifying for patients. Diagnosis is often one of exclusion; other causes of CNS events should be considered and ruled out, such as cerebrovascular events, sagittal sinus thrombosis, infections, or CNS involvement with ALL. There may be typical findings on MRI scanning.[61] In the event of this complication, the role of future MTX should be questioned. Future MTX should be discontinued when patients are also receiving cytarabine systemically. Safe rechallenge in other circumstances may possible without recurrence of toxicity, but if recurrence happens, the intrathecal regimen should be changed to cytarabine (50 mg) in association with hydrocortisone (12.5 mg). Local policy may be followed for the hydrocortisone dose if necessary.

Consolidation and Maintenance Therapy

Consolidation therapy typically consists of several cycles of treatment similar to but often less intensive than those given during induction. Consolidation is typically better tolerated than induction, although specific practices during consolidation are poorly studied. In line with pediatric style approaches, consolidation often contains one or more blocks of delayed intensification, in which the intensity of therapy is enhanced. Again, this approach has been adopted to a variable extent, although systematic study of intensification of therapy in consolidation has showed little or no evidence for benefit in adults,[62,63] suggesting that a focus on improvements to initial therapy holds more promise.

Maintenance therapy remains obligatory in those not undergoing alloHSCT. Daily mercaptopurine, weekly MTX, and pulses of vincristine and steroids for 18 to 24 months after consolidation are standard. The composition and duration of maintenance therapy has never been the subject of a specific study in adults and has not changed in approach for many years. There is now randomized controlled trial evidence, however, of the value of prolonged chemotherapy compared with a shorter, more-intensive approach in adult ALL.[64] In the Medical Research Council (MRC) UKALL12/E2993, patients without a matched sibling donor were eligible for randomization between high-dose therapy with etoposide and total body irradiation (TBI) with autologous HSCT (autoHSCT) rescue and maintenance therapy. The intent-to-treat analysis of 456 randomized patients showed that those randomized to prolonged chemotherapy had significantly superior EFS (41% vs 32%; $P = .02$) and OS (46% vs 37%; $P = .03$) at 5 years compared with those randomized to autoHSCT. The TRM did not differ between the groups. AutoHCST simply provided less-adequate disease control than prolonged chemotherapy.

Allogeneic Hematopoietic Stem Cell Transplant

alloHSCT has been extensively investigated in the treatment of ALL. Most physicians recommend alloHSCT for patients with high-risk ALL who are of suitable age and performance status where a donor is available. Patients receiving fully matched unrelated donor stem cells probably have an equivalent outcome in terms of toxicity and TRM as those receiving sibling stem cells from matched siblings—several studies have addressed this and although disease-free survival (DFS) is hard to compare with studies of sibling alloHSCT, TRM seems similar. In a single-center study of 84 patients with high-risk ALL, a considerable proportion of whom were beyond CR1, in which almost all patients received a TBI-based conditioning regimen, TRM did not differ significantly and in which almost all patients received either sibling or unrelated donor stem cells. The median age of patients in this study, however, was only 23 years and the study included children.[65] A National Marrow Donor Program study of 127 patients in 46 centers demonstrated a high TRM for unrelated donor alloHSCT. The low relapse rate, however, resulted in a 37% ± 13% DFS for patients in CR1, which compared favorably at the time to results obtained with chemotherapy alone and those after HLA-identical sibling alloHSCT.[66] A similar study in a smaller number of centers included a larger number of patients (N = 221, 72 of whom were Philadelphia positive [Ph+]) and a median age more representative of an adult population also showed no difference in TRM between matched sibling and unrelated donor alloHSCT. Again, patients beyond CR1 were included, which is likely to adversely influence the TRM, which was high (43% for sibling alloHSCT and 50% for unrelated donor alloHSCT).[67]

The succinct conclusion, however, that adults with high-risk ALL should be offered alloHSCT in ALL—although true in overarching conceptual simplicity—oversimplifies the situation considerably and does little to help with clinical management of individual patients, because as new risk factors emerge, transplant conditioning regimens and supportive care change, chemotherapy protocols develop and improve, and novel agents become available. At the same time, past data and trials involving alloHSCT cannot take into account current insights. As an example, what constitutes high risk now includes those who are MRD positive at certain time points within the protocol. Conversely, the high risk of BCR-ABL positivity may be mitigated to some extent by the use of tyrosine kinase inhibitor (TKIs)—in children, this has provoked interest in managing pediatric patients who are BCR-ABL positive without alloHSCT (discussed later, in section on "Philadelphia-positive ALL"). Furthermore, a "suitable age" for alloHSCT is also the subject of debate. As the results for chemotherapy alone regimens continue to improve outcomes for adolescents and young adults, there is increased potential for better long-term OS without the toxicity of alloHSCT. It is against this fluid background that data on alloHSCT must be interpreted and decisions made for individual patients. Many trials have been conducted incorporating autoHSCT and alloHSCT into the treatment algorithm. There are several studies of myeloablative therapy followed by sibling alloHSCT.[68–72] In all, the data indicate that in selected individuals, DFS or OS seems better than expected with treatment with chemotherapy alone. The strongest direct experimental support for alloHSCT in ALL, however, comes from 3 large studies from France, the United Kingdom and United States, and the Dutch-Belgian *Hemato-Oncology Cooperative Group* (HOVON).[64,68,73] In all the studies, the existence of an allogeneic donor among those eligible for alloHSCT was independently predictive of remission duration; demonstrations of how so-called biologic randomization or donor versus no donor analysis can be used.

The largest study of alloHSCT, UKALL12/E2993, evaluated the outcome of Philadelphia-negative patients assigned to HLA-matched sibling alloHSCT compared with patients randomized to autologous SCT or chemotherapy.[64] In a comparison of 389 patients with a donor to 530 patients without a donor, the donor groups had superior EFS (50% vs 41%; P = .009) and OS (53% vs 45%; P = .02). A similar statistically significant benefit was seen when the no donor group was restricted to those who were randomized to the chemotherapy arm only. This benefit was primarily seen in the standard-risk patients (OS 63% for donor vs 51% for no donor patients; P = .01) but not in high-risk patients (OS 40% vs 36%; P = .6). The lack of difference in outcomes between donor and no donor patients in the high-risk group was related to a high nonrelapse mortality of 39% at 2 years (20% at 2 years for the standard risk patients), which in large part was seen in older patients.

Meta-analysis of abstract data also shows an advantage for myeloablative alloHSCT.[74] An additional justification for considering alloHSCT in high-risk patients first in CR (CR1) is the dismal outcome of patients who relapse from CR1 (discussed later).

Currently, the role of myeloablative alloHSCT in adults with ALL could be considered fluid and decisions may change as new data emerge. At the time of this writing, for patients in their early 20s and 30s in whom a sibling donor is available, results achieved can be superimposed on those achieved using a young adult chemotherapy approach. Data from 2 recent studies illustrate this point. In a Spanish study group Programa para el Estudio de la Terapéutica en Hemopatía Maligna (PETHEMA) trial, a pediatric-style approach was used for adults ages 19 to 30 with standard-risk disease—a CR rate of 98% was obtained and the 3-year OS was 63%.[75] An almost identical, superimposable outcome for patients of the same age group (15–35) was shown in the UKALL12/E2993 study, in which patients received adult induction followed by sibling alloHSCT; the CR rate was 95% and 5-year OS was 62%.

Choice of Myeloablative Conditioning Regimen

The Stanford conditioning regimen of high-dose etoposide and TBI is often used because, when published, it demonstrated superior results in alloHSCT for ALL.[76] There are no randomized controlled studies, however, comparing conditioning regimens; the optimal conditioning regimen has not been demonstrated. A retrospective analysis of data from selected centers suggested that TBI-based conditioning likely results in improved DFS by comparison with non-TBI, busulfan-containing regimens.[67] The most commonly used regimens in conjuction with TBI are cyclophosphamide or etoposide. A small study suggested no difference between these 2 TBI-based regimens in childhood ALL.[77] To date, the best available evidence comes from a retrospective analysis of International Blood and Marrow Transplant Research (IBMTR) data.[78] No difference in relapse risk or OS was demonstrated between conditioning regimens containing either cyclophosphamide or etoposide when alloHSCT was performed in CR1. There was a modest advantage to using etoposide and higher doses of TBI when the alloHSCT was in second CR (CR2). The major acute toxicity of the etoposide-containing regimen is severe mucositis. One aspect of the UKALL14 study will examine whether amelioration of the mucositis[79] by using the keratinocyte growth factor pallifermin might have a beneficial effect on graft-versus-host disease by facilitating delivery of the full dose of MTX prophylaxis. A role for T-cell–depletion unrelated-donor alloHSCT has not been defined. A British Society of Blood and Marrow Transplantation study shows an excellent outcome for high-risk ALL treated with alemtuzumab in vivo as part of the conditioning regimen.[80] Conversely, an IMBTR study showed a less good outcome for those who received T-cell depletion as part of their therapy.[81] Whether the use of alternative donor options, such as haploidentical stem cells or umbilical cord blood, is justified is a relevant question in high-risk ALL,[82] but a full discussion is beyond the scope of this article.

Nonmyeloablative, Reduced-Intensity Conditioning

No prospective studies of transplant using reduced-intensity conditioning (RIC) have been reported to date. Published reports are subject to the considerable bias. To compound interpretation of the data, many series include patients beyond CR1. Only one study has compared the outcome of patients receiving reduced intensity as opposed to myeloablative conditioning—multivariate analysis showed that conditioning intensity did not affect transplantation-related mortality ($P = .92$) or relapse risk ($P = .14$), adding considerable justification for the further study of this approach. There are a plethora of reports of RIC alloHSCT in adult ALL. The European Group for Blood and Marrow Transplantation reported 97 patients who received various different RIC regimens, many of which were delivered in conjunction with some form of T-cell depletion.[83] A 2-year OS of 52% for those transplanted in CR1 was reported. A GMALL examined the outcome of a mixed group of 22 patients with high-risk ALL receiving nonmyeloablative alloHSCT,[84] 11 of whom had Ph+ disease. Half were beyond CR1. Few patients survived long term and mortality was high, but for many patients it was a second alloHSCT after relapse, making a good outcome unlikely. Another retrospective study included 27 patients from 4 different studies who had undergone nonmyeloablative alloHSCT.[85] More than 80% of the patients whose median age was 50 years were beyond CR1. Two-year OS was 31%. Treatment-related mortality was modest for such a high-risk population, at 23%. A City of Hope study[86] reported on 24 patients with adults with high-risk ALL treated with fludarabine and melphalan conditioning without T-cell depletion. Approximately half of the patients were over 50 years of age; there was a 2-year OS of 61.5% and DFS of 61.5%, with a treatment-related mortality of 21.5%. Bachanova and colleagues[87] reported a 3-year OS of 50% among 22 patients, median age 49, all with high-risk ALL. Patients received a uniform reduced-intensity approach of fludarabine, cyclophosphamide, and low-dose TBI in the University of Minnesota Transplant Program. Nonmyeloablative allogeneic HSCT approaches are promising but require careful prospective study required to define their role in Ph+ ALL. The forthcoming study from the UK National Cancer Research Institute, UKALL14, will assign all patients with ALL aged 40 or older to a nonmyeloablative approach with fludarabine, melphalan, and alemtuzumab in an attempt to reduce the high incidence of graft-versus-host disease (86%), which occurred in the City of Hope report, in which fludarabine and melphalan was used without T-cell depletion. A recent report from the Fred Hutchinson Cancer Research Center Seattle[88] underscores an important point that the level of disease at the time of alloHSCT might be of more relevance when RIC is used. In the series of 51 patients with high-risk ALL conditioned with a low-dose TBI approach, the 3-year OS rate was 62%; for the subgroup without evidence of MRD at transplantation, the OS was 73%.

SPECIFIC SCENARIOS IN ALL THERAPY
CNS Involvement

When the CNS is involved at diagnosis, specific therapy needs to be given. Systemic chemotherapy, cranial irradiation, and intrathecal therapy can all be used to help control CNS ALL. Although cranial irradiation as CNS-directed prophylaxis is arguably dispensable in the presence of prolonged intrathecal therapy,[89] it is undoubtedly an effective form of therapy for established CNS leukemia and should be given strong consideration.

MTX, cytarabine, and glucocorticoids can all be safely given by the intrathecal route. Intrathecal therapy should be given once or twice per week until resolution of any CNS signs and symptoms and clearance of blasts from the cerebrospinal fluid (CSF) has occurred. There have been no benefits demonstrated by giving triple intrathecal therapy compared with MTX alone. When administering intrathecal medication there are some practical considerations: it should be given in sufficient volume to distribute well throughout the CSF and patients should remain recumbent for at least 1 hour (some recommend 6 or even 12 hours) after treatment.[33] Because cytotoxic concentrations are not maintained in the CSF for long, frequent intrathecal administrations are needed, which can present technical difficulties. A liposomal preparation of cytarabine is available, which results in an extended concentration of cytarabine in the CSF. This should not be given during treatment with high-dose, CNS-penetrating treatment because there are reports of serious neurotoxicity.[90] Whatever standard drug or route of intrathecal administration is given, therapy should be given once or twice per week until resolution of any CNS signs and symptoms and clearance of blasts from the CSF.

High doses of MTX, cytarabine, and glucocortocoids cross the blood-brain barrier. Many regimens have used MTX at doses ranging from 0.5 g/m^2 to 5 g/m^2 and meta-analysis of 43 randomized controlled trials showed a benefit to this approach in terms of reduction in relapse risk and improved event-free survival athough only a small effect on CNS disease.[89] Rescue with folinic acid is required at an appropriate time (not too early to reduce efficacy) as is careful determination of systemic MTX levels to minimize systemic toxicity, in particular nephrotoxicity. Because systemic steroids also cross the blood-brain barrier, they may also constitute good agents for inclusion in the therapy for CNS disease—it was reported that dexamethasone was superior to prednisolone in reducing CNS relapse risk.[91] This may have been due, however, to lack of dose equivalence between the 2 agents.

What is the effect on outcome when the CNS is involved at diagnosis? In the MRC UKALL12/E2993 trial,[92] 77 of 1508 (5%) patients had CNS involvement at diagnosis. The incidence was higher in patients with T-cell ALL. Of these 77 patients, 69 (90%) achieved CR. This study demonstrated that although long-term DFS is attainable in patients who present with CNS involvement, OS at 5 years was inferior at 29% compared with 38% for patients without CNS involvement ($P = .03$).

ALL in Younger Adults

Several retrospective studies have shown that an intensive pediatric approach to therapy with high doses of steroid and L-asp can confer survival superior to an adult approach in older teenagers and young adults.[92–99] Although such retrospective studies are subject to considerable selection bias, the weight of evidence favors evaluating such a therapeutic approach carefully in older adults. As a consequence, the field has tended to become somewhat polarized, with chemotherapy and bone marrow transplant viewed as opposing therapeutic candidates. The outcome of this debate and shift in emphasis in terms of long-term OS and long-term toxicity remain to be determined and it is likely both approaches will play a role in continued improvement of outcomes.

It is becoming clearer that pediatric-style intensive therapy can be delivered to patients who are by no means adolescents—at least up to age 30—with a reasonably good outcome of approximately 60% OS at 5 years.[75] This outcome is superimposable, however, on the outcome seen for patients of the same age and risk status with a sibling donor in the UKALL12/E2993 donor versus no donor analysis.[64] To date, there are currently no data to suggest that the poor prognostic relevance of being over 40 can be overcome by a pediatric therapeutic approach but this is an active and important area of study for both chemotherapy and RIC alloHSCT approaches. Data from the French Group for Research on Adult Acute Lymphoblastic

Leukemia (GRAALL) indicate a 22% chance of death in remission when the intensive approach was used in over-40s.[98] A US intergroup study is currently evaluating a pediatric chemotherapy approach whereas the UKALL14 study from the United Kingdom evaluates RIC alloHSCT in all patients over 40 with a suitable donor.

ALL in Older Adults

Large studies have typically not included patients over age 65 and this may be one of the reasons that patients of this age are the only group in whom survival has not improved over time. The median age of adults with ALL is over 60 years, however. In the United Kingdom, the age-specific annual incidence of ALL rises from 0.45/100,000 in adults aged 35 to 39 to 0.78/100,000 in patients 60 to 64 to 1.2/100,000 cases in the over-85 group.[100] The predicted rise in the proportion of people over 65 in the United Kingdom from 16% of the population in 2009 to 23% by 2034 (UK Office for National Statistics) will result in a UK national increase in the number of older patients with ALL in the future.

There is no standard regimen for the treatment of older patients with ALL worldwide. UKALL XII shows that older patients fared poorly, with less than 15% 5-year OS.[1] For older patients with ALL, deemed unsuitable for trial entry either because of eligibility criteria or fitness, treatment is scheduled only according to prevailing local practice. It is not known whether treatment is with curative or palliative intent. It is not known whether long-term DFS equating to cure is a realistic goal. Moreover, there are no data investigating quality of life in elderly patients with ALL and its relationship with the intensity of treatment regimens and response. In the Southwest Oncology Group study, the median survival of 40 patients aged 50 years or older was 1 month versus 17.1 months for the whole cohort of 168 patients.[101] A CR rate of just 77% was reported on CALGB 9111 in 35 patients aged 60 years or older versus 85% in the whole group. Median survival in the over-60s was 12 months compared with 23 months for the cohort as a whole.[39] In an MD Anderson Cancer Center study of patients treated with hyperfractionated cyclophosphamide, vincristine, doxorubicin, and dexamethasone (hyper-CVAD), only 79% of the 44 patients aged 60 years or older achieved a CR compared with 91% in the 204 total patient cohort. Five-year survival in this study was only 17% in the over-60s versus 39% in the under 60s.[102] Recent data from the UKALL12/E2993 study also confirm significantly inferior CR, EFS, and OS rates in patients over age 55.[103] This study reported significantly more infections during phase I induction in patients aged 55 years and older versus those younger than 55 years (67% vs 45% respectively; $P<.0001$) and a need for more drug dose reductions during induction in the patients 55 years and older (47% vs 27%; $P = .0006$) compared with those younger than 55 years old. Crucially, infection during induction in addition to adverse karyotype and high white blood cell count predicted for worse EFS and this was especially significant in those who had infection in both phases of induction (6% vs 38%; $P = .007$). Overall, published data indicate a 3-times to 10-times higher high rate of induction deaths in older individuals after treatment of ALL.[47]

Two population-based registry studies (from the Northern region of the United Kingdom) report even lower response and survival rates. Taylor and colleagues[104] and Moorman and colleagues[100] reported CRs in only 10 of 49 and 20 of 39 older patients with ALL, respectively. The contrast between outcomes reported in studies and population-based surveys suggests a significant bias toward including only younger and fitter older patients in therapy trials. It is likely that the overall outcome for older patients with ALL may be poorer than are reported from published studies. The Dutch-Belgian group, HOVON, recently trialed an intensive regimen in patients up to 70 years. In the HOVON 71 study, patients between 40 and 70 years were included. CR rate in the pilot study was 85% and OS at 3 years in patients over 60 was 54% (median follow-up 30 months) but EFS was 41%. It is not clear how to predict which older persons will most benefit from intensive approaches to treatment. Formal studies of attempts to increase intensity of specific aspects of therapy, such as anthracylines, have not shown benefit in any subgroup of older people.[105]

For older patients with Ph+ ALL, there has been some recent, real progress in improving at least short-term outcomes. The understanding that CR might be achieved with less toxicity when TKIs are added to therapy has emerged from 2 studies conducted in older people. One of the early studies, by the GMALL,[106] was performed in patients older than 55 years of age and randomized participants to receive imatinib or multiagent chemotherapy for initial induction. In this randomized comparison of the 2 approaches, the overall CR in the imatinib arm was 96%, whereas in the chemotherapy arm it was 50%. The suggestion that imatinib may offer good initial responses with less toxicity is also borne out by the imatinib and steroid combination results reported in 30 elderly patients (median age 69 years) by the Gruppo Italiano Malattie Ematologiche dell'Adulto,[107] with all achieving hematologic CR with a median survival from diagnosis of 20 months, although continuing drops in the survival curves suggest that there are unlikely to be any long-term disease-free survivors. Remarkably, within this study, most patients did not require admission to hospital.

Balancing toxicity of treatment against potentially a more aggressive disease phenotype is an enormous challenge in the management of older patients with ALL—attempts to increase intensity of therapy undoubtedly result in significant increases in toxicity. Emerging novel agents, such as monoclonal antibodies, have the tremendous potential of adding independent antileukemia effect without the addition of substantial toxicity. The challenge, however, is how best to integrate these novel agents into ALL protocols for older individuals for whom a standard of care is not defined.

Philadelphia-Positive ALL

The treatment of Ph+ ALL has been revolutionized by the addition of TKIs to treatment. A detailed description of the considerable literature exploring the use of TKIs in Ph+ ALL is beyond the scope of this article—readers are referred to recent review articles by the author and others.[108–110] There are many studies published that document a higher rate of CR when the BCR-ABL–specific TKI is added to combination chemotherapy.[106,107,111–118] When used as a single agent in conjunction with steroids, CR has been demonstrated in all patients without treatment-related mortality—this was particularly impressive in a study of older patients, most of whom were treated as outpatients.[107] This, however, is not a long-term curative option for such patients, who eventually all relapse without substantive therapy. An accumulating data set demonstrates the existence of small clones with pre-existing resistance to TKIs as a result of BCR-ABL kinase domain mutations,[119,120] which undoubtedly contribute to loss of response to TKIs. For this reason, BCR-ABL quantitation showing a good initial reduction in BCR-ABL in response to TKI therapy does not correlate with a good long-term outcome[114,121–124] in the same way it was originally reported in the pre-TKI era.[122,123] Although there have been no randomized controlled trials comparing chemotherapy with chemotherapy plus imatinib in this disease, OS when imatinib is included as part of therapy has been compared with historical controls in large data sets in several studies.[111,113] There is little doubt from these studies that the overall outcome of therapy is superior with the inclusion of TKIs. It is not clear, however, whether this ultimately relates to the higher rate of alloHSCT, which also been demonstrated in these and other studies. When imatinib and chemotherapy combinations have been used followed by subsequent alloHSCT, reports of 3-year OS of up to 60% are emerging.[113,119] Although there is some evidence that Ph+ ALL in children can be treated successfully with chemotherapy and TKI combinations alone, this conclusion is based on a small study that was not designed to ask this specific question.[116]

In adults, for whom alloHSCT remains the mainstay of therapy, there are many questions of how best to use TKIs after alloHSCT. It is not clear whether TKIs are needed at all. A German study is currently investigating in a randomized fashion the relative effectiveness of an expectant approach, giving imatinib only if the BCR-ABL PCR is positive, with an approach in which all patients are given imatinib starting at 3 months post-alloHSCT. Imatinib is not always well tolerated post-alloHSCT.[115] Outside a clinical trial, administration of imatinib in this setting might be best confined to situations when a BCR-ABL signal is detected.

The agent dasatinib is less specific for brc-abl and also blocks Src kinases, which, unlike in CML, are known to play a role in Ph+ ALL.[125] In theory, this agent should result in a better outcome. It is less well tested than imatinib in Ph+ ALL but phase 2 studies have evaluated its efficacy has also been used both alone and in combination with chemotherapy.[126] Initial studies demonstrated responses to single-agent dasatinib in relapsed disease—the drug was active in situations of imatinib resistance due to BCR-ABL kinase domain mutations.[127] This agent also crosses the blood-brain barrier.[128] The occurrence of the T315I mutation confers resistance to all currently licensed TKIs and requires an experimental approach to treatment either using novel TKIs, such as ponatinib,[129] or the bispecific antibody blinatumomab.[130] The role of monoclonal antibodies in ALL treatment is discussed in a subsequent article in this issue. There is no clear evidence to date in the adult setting that Ph+ ALL can be optimally managed without alloHSCT because, even in the presence of TKIs, most patients eventually relapse without the definitive therapy for alloHSCT.

TREATMENT OF RELAPSED DISEASE

Unfortunately, at least half of adults with ALL who achieve CR later relapse. There are several studies of the outcome of relapsed disease that show poor outcomes.[131–135] The largest studies include patients who have relapsed after uniform therapy; 3 major national trials—from the United Kingdom/United States, MRC UKALL12/E2993; the French LALA-94 study; and the Spanish PETHEMA trials. UKALL12/E2993[136] examined the outcome of 609 adults with relapsed ALL. Unfortunately, data on therapy received and the achievement of CR2 was not collected. The OS at 5 years after relapse was 7% (95% CI, 4%–9%). Factors predicting a good outcome after salvage therapy were young age (OS 12% in patients <20 years vs OS 3% in patients >50 years; $2P$ <0.00005) and short duration of CR1 (OS 11% in those with CR1 >2 years vs OS 5% in those with CR1 <2 years; $2P$ <0.00005). Treatment received in CR1 did not influence outcome after relapse. In a PETHEMA study of 263 patients,[137] 45% of patients achieved CR2. The median OS was 4.5 months (95% CI, 4–5 months) with a 5-year OS of 10%. Again, younger patients and those with longer duration of first remission had a better outcome. Tavernier[138] reported on 421 patients relapsing after LALA-94 treatment. The CR2 rate was 44%. The median DFS was 5.2 months with a 5-year DFS at 12%.

In summary, most adults with relapsed ALL, whatever their prior treatment, cannot be rescued using currently available therapies. Less than one-half achieve CR2 with standard therapies. There is no standardized approach for the initial treatment of relapsed disease. AlloHSCT, however, seems the only treatment with curative potential at the present time. In the selected subgroup of patients who can receive alloHSCT after relapse, approximately 20% are expected to be long-term survivors. For patients who have relapsed after alloHSCT, the most logical strategy is participation in a study of a novel approach. Prevention of relapse by optimizing first-line therapy is the best strategy for long-term survival in adults with ALL.

LONG-TERM CONSEQUENCES OF THERAPY

Long-term consequences of therapy for ALL have been studied extensively in children but are poorly understood in adults partly because there are fewer long-term survivors. Avascular necrosis (AVN) of the bone is a serious complication of ALL therapy. The problem has been studied extensively in childhood ALL and one excellent prospective study has documented genetic and pharmacogenetic correlates in children.[139] The magnitude of this problem among adults with ALL is unclear and has been little studied. The incidence of and risk factors for AVN have been studied in 1053 patients on the UKALL12/E2993 protocol.[140] Osteonecrosis affected 99 joints in 42 patients, giving a crude incidence rate of 4.0%. Onset was at a median of 2.2 years from diagnosis. Treatment with chemotherapy (as opposed to alloHSCT) was highly significantly predictive of development of AVN. Age was also a significant predictive factor; the actuarial incidence of AVN was 29% at 10 years in patients under 20 years old compared with 8% at 10 years in those older than 20. Taken together with the pediatric data suggesting a lower age limit for AVN, these data suggest that AVN may often be a disease of adolescence and may relate to physiologic changes, such as epiphyseal closure and changes in circulating hormone levels in the maturing bones of adolescents, which may be more susceptible to steroid-induced bony changes.[141,142] It is not clear whether the move to a more pediatric approach to therapy will exacerbate the problem with AVN or whether the older age of adult patients will be protective against AVN. All studies of ALL should document the occurrence of this complication prospectively and treating clinicians should have a low threshold of suspicion.

Second malignant neoplasms are a serious complication after successful treatment of childhood ALL.[143]

The French group analyzed the incidence of second malignancies in 1494 patients enrolled in 2 successive LALA protocols from 1987 to 2002.[144] The overall cumulative risk of secondary neoplasms was 2.1% at 5 years, 4.9% at 10 years, and 9.4% at 15 years with hematological malignancies predominating in the earlier period and solid tumors predominating later. No specific cytotoxic agent could be associated with this complication. The risk of secondary or concomitant neoplasm seems higher than that of childhood ALL previously reported but it is not clear how much of this risk relates specifically to anti-ALL therapy, and there is room for considerable study in this area.

REFERENCES

1. Rowe JM, Buck G, Burnett AK, et al. Induction therapy for adults with acute lymphoblastic leukemia: results of more than 1500 patients from the international ALL trial: MRC UKALL XII/ECOG E2993. Blood 2005;106(12):3760–7.
2. Larson RA, Dodge RK, Burns CP, et al. A five-drug remission induction regimen with intensive consolidation for adults with acute lymphoblastic leukemia: cancer and leukemia group B study 8811. Blood 1995;85(8):2025–37.
3. Hoelzer D, Thiel E, Loffler H, et al. Prognostic factors in a multicenter study for treatment of acute lymphoblastic leukemia in adults. Blood 1988;71(1):123–31.

4. Chessells JM, Hall E, Prentice HG, et al. The impact of age on outcome in lymphoblastic leukaemia; MRC UKALL X and XA compared: a report from the MRC Paediatric and Adult Working Parties. Leukemia 1998;12(4):463–73.

5. Thomas DA, O'Brien S, Jorgensen JL, et al. Prognostic significance of CD20 expression in adults with de novo precursor B-lineage acute lymphoblastic leukemia. Blood 2009;113(25):6330–7.

6. Maury S, Huguet F, Leguay T, et al. Adverse prognostic significance of CD20 expression in adults with Philadelphia chromosome-negative B-cell precursor acute lymphoblastic leukemia. Haematologica 2010;95(2):324–8.

7. Pullarkat V, Slovak ML, Kopecky KJ, et al. Impact of cytogenetics on the outcome of adult acute lymphoblastic leukemia: results of Southwest Oncology Group 9400 study. Blood 2008;111(5):2563–72.

8. Moorman AV, Harrison CJ, Buck GA, et al. Karyotype is an independent prognostic factor in adult acute lymphoblastic leukemia (ALL): analysis of cytogenetic data from patients treated on the Medical Research Council (MRC) UKALLXII/Eastern Cooperative Oncology Group (ECOG) 2993 trial. Blood 2007;109(8):3189–97.

9. Mullighan CG, Miller CB, Radtke I, et al. BCR-ABL1 lymphoblastic leukaemia is characterized by the deletion of Ikaros. Nature 2008;453(7191):110–4.

10. Waanders E, van der Velden VH, van der Schoot CE, et al. Integrated use of minimal residual disease classification and IKZF1 alteration status accurately predicts 79% of relapses in pediatric acute lymphoblastic leukemia. Leukemia 2011;25(2):254–8.

11. Iacobucci I, Storlazzi CT, Cilloni D, et al. Identification and molecular characterization of recurrent genomic deletions on 7p12 in the IKZF1 gene in a large cohort of BCR-ABL1-positive acute lymphoblastic leukemia patients: on behalf of Gruppo Italiano Malattie Ematologiche dell'Adulto Acute Leukemia Working Party (GIMEMA AL WP). Blood 2009;114(10):2159–67.

12. Mullighan CG. JAK2—a new player in acute lymphoblastic leukaemia. Lancet 2008;372(9648):1448–50.

13. Mullighan CG, Goorha S, Radtke I, et al. Genome-wide analysis of genetic alterations in acute lymphoblastic leukaemia. Nature 2007;446(7137):758–64.

14. Mullighan CG, Zhang J, Kasper LH, et al. CREBBP mutations in relapsed acute lymphoblastic leukaemia. Nature 2011;471(7337):235–9.

15. Schrappe M, Aricò M, Harbott J, et al. Philadelphia chromosome-positive (Ph+) childhood acute lymphoblastic leukemia: good initial steroid response allows early prediction of a favorable treatment outcome. Blood 1998;92(8):2730–41.

16. Grosicki S, Holowiecki J, Giebel S, et al. The early reduction of leukemic blasts in bone marrow on day 6 of induction treatment is predictive for complete remission rate and survival in adult acute myeloid leukemia; the results of multicenter, prospective Polish Adult Leukemia Group study. Am J Hematol 2011;86(5):437–9.

17. Holowiecki J, Krawczyk-Kulis M, Giebel S, et al. Status of minimal residual disease after induction predicts outcome in both standard and high-risk Ph-negative adult acute lymphoblastic leukaemia. The Polish Adult Leukemia Group ALL 4-2002 MRD Study. Br J Haematol 2008;142(2):227–37.

18. Patel B, Rai L, Buck G, et al. Minimal residual disease is a significant predictor of treatment failure in non T-lineage adult acute lymphoblastic leukaemia: final results of the international trial UKALL XII/ECOG2993. Br J Haematol 2010;148(1):80–9.

19. Mortuza FY, Papaioannou M, Moreira IM, et al. Minimal residual disease tests provide an independent predictor of clinical outcome in adult acute lymphoblastic leukemia. J Clin Oncol 2002;20(4):1094–104.

20. Bruggemann M, Raff T, Flohr T, et al. Clinical significance of minimal residual disease quantification in adult patients with standard-risk acute lymphoblastic leukemia. Blood 2006;107(3):1116–23.

21. Bassan R, Spinelli O, Oldani E, et al. Improved risk classification for risk-specific therapy based on the molecular study of minimal residual disease (MRD) in adult acute lymphoblastic leukemia (ALL). Blood 2009;113(18):4153–62.

22. Schrappe M, Valsecchi MG, Bartram CR, et al. Late MRD response determines relapse risk overall and in subsets of childhood T-cell ALL: results of the AIEOP-BFM-ALL 2000 study. Blood 2011;118(8):2077–84.

23. Pulte D, Gondos A, Brenner H. Improvement in survival in younger patients with acute lymphoblastic leukemia from the 1980s to the early 21st century. Blood 2009;113(7):1408–11.

24. Peters JM, Ansari MQ. Multiparameter flow cytometry in the diagnosis and management of acute leukemia. Arch Pathol Lab Med 2011;135(1):44–54.

25. Gabert J, Beillard E, van der Velden VH, et al. Standardization and quality control studies of 'real-time' quantitative reverse transcriptase polymerase chain reaction of fusion gene transcripts for residual disease detection in leukemia—a Europe Against Cancer program. Leukemia 2003;17(12):2318–57.

26. Bruggemann M, van der Velden VH, Raff T, et al. Rearranged T-cell receptor beta genes represent powerful targets for quantification of minimal residual disease in childhood and adult T-cell acute lymphoblastic leukemia. Leukemia 2004;18(4):709–19.

27. Bruggemann M, Schrauder A, Raff T, et al. Standardized MRD quantification in European ALL trials: proceedings of the Second International Symposium on MRD assessment in Kiel, Germany, 18-20 September 2008. Leukemia 2010; 24(3):521–35.

28. Bruggemann M, Droese J, Bolz I, et al. Improved assessment of minimal residual disease in B cell malignancies using fluorogenic consensus probes for real-time quantitative PCR. Leukemia 2000;14(8):1419–25.

29. van der Velden VH, Cazzaniga G, Schrauder A, et al. Analysis of minimal residual disease by Ig/TCR gene rearrangements: guidelines for interpretation of real-time quantitative PCR data. Leukemia 2007;21(4):604–11.

30. Robillard N, Cave H, Mechinaud F, et al. Four-color flow cytometry bypasses limitations of IG/TCR polymerase chain reaction for minimal residual disease detection in certain subsets of children with acute lymphoblastic leukemia. Haematologica 2005;90(11):1516–23.

31. Coustan-Smith E, Song G, Clark C, et al. New markers for minimal residual disease detection in acute lymphoblastic leukemia. Blood 2011;117(23): 6267–76.

32. Raff T, Gokbuget N, Luschen S, et al. Molecular relapse in adult standard-risk ALL patients detected by prospective MRD monitoring during and after maintenance treatment: data from the GMALL 06/99 and 07/03 trials. Blood 2007; 109(3):910–5.

33. Pui CH, Robison LL, Look AT. Acute lymphoblastic leukaemia. Lancet 2008; 371(9617):1030–43.

34. Pui CH, Evans WE. Treatment of acute lymphoblastic leukemia. N Engl J Med 2006;354(2):166–78.

35. Styczynski J, Reusser P, Einsele H, et al. Management of HSV, VZV and EBV infections in patients with hematological malignancies and after SCT: guidelines from the Second European Conference on Infections in Leukemia. Bone Marrow Transplant 2009;43(10):757–70.

36. van Schie RM, Bruggemann RJ, Hoogerbrugge PM, et al. Effect of azole anti-fungal therapy on vincristine toxicity in childhood acute lymphoblastic leukaemia. J Antimicrob Chemother 2011;66(8):1853–6.
37. Bohme A, Ganser A, Hoelzer D. Aggravation of vincristine-induced neurotoxicity by itraconazole in the treatment of adult ALL. Ann Hematol 1995;71(6):311–2.
38. Ohno R, Tomonaga M, Ohshima T, et al. A randomized controlled study of granulocyte colony stimulating factor after intensive induction and consolidation therapy in patients with acute lymphoblastic leukemia. Japan Adult Leukemia Study Group. Int J Hematol 1993;58(1–2):73–81.
39. Larson RA, Dodge RK, Linker CA, et al. A randomized controlled trial of filgrastim during remission induction and consolidation chemotherapy for adults with acute lymphoblastic leukemia: CALGB study 9111. Blood 1998;92(5): 1556–64.
40. Giebel S, Holowiecki J, Krawczyk-Kulis M, et al. Impact of granulocyte colony stimulating factor administered during induction and consolidation of adults with acute lymphoblastic leukemia on survival: long-term follow-up of the Polish adult leukemia group 4-96 study. Leuk Lymphoma 2009;50(6):1050–3.
41. Nowak-Gottl U, Ahlke E, Fleischhack G, et al. Thromboembolic events in children with acute lymphoblastic leukemia (BFM protocols): prednisone versus dexamethasone administration. Blood 2003;101(7):2529–33.
42. Igarashi S, Manabe A, Ohara A, et al. No advantage of dexamethasone over prednisolone for the outcome of standard- and intermediate-risk childhood acute lymphoblastic leukemia in the Tokyo Children's Cancer Study Group L95-14 protocol. J Clin Oncol 2005;23(27):6489–98.
43. Takeuchi J, Kyo T, Naito K, et al. Induction therapy by frequent administration of doxorubicin with four other drugs, followed by intensive consolidation and maintenance therapy for adult acute lymphoblastic leukemia: the JALSG-ALL93 study. Leukemia 2002;16(7):1259–66.
44. Kantarjian H, Thomas D, O'Brien S, et al. Long-term follow-up results of hyperfractionated cyclophosphamide, vincristine, doxorubicin, and dexamethasone (Hyper-CVAD), a dose-intensive regimen, in adult acute lymphocytic leukemia. Cancer 2004;101(12):2788–801.
45. Gokbuget N, Hoelzer D, Arnold R, et al. Treatment of Adult ALL according to protocols of the German Multicenter Study Group for Adult ALL (GMALL). Hematol Oncol Clin North Am 2000;14(6):1307–25, ix.
46. Fiere D, Lepage E, Sebban C, et al. Adult acute lymphoblastic leukemia: a multicentric randomized trial testing bone marrow transplantation as postremission therapy. The French Group on Therapy for Adult Acute Lymphoblastic Leukemia. J Clin Oncol 1993;11(10):1990–2001.
47. Annino L, Vegna ML, Camera A, et al. Treatment of adult acute lymphoblastic leukemia (ALL): long-term follow-up of the GIMEMA ALL 0288 randomized study. Blood 2002;99(3):863–71.
48. Thomas D, O'Brien S, Faderl S, et al. Anthracycline dose intensification in adult acute lymphoblastic leukemia: lack of benefit in the context of the fractionated cyclophosphamide, vincristine, doxorubicin, and dexamethasone regimen. Cancer 2010;116(19):4580–9.
49. Stock W, Douer D, Deangelo DJ, et al. Prevention and management of asparaginase/pegasparaginase-associated toxicities in adults and older adolescents: recommendations of an expert panel. Leuk Lymphoma 2011. [Epub ahead of print].

50. Steiner M, Attarbaschi A, Haas OA, et al. Fresh frozen plasma contains free asparagine and may replace the plasma asparagine pool during L-asparaginase therapy. Leukemia 2008;22(6):1290.

51. Hunault-Berger M, Chevallier P, Delain M, et al. Changes in antithrombin and fibrinogen levels during induction chemotherapy with L-asparaginase in adult patients with acute lymphoblastic leukemia or lymphoblastic lymphoma. Use of supportive coagulation therapy and clinical outcome: the CAPELAL study. Haematologica 2008;93(10):1488–94.

52. Avramis VI, Panosyan EH. Pharmacokinetic/pharmacodynamic relationships of asparaginase formulations: the past, the present and recommendations for the future. Clin Pharmacokinet 2005;44(4):367–93.

53. Avramis VI, Sencer S, Periclou AP, et al. A randomized comparison of native Escherichia coli asparaginase and polyethylene glycol conjugated asparaginase for treatment of children with newly diagnosed standard-risk acute lymphoblastic leukemia: a Children's Cancer Group study. Blood 2002;99(6):1986–94.

54. Silverman LB, Supko JG, Stevenson KE, et al. Intravenous PEG-asparaginase during remission induction in children and adolescents with newly diagnosed acute lymphoblastic leukemia. Blood 2010;115(7):1351–3.

55. Wetzler M, Sanford BL, Kurtzberg J, et al. Effective asparagine depletion with pegylated asparaginase results in improved outcomes in adult acute lymphoblastic leukemia—Cancer and Leukemia Group B Study 9511. Blood 2007; 109(10):4164–7.

56. Piatkowska-Jakubas B, Krawczyk-Kulis M, Giebel S, et al. Use of L-asparaginase in acute lymphoblastic leukemia: recommendations of the Polish Adult Leukemia Group. Pol Arch Med Wewn 2008;118(11):664–9.

57. Kearney SL, Dahlberg SE, Levy DE, et al. Clinical course and outcome in children with acute lymphoblastic leukemia and asparaginase-associated pancreatitis. Pediatr Blood Cancer 2009;53(2):162–7.

58. Hill FG, Richards S, Gibson B, et al. Successful treatment without cranial radiotherapy of children receiving intensified chemotherapy for acute lymphoblastic leukaemia: results of the risk-stratified randomized central nervous system treatment trial MRC UKALL XI (ISRC TN 16757172). Br J Haematol 2004;124(1): 33–46.

59. Tubergen DG, Gilchrist GS, O'Brien RT, et al. Prevention of CNS disease in intermediate-risk acute lymphoblastic leukemia: comparison of cranial radiation and intrathecal methotrexate and the importance of systemic therapy: a Childrens Cancer Group report. J Clin Oncol 1993;11(3):520–6.

60. Aradillas E, Arora R, Gasperino J. Methotrexate-induced posterior reversible encephalopathy syndrome. J Clin Pharm Ther 2011;36(4):529–36.

61. Inaba H, Khan RB, Laningham FH, et al. Clinical and radiological characteristics of methotrexate-induced acute encephalopathy in pediatric patients with cancer. Ann Oncol 2008;19(1):178–84.

62. Jinnai I, Sakura T, Tsuzuki M, et al. Intensified consolidation therapy with dose-escalated doxorubicin did not improve the prognosis of adults with acute lymphoblastic leukemia: the JALSG-ALL97 study. Int J Hematol 2010;92(3): 490–502.

63. Ribera JM, Ortega JJ, Oriol A, et al. Late intensification chemotherapy has not improved the results of intensive chemotherapy in adult acute lymphoblastic leukemia. Results of a prospective multicenter randomized trial (PETHEMA ALL-89). Spanish Society of Hematology. Haematologica 1998;83(3):222–30.

64. Goldstone AH, Richards SM, Lazarus HM, et al. In adults with standard-risk acute lymphoblastic leukemia, the greatest benefit is achieved from a matched sibling allogeneic transplantation in first complete remission, and an autologous transplantation is less effective than conventional consolidation/maintenance chemotherapy in all patients: final results of the International ALL Trial (MRC UKALL XII/ECOG E2993). Blood 2008;111(4):1827–33.

65. Dahlke J, Kroger N, Zabelina T, et al. Comparable results in patients with acute lymphoblastic leukemia after related and unrelated stem cell transplantation. Bone Marrow Transplant 2006;37(2):155–63.

66. Cornelissen JJ, Carston M, Kollman C, et al. Unrelated marrow transplantation for adult patients with poor-risk acute lymphoblastic leukemia: strong graft-versus-leukemia effect and risk factors determining outcome. Blood 2001;97(6):1572–7.

67. Kiehl MG, Kraut L, Schwerdtfeger R, et al. Outcome of allogeneic hematopoietic stem-cell transplantation in adult patients with acute lymphoblastic leukemia: no difference in related compared with unrelated transplant in first complete remission. J Clin Oncol 2004;22(14):2816–25.

68. Dombret H, Gabert J, Boiron JM, et al. Outcome of treatment in adults with Philadelphia chromosome-positive acute lymphoblastic leukemia—results of the prospective multicenter LALA-94 trial. Blood 2002;100(7):2357–66.

69. Forman SJ, O'Donnell MR, Nademanee AP, et al. Bone marrow transplantation for patients with Philadelphia chromosome-positive acute lymphoblastic leukemia. Blood 1987;70(2):587–8.

70. Chao NJ, Blume KG, Forman SJ, et al. Long-term follow-up of allogeneic bone marrow recipients for Philadelphia chromosome-positive acute lymphoblastic leukemia. Blood 1995;85(11):3353–4.

71. Barrett AJ, Horowitz MM, Ash RC, et al. Bone marrow transplantation for Philadelphia chromosome-positive acute lymphoblastic leukemia. Blood 1992;79(11):3067–70.

72. Snyder DS, Nademanee AP, O'Donnell MR, et al. Long-term follow-up of 23 patients with Philadelphia chromosome-positive acute lymphoblastic leukemia treated with allogeneic bone marrow transplant in first complete remission. Leukemia 1999;13(12):2053–8.

73. Cornelissen J, Van Der Holt B, Verhoef G, et al. Myeloablative allogeneic versus autologous stem cell transplantation in adult patients with acute lymphoblastic leukemia in first remission: a prospective sibling donor versus no-donor comparison. Blood 2009;113(6):1375–82.

74. Yanada M, Matsuo K, Suzuki T, et al. Allogeneic hematopoietic stem cell transplantation as part of postremission therapy improves survival for adult patients with high-risk acute lymphoblastic leukemia: a metaanalysis. Cancer 2006;106(12):2657–63.

75. Ribera JM, Oriol A, Sanz MA, et al. Comparison of the results of the treatment of adolescents and young adults with standard-risk acute lymphoblastic leukemia with the Programa Espanol de Tratamiento en Hematologia pediatric-based protocol ALL-96. J Clin Oncol 2008;26(11):1843–9.

76. Blume KG, Schmidt GM, Chao NJ, et al. Bone marrow transplantation from histocompatible sibling donors for patients with acute lymphoblastic leukemia. Haematol Blood Transfus 1990;33:636–7.

77. Gassas A, Sung L, Saunders EF, et al. Comparative outcome of hematopoietic stem cell transplantation for pediatric acute lymphoblastic leukemia following cyclophosphamide and total body irradiation or VP16 and total body irradiation conditioning regimens. Bone Marrow Transplant 2006;38(11):739–43.

78. Marks DI, Forman SJ, Blume KG, et al. A comparison of cyclophosphamide and total body irradiation with etoposide and total body irradiation as conditioning regimens for patients undergoing sibling allografting for acute lymphoblastic leukemia in first or second complete remission. Biol Blood Marrow Transplant 2006;12(4):438–53.
79. Worthington HV, Clarkson JE, Eden OB, et al. Interventions for preventing oral mucositis for patients with cancer receiving treatment. Cochrane Database Syst Rev 2011;4:CD000978.
80. Patel B, Kirkland KE, Szydlo R, et al. Favorable outcomes with alemtuzumab-conditioned unrelated donor stem cell transplantation in adults with high-risk Philadelphia chromosome-negative acute lymphoblastic leukemia in first complete remission. Haematologica 2009;94(10):1399–406.
81. Marks DI, Perez WS, He W, et al. Unrelated donor transplants in adults with Philadelphia-negative acute lymphoblastic leukemia in first complete remission. Blood 2008;112(2):426–34.
82. Marks DI, Aversa F, Lazarus HM. Alternative donor transplants for adult acute lymphoblastic leukaemia: a comparison of the three major options. Bone Marrow Transplant 2006;38(7):467–75.
83. Mohty M, Labopin M, Tabrizzi R, et al. Reduced intensity conditioning allogeneic stem cell transplantation for adult patients with acute lymphoblastic leukemia: a retrospective study from the European Group for Blood and Marrow Transplantation. Haematologica 2008;93(2):303–6.
84. Arnold R, Massenkeil G, Bornhauser M, et al. Nonmyeloablative stem cell transplantation in adults with high-risk ALL may be effective in early but not in advanced disease. Leukemia 2002;16(12):2423–8.
85. Martino R, Giralt S, Caballero MD, et al. Allogeneic hematopoietic stem cell transplantation with reduced-intensity conditioning in acute lymphoblastic leukemia: a feasibility study. Haematologica 2003;88(5):555–60.
86. Stein A, O'Donnell M, Snyder DS, et al. Reduced-intensity stem cell tansplantation for high-risk acute lymphoblastic leukaemia. Biol Blood Marrow Transplant 2007;13:134.
87. Bachanova V, Verneris MR, DeFor T, et al. Prolonged survival in adults with acute lymphoblastic leukemia after reduced-intensity conditioning with cord blood or sibling donor transplantation. Blood 2009;113(13):2902–5.
88. Ram R, Storb R, Sandmaier BM, et al. Non-myeloablative conditioning with allogeneic hematopoietic cell transplantation for the treatment of high-risk acute lymphoblastic leukemia. Haematologica 2011;96(8):1113–20.
89. Clarke M, Gaynon P, Hann I, et al. CNS-directed therapy for childhood acute lymphoblastic leukemia: Childhood ALL Collaborative Group overview of 43 randomized trials. J Clin Oncol 2003;21(9):1798–809.
90. Jabbour E, O'Brien S, Kantarjian H, et al. Neurologic complications associated with intrathecal liposomal cytarabine given prophylactically in combination with high-dose methotrexate and cytarabine to patients with acute lymphocytic leukemia. Blood 2007;109(8):3214–8.
91. Mitchell CD, Richards SM, Kinsey SE, et al. Benefit of dexamethasone compared with prednisolone for childhood acute lymphoblastic leukaemia: results of the UK Medical Research Council ALL97 randomized trial. Br J Haematol 2005;129(6):734–45.
92. Lazarus HM, Richards SM, Chopra R, et al. Central nervous system involvement in adult acute lymphoblastic leukemia at diagnosis: results from the international ALL trial MRC UKALL XII/ECOG E2993. Blood 2006;108(2):465–72.

93. de Bont JM, Holt B, Dekker AW, et al. Significant difference in outcome for adolescents with acute lymphoblastic leukemia treated on pediatric vs adult protocols in the Netherlands. Leukemia 2004;18(12):2032–5.

94. Hallbook H, Gustafsson G, Smedmyr B, et al. Treatment outcome in young adults and children >10 years of age with acute lymphoblastic leukemia in Sweden: a comparison between a pediatric protocol and an adult protocol. Cancer 2006;107(7):1551–61.

95. Ramanujachar R, Richards S, Hann I, et al. Adolescents with acute lymphoblastic leukaemia: Emerging from the shadow of paediatric and adult treatment protocols. Pediatr Blood Cancer 2006;47(6):748–56.

96. Rijneveld AW, van der Holt B, Daenen SM, et al. Intensified chemotherapy inspired by a pediatric regimen combined with allogeneic transplantation in adult patients with acute lymphoblastic leukemia up to the age of 40. Leukemia 2011. [Epub ahead of print].

97. Boissel N, Auclerc MF, Lheritier V, et al. Should adolescents with acute lymphoblastic leukemia be treated as old children or young adults? Comparison of the French FRALLE-93 and LALA-94 trials. J Clin Oncol 2003;21(5):774–80.

98. Huguet F, Leguay T, Raffoux E, et al. Pediatric-inspired therapy in adults with Philadelphia chromosome-negative acute lymphoblastic leukemia: the GRAALL-2003 study. J Clin Oncol 2009;27(6):911–8.

99. Stock W, La M, Sanford B, et al. What determines the outcomes for adolescents and young adults with acute lymphoblastic leukemia treated on cooperative group protocols? A comparison of Children's Cancer Group and Cancer and Leukemia Group B studies. Blood 2008;112(5):1646–54.

100. Moorman AV, Chilton L, Wilkinson J, et al. A population-based cytogenetic study of adults with acute lymphoblastic leukemia. Blood 2010;115(2):206–14.

101. Hussein KK, Dahlberg S, Head D, et al. Treatment of acute lymphoblastic leukemia in adults with intensive induction, consolidation, and maintenance chemotherapy. Blood 1989;73(1):57–63.

102. Kantarjian HM, O'Brien S, Smith TL, et al. Results of treatment with hyper-CVAD, a dose-intensive regimen, in adult acute lymphocytic leukemia. J Clin Oncol 2000;18(3):547–61.

103. Sive JI, Buck G, Fielding AK, et al. Inability to tolerate standard therapy is a major reason for poor outcome in older adults with Acute Lymphoblastic Leukemia (ALL): results from the international MRC/ECOG trial. Blood 2010;116:493.

104. Taylor PR, Reid MM, Bown N, et al. Acute lymphoblastic leukemia in patients aged 60 years and over: a population-based study of incidence and outcome. Blood 1992;80(7):1813–7.

105. Hunault-Berger M, Leguay T, Thomas X, et al. A randomized study of pegylated liposomal doxorubicin versus continuous-infusion doxorubicin in elderly patients with acute lymphoblastic leukemia: the GRAALL-SA1 study. Haematologica 2011;96(2):245–52.

106. Wassmann B, Pfeifer H, Goekbuget N, et al. Alternating versus concurrent schedules of imatinib and chemotherapy as front-line therapy for Philadelphia-positive acute lymphoblastic leukemia (Ph+ ALL). Blood 2006;108(5):1469–77.

107. Vignetti M, Fazi P, Cimino G, et al. Imatinib plus steroids induces complete remissions and prolonged survival in elderly Philadelphia chromosome-positive patients with acute lymphoblastic leukemia without additional chemotherapy: results of the Gruppo Italiano Malattie Ematologiche dell'Adulto (GIMEMA) LAL0201-B protocol. Blood 2007;109(9):3676–8.

108. Fielding AK. Current treatment of Philadelphia chromosome-positive acute lymphoblastic leukemia. Haematologica 2010;95(1):8–12.
109. Fielding AK. How I treat Philadelphia chromosome-positive acute lymphoblastic leukemia. Blood 2010;116(18):3409–17.
110. Gruber F, Mustjoki S, Porkka K. Impact of tyrosine kinase inhibitors on patient outcomes in Philadelphia chromosome-positive acute lymphoblastic leukaemia. Br J Haematol 2009;145(5):581–97.
111. Bassan R, Rossi G, Pogliani EM, et al. Chemotherapy-phased imatinib pulses improve long-term outcome of adult patients with Philadelphia chromosome-positive acute lymphoblastic leukemia: Northern Italy Leukemia Group protocol 09/00. J Clin Oncol 2010;28(22):3644–52.
112. Chalandon Y, Thomas X, Hayette S, et al. First results of the GRAAPH-2005 study in younger adult patients with de novo Philadelphia positive acute lymphoblastic leukemia. Blood 2008;112 [abstract 12].
113. Fielding AK, Buck G, Lazarus H, et al. Imatinib significantly enhances long-term outcomes in Philadelphia positive acute lymphoblastic leukaemia; final results of the UKALLXII/ECOG2993 Trial. Blood 2010;116:493.
114. Ottmann OG, Wassmann B, Pfeifer H, et al. Imatinib compared with chemotherapy as front-line treatment of elderly patients with Philadelphia chromosome-positive acute lymphoblastic leukemia (Ph+ALL). Cancer 2007; 109(10):2068–76.
115. Ribera JM, Oriol A, Gonzalez M, et al. Concurrent intensive chemotherapy and imatinib before and after stem cell transplantation in newly diagnosed Philadelphia chromosome-positive acute lymphoblastic leukemia. Final results of the CSTIBES02 trial. Haematologica 2010;95(1):87–95.
116. Schultz K, Bowman W, Aledo A, et al. Improved early event-free survival with imatinib in Philadelphia chromosome-positive acute lymphoblastic leukemia: a children's oncology group study. J Clin Oncol 2009;27(31):5175–81.
117. Thomas DA, Faderl S, Cortes J, et al. Treatment of Philadelphia chromosome-positive acute lymphocytic leukemia with hyper-CVAD and imatinib mesylate. Blood 2004;103(12):4396–407.
118. Yanada M, Takeuchi J, Sugiura I, et al. High complete remission rate and promising outcome by combination of imatinib and chemotherapy for newly diagnosed BCR-ABL-positive acute lymphoblastic leukemia: a phase II study by the Japan Adult Leukemia Study Group. J Clin Oncol 2006;24(3):460–6.
119. Pfeifer H, Goekbuget N, Volp C, et al. Long-term outcome of 335 adult patients receiving Different schedules of imatinib and chemotherapy as front-line treatment for Philadelphia-positive acute lymphoblastic leukemia (Ph+ ALL). Blood 2010;116:173.
120. Soverini S, Vitale A, Poerio A, et al. Philadelphia-positive acute lymphoblastic leukemia patients already harbor BCR-ABL kinase domain mutations at low levels at the time of diagnosis. Haematologica 2011;96(4):552–7.
121. Lee S, Kim DW, Cho B, et al. Risk factors for adults with Philadelphia-chromosome-positive acute lymphoblastic leukaemia in remission treated with allogeneic bone marrow transplantation: the potential of real-time quantitative reverse-transcription polymerase chain reaction. Br J Haematol 2003;120(1):145–53.
122. Pane F, Cimino G, Izzo B, et al. Significant reduction of the hybrid BCR/ABL transcripts after induction and consolidation therapy is a powerful predictor of treatment response in adult Philadelphia-positive acute lymphoblastic leukemia. Leukemia 2005;19(4):628–35.

123. Preudhomme C, Henic N, Cazin B, et al. Good correlation between RT-PCR analysis and relapse in Philadelphia (Ph1)-positive acute lymphoblastic leukemia (ALL). Leukemia 1997;11(2):294–8.

124. Yanada M, Sugiura I, Takeuchi J, et al. Prospective monitoring ofBCR-ABL1transcript levels in patients with Philadelphia chromosome-positive acute lymphoblastic leukaemia undergoing imatinib-combined chemotherapy. Br J Haematol 2008;143(3):503–10.

125. Hu Y, Liu Y, Pelletier S, et al. Requirement of Src kinases Lyn, Hck and Fgr for BCR-ABL1-induced B-lymphoblastic leukemia but not chronic myeloid leukemia. Nat Genet 2004;36(5):453–61.

126. Ravandi F, O'Brien S, Thomas D, et al. First report of phase 2 study of dasatinib with hyper-CVAD for the frontline treatment of patients with Philadelphia chromosome-positive (Ph+) acute lymphoblastic leukemia. Blood 2010; 116(12):2070–7.

127. Ottmann O, Dombret H, Martinelli G, et al. Dasatinib induces rapid hematologic and cytogenetic responses in adult patients with Philadelphia chromosome positive acute lymphoblastic leukemia with resistance or intolerance to imatinib: interim results of a phase 2 study. Blood 2007;110(7):2309–15.

128. Porkka K, Koskenvesa P, Lundan T, et al. Dasatinib crosses the blood-brain barrier and is an efficient therapy for central nervous system Philadelphia chromosome-positive leukemia. Blood 2008;112(4):1005–12.

129. Cortes J, Talpaz M, Bixby D, et al. A phase 1 trial of oral ponatinib (AP24534) in patients with refractory chronic myelogenous leukemia (CML) and other hematologic malignancies: emerging safety and clinical response findings. Blood 2010;116(21):210.

130. Topp MS, Kufer P, Gokbuget N, et al. Targeted therapy with the T-cell-engaging antibody blinatumomab of chemotherapy-refractory minimal residual disease in B-lineage acute lymphoblastic leukemia patients results in high response rate and prolonged leukemia-free survival. J Clin Oncol 2011;29(18):2493–8.

131. Garcia-Manero G, Thomas DA. Salvage therapy for refractory or relapsed acute lymphocytic leukemia. Hematol Oncol Clin North Am 2001;15(1):163–205.

132. Giona F, Annino L, Rondelli R, et al. Treatment of adults with acute lymphoblastic leukaemia in first bone marrow relapse: results of the ALL R-87 protocol. Br J Haematol 1997;97(4):896–903.

133. Koller CA, Kantarjian HM, Thomas D, et al. The hyper-CVAD regimen improves outcome in relapsed acute lymphoblastic leukemia. Leukemia 1997;11(12): 2039–44.

134. Montillo M, Tedeschi A, Centurioni R, et al. Treatment of relapsed adult acute lymphoblastic leukemia with fludarabine and cytosine arabinoside followed by granulocyte colony-stimulating factor (FLAG-GCSF). Leuk Lymphoma 1997; 25(5–6):579–83.

135. Thomas DA, Kantarjian H, Smith TL, et al. Primary refractory and relapsed adult acute lymphoblastic leukemia: characteristics, treatment results, and prognosis with salvage therapy. Cancer 1999;86(7):1216–30.

136. Fielding AK, Richards SM, Chopra R, et al. Outcome of 609 adults after relapse of acute lymphoblastic leukemia (ALL); an MRC UKALL12/ECOG 2993 study. Blood 2007;109(3):944–50.

137. Oriol A, Vives S, Hernandez-Rivas JM, et al. Outcome after relapse of acute lymphoblastic leukemia in adult patients included in four consecutive risk-adapted trials by the PETHEMA Study Group. Haematologica 2010;95(4): 589–96.

138. Tavernier E, Boiron JM, Huguet F, et al. Outcome of treatment after first relapse in adults with acute lymphoblastic leukemia initially treated by the LALA-94 trial. Leukemia 2007;21(9):1907–14.

139. Kawedia JD, Kaste SC, Pei D, et al. Pharmacokinetic, pharmacodynamic, and pharmacogenetic determinants of osteonecrosis in children with acute lympho-blastic leukemia. Blood 2011;117(8):2340–7 [quiz: 2556].

140. Patel B, Richards SM, Rowe JM, et al. High incidence of avascular necrosis in adolescents with acute lymphoblastic leukaemia: a UKALL XII analysis. Leukemia 2008;22(2):308–12.

141. Haajanen J, Saarinen O, Laasonen L, et al. Steroid treatment and aseptic necrosis of the femoral head in renal transplant recipients. Transplant Proc 1984;16(5):1316–9.

142. Ruderman RJ, Poehling GG, Gray R, et al. Orthopedic complications of renal transplantation in children. Transplant Proc 1979;11(1):104–6.

143. Neglia JP, Meadows AT, Robison LL, et al. Second neoplasms after acute lymphoblastic leukemia in childhood. N Engl J Med 1991;325(19):1330–6.

144. Tavernier E, Le QH, de Botton S, et al. Secondary or concomitant neoplasms among adults diagnosed with acute lymphoblastic leukemia and treated ac-cording to the LALA-87 and LALA-94 trials. Cancer 2007;110(12):2747–55.

Cellular Therapies in Acute Lymphoblastic Leukemia

Jae H. Park, MD[a,b], Craig Sauter, MD[b,c],
Renier Brentjens, MD, PhD[b,d],*

KEYWORDS

- Acute lymphoblastic leukemia • Adoptive cellular therapy
- Hematopoietic stem cell transplants
- Chimeric antigen receptor

In general, adult patients diagnosed with acute lymphoblastic leukemia (ALL) have a poor prognosis. Overall, more than 6 of 10 adult patients diagnosed with ALL will ultimately die of the disease.[1] The prognosis is more favorable in the pediatric population, with greater than 8 of 10 patients experiencing long-term survival.[1,2] In most cases, up-front therapy involves long-term, toxic, and complex chemotherapy regimens. However, for adult and pediatric patients, failure to experience response to up-front chemotherapy or disease relapse after remission portends a dismal prognosis.[3–5] These findings suggest that novel approaches to adoptive cell therapies are needed to improve the outcome of patients with ALL. Recent advances in the understanding of tumor biology and immunology, combined with enhanced gene transfer technologies, have increased the interest in the field of adoptive cell therapy among investigators seeking alternative treatment approaches for this disease.

HEMATOPOIETIC STEM CELL TRANSPLANTATION

Allogeneic hematopoietic stem cell transplantation (allo-HSCT) is the earliest and most studied form of adoptive cell therapy for leukemia. The original guiding principle of

Drs Park and Sauter contributed equally to this publication.
The authors disclose no competing financial interests.
[a] Leukemia Service, Department of Medicine, Memorial Sloan-Kettering Cancer Center, 1275 York Avenue, Box 569, New York, NY 10065, USA
[b] Department of Medicine, Weill Cornell Medical College, 1300 York Avenue New York, NY 10065, USA
[c] Bone Marrow Transplant Service, Department of Medicine, Memorial Sloan-Kettering Cancer Center, 1275 York Avenue, Box 276, New York, NY 10065, USA
[d] Leukemia Service, Department of Medicine, Memorial Sloan-Kettering Cancer Center, 410 East, 68th Street, Box 242, New York, NY 10065, USA
* Corresponding author. Leukemia Service, Department of Medicine, Memorial Sloan-Kettering Cancer Center, 410 East, 68th Street, Box 242, New York, NY 10065.
E-mail address: brentjer@mskcc.org

Hematol Oncol Clin N Am 25 (2011) 1281–1301
doi:10.1016/j.hoc.2011.09.015
0889-8588/11/$ – see front matter © 2011 Elsevier Inc. All rights reserved.

allo-HSCT was that it allows for higher-dose chemotherapy with or without additional total body irradiation, ideally resulting in consequent ablation of both tumor and normal bone marrow stem cells, the latter of which is subsequently rescued by the infusion of nonmalignant hematopoietic stem cells from a healthy allogeneic donor. Clinical studies of allo-HSCT illustrate an additional immunologic benefit of this approach, wherein donor T cells may mediate a beneficial graft-versus-leukemia (GvL) effect through donor T cells recognizing antigens present on residual tumor cells. This GvL effect was first described in patients with acute leukemia, including ALL,[6] and is best illustrated by higher relapse rates in patients who have received donor grafts from identical twin siblings and patients treated with T-cell–depleted grafts designed to minimize graft-versus-host disease (GvHD).[7] Consistent with this donor T-cell–mediated GvL effect is the finding that patients who experience acute or chronic GvHD after allo-HSCT are less likely to experience disease relapse compared with those who experience little or no GvHD after treatment.[7] Unfortunately, because this GvL benefit is met with the untoward consequences of GvHD and associated morbidity and mortality, the benefit of allo-HSCT remains debatable.

Human Leukocyte Antigen–Matched Donor Allo-HSCT in ALL as First Remission Therapy

Although a large body of clinical data exists using myeloablative, matched related donor allo-HSCT in patients with ALL, debate remains regarding the use of matched related donor allo-HSCT as a postremission therapy in the setting of adult patients with ALL. Based on the poor overall prognosis of this disease, the contention remains that all patients with a suitable matched related donor should undergo allo-HSCT. However, this contention should take into account the significant treatment-related mortality of 20% to 30% associated with allo-HSCT[8] in addition to quality-of-life considerations. Moreover, patients' age and comorbidities must be carefully considered when determining transplant eligibility to achieve the potential benefit of this modality in terms of overall survival.

Most patients with ALL (>80%), adult and pediatric, will experience disease remission after one or two cycles of induction chemotherapy.[1] Whether patients in first complete remission benefit with matched related donor HSCT versus chemotherapy alone in the adult ALL setting is a critical question with conflicting answers. Adult patients with ALL traditionally have been divided into standard- and high-risk groups based on several clinical and genetic criteria. High-risk patients are variably defined as those older than 35 years, with an elevated white blood cell count at diagnosis, a delayed response (>28 days) after initial induction chemotherapy, and with genetically adverse features, including the presence of the Philadelphia chromosome (Ph+), t(1;19), and t(4;11). In high-risk transplant-eligible patients, myeloablative matched related donor allo-HSCT is currently the preferred consolidation treatment in the setting of first complete remission,[9] given several large clinical trials and a meta-analysis showing benefit compared with either chemotherapy alone or autologous HSCT.[10–13] However, in contrast to these findings, data from the PETHEMA ALL-93 trial and the international collaborative trial conducted by the Medical Research Council (MRC) and the Eastern Cooperative Oncology Group (ECOG), MRC UKALL XII/ECOG E2993, failed to show a similar advantage for patients with high risk disease, again placing the role of matched related donor HSCT for high-risk patients into question.[14,15]

The high-risk category of patients with ALL harboring Ph+ deserves a separate discussion for several reasons, including (1) poor prognosis predominately secondary to relative chemoinsensitivity,[16] (2) predilection for older patients who may not be able to tolerate intensive therapy, and (3) opportunity for targeted tyrosine kinase inhibitor (TKI) therapy (imatinib, dasatinib, and nilotinib). Before the incorporation of TKIs into treatment regimens, patients with Ph⁺ ALL fared poorly in the setting of matched related donor HSCT. However, one recently published report of data generated by the MRC UKALL XII/ECOG E2993 showed a significantly improved relapse-free survival in patients with Ph⁺ ALL after matched unrelated donor or matched related donor HSCT when compared with chemotherapy alone, before the use of a TKI.[16] Although this is the largest prospective study evaluating chemotherapy versus allo-HSCT as postremission consolidation for Ph+ ALL, it has important limitations. Given the age restriction for allo-HSCT on the study (of patients receiving allo-HSCT, 95% were younger than 50 years), the patients who received chemotherapy alone were significantly older than those that received allo-HSCT ($P = .004$), which may introduce a potentially large confounder effect, because age was a significant prognostic factor in the multivariate analysis. Additionally, further analysis through intent-to-treat showed nonsignificant differences between the groups, again speaking to the relative chemo-insensitive nature of Ph⁺ ALL and the intolerance of therapy among advanced-age patients with this disease phenotype.

TKIs in combination with chemotherapy has become an accepted standard of care for inducing remission in patients with Ph⁺ ALL, showing significant improvements in complete remission rates compared with chemotherapy-only historical controls.[17] The low toxicity of an adjunctive TKI with combination chemotherapy seems to offer access to allo-HSCT for this high-risk and typically advanced-age patient cohort. Considering intent-to-treat models, the efficacy of TKI therapy for patients with Ph⁺ ALL necessitates reevaluation of the role of allo-HSCT in this disease phenotype. Early results of allo-HSCT in patients with high-risk Ph⁺ disease treated with a TKI during induction and consolidation before transplantation suggest that adding imatinib before allo-HSCT results in favorable complete remission rates and seems to offer improved disease-free and overall survivals after allo-HSCT transplantation compared with historical controls.[18,19] More recent studies of a larger Ph⁺ patient cohorts have confirmed favorable outcomes of TKI in combination with chemotherapy followed by transplantation. In the MRC UKALL XII/ECOG E2993 series, patients randomized to allo-HSCT in the post-TKI era had improved 3-year overall survival compared with patients randomized to allo-HCT pre-TKI based on the same complete remission criteria (56% vs 40%).[20] Lastly, a study from Japan showed added efficacy of TKI in patients experiencing first complete remission before myeloablative allo-HSCT compared with pre-TKI historic controls (3-year overall survival, 65% and 44%, respectively; $P = .005$).[21]

The more contentious debate has been the role of allo-HSCT in standard-risk adult patients experiencing first complete remission. The largest prospective randomized trial to attempt to answer this question was the MRC UKALL XII/ECOG E2993. In this trial, 1646 patients with Ph-negative ALL underwent a standardized induction, and those that experienced complete remission were biologically randomized to allo-HSCT if a matched related donor was identified and the patient was of appropriate myeloablative versus allo-HSCT age, either younger than 50 (ECOG) or 55 years (MRC), or chemotherapy/autologous HSCT if no matched related donor was identified. The standard-risk matched related donor allo-HSCT arm showed a 5-year overall survival of 62%, which was significantly better than 52% in the no-donor arm ($P = .02$).[14] Paradoxically, the high-risk Ph-negative patients did not derive significant advantage from allo-HSCT. In both high- and standard-risk groups, the relapse risk was significantly abrogated in the matched related donor allo-HSCT arm, lending credence to a GvL effect. Thus, this study may pose more questions than it answers, such as whether intensifying consolidation with allo-HSCT truly overcomes the poor prognosis of traditionally defined Ph-negative high-risk patients. Additionally, one could argue that, given the relative success of intensified pediatric-inspired chemotherapy programs,[22] the control chemotherapy group in this large randomized intent-to-treat study may have been suboptimally treated. Lastly, prognostic modeling has improved in the modern era. Thus, strategies to better risk-adapt patients in the hope of potentiating benefit from the toxicity of allo-HSCT consolidation based on clinical response to induction chemotherapy (ie, time to complete remission and minimal residual disease after completion of induction) are being largely adapted in clinical trials in Europe.[23–25] In addition to identifying the appropriate standard-risk patients in whom to escalate therapy with allo-HSCT,[26] high-risk patients may be afforded the opportunity to be spared allo-HSCT if prompt minimal residual disease-negative status is attained.[27] Thus, despite MRC/ECOG randomized data, the role of allo-HSCT in the contemporary era remains a point of discussion.

Unrelated Allo-HSCT and ALL

Overall, adult patients with ALL experiencing first complete remission seem to benefit from allo-HSCT from a matched related donor; unfortunately, only approximately one-third of these patients have an appropriate matched related donor. Therefore, most patients rely on identification of either an unrelated donor, an umbilical cord blood (UCB) donor, or a haploidentical donor. In all of these settings, one would expect that the risk of transplant-related mortality secondary to GvHD would be increased but with a consequently enhanced GvL effect. However, these presumptions are challenged by published data.

Historically, in the myeloablative setting, patients with a matched unrelated donor have fared poorly compared with those transplanted from a matched related donor secondary to increased transplant-related mortality associated with GvHD.[28,29] In the contemporary allo-HSCT era of more-resolute human leukocyte antigen (HLA)– matching criteria[30] and improved supportive care,[31] the differences in clinical outcome have become less appreciable between allo-HSCT from a matched related donor and that from a matched unrelated donor.[32–34] Several studies have addressed this question specifically in the setting of myeloablative allo-HSCT for ALL in first complete remission, showing similar transplant-related mortality, relapse rate, and ultimately overall survival when comparing patients with ALL who underwent either a matched related donor or a matched unrelated donor HSCT.[35–37] A recent study from Japan showed the traditionally increased risk of transplant-related mortality but concurrently reduced relapse rate in matched unrelated donor HSCT compared with matched related donor HSCT, illustrating the enhanced GvL and GvHD effects, resulting in comparable overall survival.[38] These data support the recommendation that eligible patients in first complete remission, with either a matched related donor or matched unrelated donor available, be considered for an allo-HSCT.

Alternative-Donor Allo-HSCT

Advances in alternative donor transplantation (ie, UCB and haploidentical allo-HSCT) offer another option for patients lacking a suitably matched related or unrelated donor. With increasing numbers of public cord blood banks, UCB in adults is becoming an increasingly viable option, with burgeoning data emerging in only the past 7 years.[39] The early experience showed lower than anticipated degrees of GvHD across greater HLA-barriers compared with traditional volunteer unrelated donor grafts.[40–42] A significant factor in transplant-related mortality is the total nucleated cell dose infused, with patients receiving less than 2×10^7/kg total nucleated cells exhibiting a higher incidence of graft failure and greater transplant-related mortality compared with those receiving grafts with greater than 2×10^7/kg total nucleated cells.[43,44] To overcome this limitation, many centers have adopted double-unit UCB transplants.[43,45] Studies have found that double-unit recipients seem to fare better than single-unit historical controls, despite most patients engrafting with only one of the two infused UCB units.[46] Theories of this benefit include reduced transplant-related mortality related to larger cell dose and brisk myeloid engraftment,[45] and enhanced GvL and subsequent protection from progression of primary hematologic malignancy.[47]

Because the field of UCB transplantation is new, most reports pool acute myeloid leukemia and ALL into a single category of patients with acute leukemia, causing recommendations regarding this modality in the specific setting of ALL to be difficult to make. However, recently reported outcomes of UCB HSCT in a large registry series compared favorably with bone marrow or peripheral blood stem cell allo-HSCT transplants in adult patients with acute leukemia.[48] In this series of more than 1500 patients, leukemia-free survival in patients who received UCB transplant mismatched at zero to two HLA loci was comparable to that of patients who received matched (8/8 HLA-allele matched) or mismatched (7/8 HLA-allele matched) volunteer unrelated donor transplants. Transplant-related mortality was significantly greater for patients who received UCB compared with 8/8 HLA-matched unrelated donors with both peripheral blood stem cell (hazard ratio [HR], 1.62; 95% CI, 1.18–2.23; $P = .003$) and bone marrow (HR, 1.69; 95% CI, 1.19–2.39; $P = .003$).

More recent published studies of UCB HSCTs have specifically focused on patients with ALL. In a large retrospective study recently published from Japan, no difference in transplant-related mortality or leukemia-free survival was seen between adult patients with ALL who received an UCB graft mismatched at up to two loci and matched or mismatched bone marrow grafts.[49] Kumar and colleagues[50] compared outcomes of patients with ALL receiving matched related donor HSCT, unrelated matched HSCT, mismatched HSCT, and matched or mismatched UCB transplants. The investigators surprisingly found superior 3-year overall survival rates in the UCB transplant group compared with all other treatment groups, and improved leukemia-free survival, lower relapse rates, and lower treatment-related mortality. The authors reported a statistically significant overall survival in patients with ALL treated with UCB transplant compared with those treated with unrelated donor HSCTs ($P = .01$). However, as the authors acknowledge, interpretation of these findings should be tempered by the low numbers of patients analyzed.

A final option for allo-HSCT in patients lacking related, unrelated, or UCB HSCT donors is a haploidentical donor HSCT. In this setting, virtually every patient has a suitable related donor (a parent or sibling). Not surprisingly, early studies using haploidentical HSCTs were hampered by significant incidences of GvHD and graft failure.[51] Over time, modifications in preparative conditioning regimens designed to optimize myeloablation and host immunosuppression, combined with enhanced techniques of T-cell depletion of the graft, and the infusion of markedly high doses of hematopoietic stem cells generated from the donor through mobilization with recombinant human granulocyte colony-stimulating factor, have led to a high rate of engraftment (>95%) with minimal GvHD even in the absence of immune suppression prophylaxis.[51–54] In a recently published report, patients with high-risk acute leukemias were evaluated after haploidentical HSCT. In patients with high-risk ALL treated with haploidentical HSCTs, Ciceri and colleagues[55] report a leukemia-free 2-year survival rate of 13% for those undergoing transplantation in first complete remission, 30% for those undergoing HSCT in second or further complete remission, and 7% in those undergoing HSCT in nonremission.

Enhanced survival of patients with ALL was recently reported in the setting of unmanipulated, non–T-cell depleted haploidentical HSCTs. Huang and colleagues[56] report more favorable leukemia-free survival in patients with ALL treated with unmanipulated haploidentical grafts, with a 3-year leukemia-free survival of 60% and 25% in those with standard-risk and high-risk disease, respectively. However, these improved survival rates were associated with increased incidences of GvHD. Debate continues regarding the use of haploidentical graft source as opposed to UCB, and vice versa.[57,58]

Reduced-Intensity Conditioning Allo-HSCT for Adult ALL

Given the typically higher-risk disease in a growing population of older, more-infirm patients with ALL, wherein myeloablative conditioning is prohibitively associated with exceedingly high transplant-related mortality, the need for extending allo-HSCT options with reduced-intensity conditioning has never been greater. This modality sacrifices disease control with reduced intensity of conditioning to minimize transplant-related mortality, thus relying more heavily on GvL. Thus, the gravity of disease control before allo-HSCT carries greater value to outcomes. The feasibility of this approach has been met with somewhat encouraging results given this high-risk patient population.[59–62] In a recent large retrospective series comparing reduced-intensity conditioning and myeloablative conditioning for Ph-negative ALL, although a trend was seen toward more frequent relapse with reduced-intensity conditioning (35% vs 28% for myeloablative conditioning; $P = .08$), no difference was seen in overall survival in multivariate analysis ($P = .92$).[63] The European Group for Blood and Marrow Transplantation registry data showed decreased nonrelapse mortality with reduced-intensity conditioning compared with myeloablative conditioning (21% vs 29%; $P = .03$), with an associated increased frequency of relapse (47% vs 31%; $P<.001$), resulting in a trend toward improved estimated 2-year leukemia-free survival with myeloablative compared with reduced-intensity conditioning ($P = .07$).[64] These data illustrate the improved safety of reduced-intensity conditioning at the expense of diminished disease control. Application of reduced-intensity conditioning with UCB transplantation to the older patient population with ALL may be feasible given data from Brunstein and colleagues[65] reporting on predominately double UCB transplants in older patients with hematologic malignancies. Overall, this approach was well tolerated, with modest treatment-related mortality at 3-year follow-up (26%) and promising overall and event-free survival rates (45% and 38%, respectively). A more recent publication from the same institution reported the results of 22 patients with ALL (21 in first complete remission) treated with the same reduced intensity conditioning regimen, followed by 4 of 22 patients receiving a matched related donor HSCT, whereas the remaining 18 patients received UCB donor grafts. Collectively, these older (median age, 49 years) high-risk patients (defined as Ph$^+$ [n = 14], and in second or further complete response [n = 10]) tolerated therapy well, with a treatment-related mortality rate of 27%, disease relapse rate of 36%, and promising overall survival rate at 3 years of 50%.[66] Interpretation of these data must be tempered by the small number of patients reported in this study, and requires further confirmation in larger prospective studies.

Novel Approaches to Lowering Risk of GvHD: T-Cell Depletion

With GvHD as the leading cause of transplant-related mortality in allo-HSCT, several groups have studied T-cell depletion of a conventional donor graft as a means of lowering the frequency of this often-fatal complication. The potential risks associated with this approach include increased risk of relapse with reduced GvL effect, and impaired immune reconstitution[67] leading to increased risk of infectious complications post–allo-HSCT. The group at Memorial Sloan-Kettering Cancer Center (MSKCC) recently reported results of 35 adult patients receiving unrelated donor allo-HSCT with ex vivo T-cell depletion for hematologic malignancies, including 13 patients with ALL in remission (3 in first remission, 7 in second complete remission, and 3 in third or further complete remission).[68] Eighteen donors were HLA disparate at 1 to 3 of 10 loci. Despite a large proportion of patients with high-risk ALL (complete remission >1), only one patient with ALL experienced relapse, and the relapse incidence of the entire cohort was 6%. The incidences of acute grade II through IV and chronic GvHD (9% and 29%, respectively) were much lower than historical controls with a non–T-cell depleted allo-HSCT, especially considering the proportion of mismatched donors in the cohort. Among the 35 patients, 5 deaths occurred.[68]

A British group recently reported on their experience with the use of the anti-CD52 antibody alemtuzumab as an in vivo T-cell depleted allo-HSCT in 48 high-risk Ph-negative patients in first complete remission, with one-third of the patients receiving HLA mismatched grafts.[69] The incidences of acute grade II through IV GvHD and extensive chronic GvHD were 27% and 22%, respectively. The overall survival rate for the entire group was 61% at 5 years. Both of these key studies show favorable disease-specific outcomes compared with conventional, non–T-cell depleted allo-HSCT, with a decreased incidence of GvHD. These encouraging results, however, still need to be validated in a randomized prospective fashion.

Allo-HSCT for Relapsed and Refractory Disease

Unfortunately, most patients with relapsed or refractory disease have a less than 50% chance of responding to salvage chemotherapy,[70] and their prognosis is extremely poor.[3] In patients with relapsed disease who have not previously received an allo-HSCT, have chemosensitive disease, have an appropriate HLA-matched donor, and lack prohibitive comorbidities, an allo-HSCT provides the only chance for long-term disease-free survival. For a multitude of reasons, the ability to match these conditions diminishes steeply in the relapsed and refractory setting. In a subset analysis from the MRC UKALL XII/ECOG E2993 study, patients with relapsed disease receiving an allo-HSCT from related or unrelated donors had improved overall survival at 5 years (23% and 16%, respectively) compared with those that did not proceed to allo-HSCT (4% overall survival at 5 years).[3] Despite the high potential of obvious confounders in this carefully selected subset of patients, the accepted standard is to proceed to allo-HSCT in chemosensitive relapsed and refractory ALL in those who are eligible, considering the incurability with chemotherapy alone.

NOVEL ADOPTIVE CELLULAR THERAPIES

Because of conflicting results of these clinical trials, the role of allo-HSCT for patients with ALL remains controversial. Furthermore, novel, less-tested approaches to allo-HSCT in ALL, including reduced-intensity conditioning, UCB, and haploidentical HSCTs, lack sufficient numbers or prospective studies to allow for definitive recommendations. Although these latter approaches and unrelated donor HSCT offer viable alternatives for patients requiring allo-HSCT but lacking a matched related donor, what is equally apparent is the fact that currently none of these alternative options offers improved outcomes. Therefore, alternative approaches to cell therapies are required for this patient population.

Donor Lymphocyte Infusion

Donor lymphocyte infusion has been shown to elicit a good response, mediated through a GvL effect, in patients with chronic myelogenous leukemia (CML) who experience relapse after allo-HSCT. However, this technique is rarely successful in relapsed ALL, with a reported long-term disease-free survival ranging from 0% to 13%.[71–75]

The reasons for the suboptimal response with donor lymphocyte infusion in ALL likely stem from several factors: a lack of adequate T-cell–mediated GvL, the delayed effects of donor lymphocyte infusion in patients with aggressive disease, or a lack of costimulatory molecule on the tumor.[73] Porter and colleagues[76] addressed the latter issue through treating seven patients with relapsed ALL post–allo-HSCT with donor lymphocytes that have been activated and costimulated ex vivo using CD3/CD28 agonist antibodies. In this phase I trial, four of the patients experienced a complete remission, but three of four patients experienced relapse, with only one patient alive in complete remission at more than 11 months, showing the limitation of the conventional donor lymphocyte infusion in relapsed ALL.

A modified approach to donor lymphocyte infusion is the enrichment of donor T cells targeted to antigens overexpressed on tumor cells. Wilms tumor 1 antigen (WT-1) is one antigen that is overexpressed on both acute myelogenous leukemia and ALL tumor cells.[77,78] WT-1 is immunogenic and may represent an attractive target for adoptive T-cell therapy, as suggested by a recent study by Rezvani and colleagues,[79] who reported WT-1 specific $CD8^+$ T-cell responses after allo-HSCT in five of seven patients, and a subsequent molecular disease relapse (ie, recurrent WT-1 transcript detection) associated with loss of detectable WT-1–specific $CD8^+$ T cells. Similarly, investigators at MSKCC and the Fred Hutchinson Cancer Research Center (FHCRC) have developed a way to enrich for WT-1–specific donor T-cell populations through co-culture of donor T cells on antigen-presenting cells pulsed with WT-1 peptides. Currently, both MSKCC (NCT00620633) and the FHCRC (NCT00052520) have open phase I clinical trials treating relapsed acute leukemias and myelodysplastic syndromes after allo-HSCT with WT-1–specific donor T cells. The completion of these trials will provide more information on the efficacy of tumor-specific alloreactive T cells in ALL.

Genetically Modified Tumor-Targeted T Cells

Given the limited GvL effect shown with donor T cells in ALL, several investigators have studied a novel form of adoptive cellular therapy through genetically modifying autologous T cells to target specific tumor antigens. One way of genetically modifying T cells is through gene transfer of the α and β chain subunits of the T-cell receptors derived from T-cell clones specific to tumor antigens.[80–82] This approach has been shown to be feasible in clinical trials of metastatic melanoma,[83,84] but published data using this approach in hematologic malignancies are limited.[85,86] Moreover, because the T-cell receptor gene transfer approach can only recognize tumor antigens that are processed and presented by HLA molecules, specificity of the T-cell receptor is restricted to specific patient HLA phenotypes and therefore lacks universal applicability. In addition, many tumor cells downregulate HLA molecules or have dysfunctional antigen-presenting machinery, so that the targeted tumor-derived peptides are often not adequately presented on the tumor cell surface.[87,88]

One way to circumvent these limitations of T-cell receptor gene transfer is the use of chimeric antigen receptors (CARs). CARs are composed of a single-chain variable-fragment (scFv) antibody specific to tumor antigen, fused to a transmembrane domain and a T-cell signaling moiety, most commonly either the CD3-ζ or Fc receptor γ cytoplasmic signaling domains.[89] The resulting receptor, when expressed on the surface of the T cell, mediates binding to the target tumor antigen through the scFv domain, which subsequently mediates an activating signal to the T cell, inducing target cell lysis.

The use of T cells engineered to express CARs has several advantages over conventional allo-HSCT. First, because this approach uses autologous patient-derived T cells, no risk of GvHD exists. Second, tumor-specific T cells may be rapidly generated ex vivo in the laboratory.[90] Third, because CAR recognition of target tumor antigen is HLA-independent, CAR-modified T cells can be applied to all HLA types and are less likely to generate resistant tumor cells through downregulation of HLA molecules. And lastly, CARs can be further modified to insert additional genes to express T-cell costimulatory molecules or proinflammatory cytokines to enhance antitumor efficacy.[91–95]

Genetically Modified T Cells in ALL

Although data are limited regarding the use of T-cell receptor gene transfer for genetic targeting of T cells in ALL, several groups, including the authors', have investigated the use of CARs as a method of adoptive cellular therapy for ALL.

The first requirement to redirect CAR-modified T cells toward a selected tumor cell is identification of an appropriate target molecule that is selectively expressed on cancer cells. With regard to ALL of B-cell origin, CD19 is an ideal target for several reasons: (1) in contrast to CD20, which is the target of current antibody-based immunotherapy, CD19 is expressed on the earliest B-precursor lymphocytes; (2) CD19 expression is retained during the process of neoplastic transformation; and (3) CD19 is absent on pluripotent hematopoietic stem cells.[93,96–103] Furthermore, a recent report showing the efficacy of bispecific single-chain antibody targeting the CD19 antigen (blinatumomab) suggests that CD19 is an attractive target for cellular immunotherapy in ALL.[104]

In fact, human T cells retrovirally modified to express CD19-targeted CAR have been shown to effectively lyse CD19+ tumor cells in vitro and eradicate systemic CD19+ tumors in SCID Beige mice.[96] Further studies in the authors' laboratory have shown in vivo that efficacy and persistence of these modified T cells is enhanced through costimulation.[96,97] Because most B-cell tumors fail to express costimulatory ligands (CD80 and CD86) required to generate optimal activation and proliferation of T cells, the authors and others have further modified the CAR to include the signaling domain of the T-cell costimulatory receptors (eg, CD28, 4-1BB, OX40). The resulting second-generation CARs exhibit in vitro activation and proliferation in the absence of exogenous costimulatory ligands, and enhanced in vivo antitumor efficacy in immunodeficient mice bearing systemic human pre–B-cell ALL tumors lacking costimulatory CD80 and CD86 ligands.[93,97,101,102,105] More recently, several investigators constructed and tested third-generation CARs containing tandem cytoplasmic signaling domains from two costimulatory receptors (ie, CD28-4-1BB or CD28-OX40) showing potentially enhanced T-cell signaling capacity when compared with second-generation CARs,[92,105–107] but these have yet to be studied in the clinical setting.

Clinical Trials with CD19-Targeted Modified T Cells in ALL

These promising preclinical data have led to a robust translation of CD19-targeted CAR+ T cells to the clinical setting for various B-cell hematologic malignancies. Currently, 11 active and 3 soon-to-open phase I clinical trials are targeting CD19 (**Table 1**). Although many of these trials have recently opened, several published preliminary results suggest that adoptive cellular therapy using autologous CD19-targeted CAR+ T cells is a promising treatment approach for B-cell malignancies. For example, investigators at the National Cancer Institute reported a dramatic regression of lymphadenopathy lasting 32 weeks in a patient with advanced follicular lymphoma who was treated with a preparative chemotherapy

Table 1
Summary of open and planned clinical trials with CD19-targeted chimeric T cells

Cell Source	Patient Population	Trial Design	Accompanying Lymphodepleting Cytotoxic Therapy	Trial Status	Trial Site
Autologous T cells	Relapsed or refractory CLL	Phase I dose-escalation trial	Cy	Open	United States, New York
Autologous T cells	Relapsed or refractory, or MRD⁺ ALL	Phase I dose-escalation trial	Cy	Open	United States, New York
Autologous T cells	MRD⁺ or residual disease after frontline CLL therapy	Phase I dose-escalation trial; consolidation therapy after up-front chemotherapy	Cy	Open	United States, New York
Autologous T cells	Relapsed or refractory low-to intermediate-grade NHL and CLL	Phase I dose-escalation trial	None	Open	United States, Texas
Autologous T cells	Relapsed or refractory B-cell leukemia/lymphoma (ALL, CLL, FL, MCL, DLBCL)	Phase I dose-escalation trial	None	Open	United States, Pennsylvania
Autologous T cells	Relapsed or refractory FL	Phase I	Fludarabine + rituximab	Open	United States, California
Autologous T cells	CD19-expressing B-cell malignancy of any type	Phase I	Fludarabine + Cy	Open	United States, National Institutes of Health

Autologous T cells	Relapsed or refractory low- to intermediate-grade NHL and CLL	Phase I; modified T-cell infusion after autologous HSCT	Autologous HSCT regimen (carmustine, etoposide, cytarabine, melphalan, rituximab)	Open	United States, Texas
Donor-derived EBV-specific T cells	MRD+ or relapsed ALL after allo-HSCT	Phase I dose-escalation trial	Cy	Open	United States, New York
Donor-derived multivirus-specific T cells	Relapsed B-ALL after allo-HSCT	Phase I dose-escalation trial	None	Open	United States, Texas
Donor-derived T cells	Relapsed B-cell leukemia/lymphoma after allo-HSCT	Phase I dose-escalation trial	N/A	Open	United States, NIH
UCB-derived T cells	Relapsed or refractory ALL, NHL, SLL, CLL	N/A	N/A	Pending	United States, Texas
Autologous T cells	High-risk, intermediate-grade NHL	Phase I/II trial; modified T-cell infusion after auto-HSCT	N/A	Pending	United States, California
Donor-derived EBV-specific T cells	High-risk or relapsed B-ALL after allo-HSCT	Phase I	N/A	Pending	Europe (France, Germany, Italy, United Kingdom)

Abbreviations: B-ALL, B cell acute lymphoblastic leukemia; CLL, chronic lymphocytic leukemia; Cy, cyclophosphamide; DLBCL, diffuse large B-cell lymphoma; FL, follicular lymphoma; MCL, mantle cell lymphoma; MRD, minimal residual disease; N/A, not available; NHL, non-Hodgkin's lymphoma; SLL, small lymphocytic lymphoma.

(60 mg/kg of cyclophosphamide for 2 days and 25 mg/m^2 of fludarabine for 5 days) followed by autologous CD19-targeted CAR$^+$ T cells and interleukin (IL)-2.[108] The authors also have observed a dramatic reduction of lymphadenopathy that lasted for 9 months in one patient and stable disease in two patients with chemotherapy-refractory relapsed chronic lymphocytic leukemia who were treated with 1.5 g/m^2 of cyclophosphamide conditioning one day before infusion of autologous CD19-targeted CAR$^+$ T cells.[109] Investigators from the University of Pennsylvania recently reported complete responses in three patients with advanced stages of indolent B-cell lymphomas and chronic lymphocytic leukemia, all treated with autologous CD19-targeted CAR$^+$ T cells.[110,111]

Although most clinical experience using CD19-targeted CARs has been in the setting of indolent or chronic B-cell malignancies, 8 of the 14 clinical trials involve patients with ALL: 3 using autologous T cells, 4 using donor-derived T cells, and 1 using UCB-modified T cells. The authors' center is currently conducting a phase I clinical trial in ALL wherein patients with relapsed disease or with minimal residual disease after the initial induction chemotherapy will be treated with cyclophosphamide conditioning followed by autologous CD19-targeted CAR$^+$ T cells (NCT01044069). To date, three patients have been enrolled and two have been treated. A persistent B-cell aplasia was observed in the first treated patient despite prompt recovery of other blood cell counts, which lasted for 8 weeks before the patient underwent allo-HSCT from a related sibling.[109] The second patient recently received the modified T cells, and the results of the peripheral blood analysis are not yet available. Similarly, investigators at the University of Pennsylvania are conducting a phase I clinical trial with autologous CD19-targeted T cells in patients with B-cell malignancies, including ALL (NCT01029366).

Other investigators have examined the use of a CD19-targeted CAR to modify donor-derived T cells for patients with relapsed ALL after allo-HSCT. To reduce the risk of GvHD associated with infusion of donor-derived T cells and to offer protection against common posttransplant virus infections, the approach using virus-specific T cells has been commonly used in this setting. Specifically, investigators at Baylor College of Medicine are conducting a phase I/II dose-escalation trial in ALL, wherein patients after allo-HSCT will be infused with allogeneic multivirus targeted T cells, specific to cytomegalovirus, Epstein-Barr virus (EBV), and adenovirus, further modified to express a CD19-targeted CAR[112] (NCT00840853). MSKCC has an open phase I dose-escalation clinical trial, wherein patients with relapsed or minimal residual disease-positive ALL will be treated with donor-derived EBV-specific CAR-modified T cells (NCT01430390). Finally, investigators in Europe (NCT01195480) will soon open a phase I trial to evaluate the safety of donor-derived EBV-specific CAR-modified T cells in patients with high-risk or relapsed B-cell ALL after allo-HSCT.

Similarly, UCB cells can be modified to express a CD19-targeted CAR, and preclinical data exploring the CAR-modified UCB cells have been published.[113,114] Based on these preclinical data, investigators at MD Anderson Cancer Center are planning a phase I clinical trial, wherein patients with B-cell malignancies will be infused with CD19-targeted CAR$^+$ T cells derived from UCB at 49 days ($\pm$7 days) after UCB transplantation (NCT01362452).

Genetically Modified CD19-Targeted Natural Killer Cells

Natural killer (NK) cells are lymphoid cells of the innate immune system that express CD56 and CD16 but fail to express a T-cell receptor (CD3$^-$). NK cells express killer immunoglobulin-like receptors (KIRs) that predominantly serve as inhibitory receptors that bind specific matched HLA class I molecules (KIR ligands) on target cells.

Expression by target cells of cognate KIR ligands induces a KIR-mediated inhibitory signal to the autologous NK cell, sparing the target cell from NK cell–mediated lysis. In the allogeneic setting, however, NK cells encounter target cells with mismatched KIR ligands and as a result trigger NK cell alloreactivity.[115]

NK cell alloreactivity does not seem to be of benefit in the setting of ALL.[116] However, genetic modification of NK cells may be a means of overcoming ALL tumor cell resistance to NK cell–mediated lysis. To this end, several investigators have successfully expanded large numbers of NK cells through co-culture of peripheral blood mononuclear cells on an irradiated K562 leukemia cell line genetically modified to express the NK cell stimulatory 4-1BB ligand and membrane bound IL-15 (K562-mb15-41BBL),[117] and generated ALL-targeted NK cells either through retroviral transduction[118] or electroporation[119] of a CD19-targeted CAR. These CD19-targeted NK cells effectively lysed NK cell–resistant ALL tumor cells, and further modification of the CAR through incorporation of the 4-1BB receptor cytoplasmic signaling domain enhanced NK cell killing of CD19+ ALL tumor cell lines and patient-derived ALL cells.[118] Significantly, these investigators at St. Jude Children's Research Hospital successfully modified the NK cell transduction and expansion protocol to large-scale cGMP conditions, and have opened a phase I dose-escalating clinical trial, wherein children with refractory or relapsed ALL are treated with CD19-targeted NK cells from a haploidentical donor. To date, they have enrolled two patients at the lowest dose cohort (D. Campana, personal communication, 2011).

SUMMARY

ALL remains a difficult disease to treat. In the adult setting, most patients will ultimately die of their disease, whereas in the pediatric setting, relapsed and refractory disease remains a therapeutic challenge. Cellular therapy through allo-HSCT remains an option for these patients, and recent advances in alternative forms of allo-HSCT, including unrelated donor transplants, UCB transplants, and haploidentical transplants, have expanded the numbers of patients eligible for allo-HSCT but have not improved outcomes when compared with HLA-matched related allo-HSCTs. In light of this persistent failure, several novel adoptive cellular approaches are being investigated to treat patients with ALL. The use of enriched WT-1–specific donor T cells to treat patients with ALL is currently under investigation in phase I trials at several centers. Treatment of ALL with genetically modified T cells targeted to the CD19 antigen through the expression of a CD19-specific CAR also have entered phase I clinical trials at several centers. Similarly, a clinical trial treating patients with ALL with genetically modified NK cells targeted to the CD19 antigen has recently opened for accrual. Collectively, these ongoing and anticipated trials provide a promising role for adoptive cellular therapies in the treatment of ALL. What remains to be seen is whether this promise will either translate into improved outcomes for these patients or provide significant insights on which to design second-generation adoptive cell therapeutic clinical trials for ALL in the future.

REFERENCES

1. Pui CH, Evans WE. Treatment of acute lymphoblastic leukemia. N Engl J Med 2006;354(2):166–78.
2. Pui CH, Robison LL, Look AT. Acute lymphoblastic leukaemia. Lancet 2008; 371(9617):1030–43.
3. Fielding AK, Richards SM, Chopra R, et al. Outcome of 609 adults after relapse of acute lymphoblastic leukemia (ALL); an MRC UKALL12/ECOG 2993 study. Blood 2007;109(3):944–50.

4. Gaynon PS. Childhood acute lymphoblastic leukaemia and relapse. Br J Haematol 2005;131(5):579–87.

5. Tavernier E, Boiron JM, Huguet F, et al. Outcome of treatment after first relapse in adults with acute lymphoblastic leukemia initially treated by the LALA-94 trial. Leukemia 2007;21(9):1907–14.

6. Weiden PL, Flournoy N, Thomas ED, et al. Antileukemic effect of graft-versus-host disease in human recipients of allogeneic-marrow grafts. N Engl J Med 1979;300(19):1068–73.

7. Porter DL, Antin JH. The graft-versus-leukemia effects of allogeneic cell therapy. Annu Rev Med 1999;50:369–86.

8. Gokbuget N, Hoelzer D. Treatment of adult acute lymphoblastic leukemia. Semin Hematol 2009;46(1):64–75.

9. Larson R. Allogeneic hematopoietic cell transplantation for adults with ALL. Bone Marrow Transplant 2008;42(Suppl 1):S18–24.

10. Hahn T, Wall D, Camitta B, et al. The role of cytotoxic therapy with hematopoietic stem cell transplantation in the therapy of acute lymphoblastic leukemia in adults: an evidence-based review. Biol Blood Marrow Transplant 2006;12(1): 1–30.

11. Thiebaut A, Vernant JP, Degos L, et al. Adult acute lymphocytic leukemia study testing chemotherapy and autologous and allogeneic transplantation. A follow-up report of the French protocol LALA 87. Hematol Oncol Clin North Am 2000; 14(6):1353–66, x.

12. Thomas X, Boiron JM, Huguet F, et al. Outcome of treatment in adults with acute lymphoblastic leukemia: analysis of the LALA-94 trial. J Clin Oncol 2004;22(20): 4075–86.

13. Yanada M, Matsuo K, Suzuki T, et al. Allogeneic hematopoietic stem cell transplantation as part of postremission therapy improves survival for adult patients with high-risk acute lymphoblastic leukemia: a metaanalysis. Cancer 2006; 106(12):2657–63.

14. Goldstone AH, Richards SM, Lazarus HM, et al. In adults with standard-risk acute lymphoblastic leukemia, the greatest benefit is achieved from a matched sibling allogeneic transplantation in first complete remission, and an autologous transplantation is less effective than conventional consolidation/maintenance chemotherapy in all patients: final results of the International ALL Trial (MRC UKALL XII/ECOG E2993). Blood 2008;111(4):1827–33.

15. Ribera JM, Oriol A, Bethencourt C, et al. Comparison of intensive chemotherapy, allogeneic or autologous stem cell transplantation as post-remission treatment for adult patients with high-risk acute lymphoblastic leukemia. Results of the PE-THEMA ALL-93 trial. Haematologica 2005;90(10):1346–56.

16. Fielding AK, Rowe JM, Richards SM, et al. Prospective outcome data on 267 unselected adult patients with Philadelphia chromosome-positive acute lympho-blastic leukemia confirms superiority of allogeneic transplantation over chemo-therapy in the pre-imatinib era: results from the International ALL Trial MRC UKALLXII/ECOG2993. Blood 2009;113(19):4489–96.

17. Lee HJ, Thompson JE, Wang ES, et al. Philadelphia chromosome-positive acute lymphoblastic leukemia: current treatment and future perspectives. Cancer 2011;117(8):1583–94.

18. de Labarthe A, Rousselot P, Huguet-Rigal F, et al. Imatinib combined with induction or consolidation chemotherapy in patients with de novo Philadelphia chromosome-positive acute lymphoblastic leukemia: results of the GRAAPH-2003 study. Blood 2007;109(4):1408–13.

19. Lee S, Kim DW, Kim YJ, et al. Minimal residual disease-based role of imatinib as a first-line interim therapy prior to allogeneic stem cell transplantation in Philadelphia chromosome-positive acute lymphoblastic leukemia. Blood 2003; 102(8):3068–70.

20. Fielding AK, Buck G, Lazarus HM, et al. Imatinib significantly enhances long-term outcomes in Philadelphia positive acute lymphoblastic leukaemia; final results of the UKALL XII/ECOG 2993 Trial. Blood 2010;16(21):77.

21. Mizuta S, Matsuo K, Yagasaki F, et al. Pre-transplant imatinib-based therapy improves the outcome of allogeneic hematopoietic stem cell transplantation for BCR-ABL-positive acute lymphoblastic leukemia. Leukemia 2011;25(1): 41–7.

22. Huguet F, Leguay T, Raffoux E, et al. Pediatric-inspired therapy in adults with Philadelphia chromosome-negative acute lymphoblastic leukemia: the GRAALL-2003 study. J Clin Oncol 2009;27(6):911–8.

23. Bruggemann M, Raff T, Flohr T, et al. Clinical significance of minimal residual disease quantification in adult patients with standard-risk acute lymphoblastic leukemia. Blood 2006;107(3):1116–23.

24. Bassan R, Spinelli O, Oldani E, et al. Improved risk classification for risk-specific therapy based on the molecular study of minimal residual disease (MRD) in adult acute lymphoblastic leukemia (ALL). Blood 2009;113(18):4153–62.

25. Goekbuget N, Brueggemann M, Arnold R, et al. New definition of treatment response in adult acute lymphoblastic leukemia (ALL): use of molecular marker s for minimal residual disease (MRD). Blood 2009;114(22):42.

26. Beldjord K, Lheritier V, Boulland ML, et al. Post-induction minimal residual disease (MRD) defines a large subset of adults with favorable Philadelphia negative acute lymphoblastic leukemia (ALL), who do not benefit from allogeneic stem cell transplantation (SCT) in first complete remission: a GRAALL study. Blood 2009;114(22):239.

27. Ribera JM, Oriol A, Morgades M, et al. Treatment of high-risk (HR) Philadelphia chromosome-negative (Ph-) adult acute lymphoblastic leukemia (ALL) according to baseline risk factors and minimal residual disease (MRD): Results of the PETHEMA ALL-AR-03 trial including the use of propensity score (PS) method to reduce assignment bias. Blood 2009;114(22):136.

28. Marks DI, Cullis JO, Ward KN, et al. Allogeneic bone marrow transplantation for chronic myeloid leukemia using sibling and volunteer unrelated donors. A comparison of complications in the first 2 years. Ann Intern Med 1993;119(3): 207–14.

29. Beatty PG, Anasetti C, Hansen JA, et al. Marrow transplantation from unrelated donors for treatment of hematologic malignancies: effect of mismatching for one HLA locus. Blood 1993;81(1):249–53.

30. Petersdorf EW, Gooley TA, Anasetti C, et al. Optimizing outcome after unrelated marrow transplantation by comprehensive matching of HLA class I and II alleles in the donor and recipient. Blood 1998;92(10):3515–20.

31. Gooley TA, Chien JW, Pergam SA, et al. Reduced mortality after allogeneic hematopoietic-cell transplantation. N Engl J Med 2010;363(22):2091–101.

32. Ottinger HD, Ferencik S, Beelen DW, et al. Hematopoietic stem cell transplantation: contrasting the outcome of transplantations from HLA-identical siblings, partially HLA-mismatched related donors, and HLA-matched unrelated donors. Blood 2003;102(3):1131–7.

33. Walter RB, Pagel JM, Gooley TA, et al. Comparison of matched unrelated and matched related donor myeloablative hematopoietic cell transplantation

for adults with acute myeloid leukemia in first remission. Leukemia 2010;24(7):
1276–82.

34. Yakoub-Agha I, Mesnil F, Kuentz M, et al. Allogeneic marrow stem-cell transplantation from human leukocyte antigen-identical siblings versus human
leukocyte antigen-allelic-matched unrelated donors (10/10) in patients with
standard-risk hematologic malignancy: a prospective study from the French
Society of Bone Marrow Transplantation and Cell Therapy. J Clin Oncol 2006;
24(36):5695–702.

35. Chim CS, Lie AK, Liang R, et al. Long-term results of allogeneic bone marrow
transplantation for 108 adult patients with acute lymphoblastic leukemia: favorable outcome with BMT at first remission and HLA-matched unrelated donor.
Bone Marrow Transplant 2007;40(4):339–47.

36. Dahlke J, Kroger N, Zabelina T, et al. Comparable results in patients with acute
lymphoblastic leukemia after related and unrelated stem cell transplantation.
Bone Marrow Transplant 2006;37(2):155–63.

37. Kiehl MG, Kraut L, Schwerdtfeger R, et al. Outcome of allogeneic hematopoietic
stem-cell transplantation in adult patients with acute lymphoblastic leukemia: no
difference in related compared with unrelated transplant in first complete remission. J Clin Oncol 2004;22(14):2816–25.

38. Nishiwaki S, Inamoto Y, Sakamaki H, et al. Allogeneic stem cell transplantation for adult Philadelphia chromosome-negative acute lymphocytic leukemia:
comparable survival rates but different risk factors between related and
unrelated transplantation in first complete remission. Blood 2010;116(20):
4368–75.

39. Sauter C, Barker JN. Unrelated donor umbilical cord blood transplantation for
the treatment of hematologic malignancies. Curr Opin Hematol 2008;15(6):
568–75.

40. Laughlin MJ, Eapen M, Rubinstein P, et al. Outcomes after transplantation of
cord blood or bone marrow from unrelated donors in adults with leukemia.
N Engl J Med 2004;351(22):2265–75.

41. Rocha V, Labopin M, Sanz G, et al. Transplants of umbilical-cord blood or bone
marrow from unrelated donors in adults with acute leukemia. N Engl J Med
2004;351(22):2276–85.

42. Takahashi S, Iseki T, Ooi J, et al. Single-institute comparative analysis of unrelated bone marrow transplantation and cord blood transplantation for adult
patients with hematologic malignancies. Blood 2004;104(12):3813–20.

43. Barker JN, Rocha V, Scaradavou A. Optimizing unrelated donor cord blood
transplantation. Biol Blood Marrow Transplant 2008;15(Suppl 1):154–61.

44. Barker JN, Byam C, Scaradavou A. How I treat: the selection and acquisition of
unrelated cord blood grafts. Blood 2011;117(8):2332–9.

45. Barker JN, Weisdorf DJ, DeFor TE, et al. Transplantation of 2 partially HLA-
matched umbilical cord blood units to enhance engraftment in adults with
hematologic malignancy. Blood 2005;105(3):1343–7.

46. Haspel RL, Ballen KK. Double cord blood transplants: filling a niche? Stem Cell
Rev 2006;2(2):81–6.

47. Verneris MR, Brunstein CG, Barker J, et al. Relapse risk after umbilical cord
blood transplantation: enhanced graft-versus-leukemia effect in recipients of 2
units. Blood 2009;114(19):4293–9.

48. Eapen M, Rocha V, Sanz G, et al. Effect of graft source on unrelated donor haemopoietic stem-cell transplantation in adults with acute leukaemia: a retrospective analysis. Lancet Oncol 2010;11(7):653–60.

49. Atsuta Y, Suzuki R, Nagamura-Inoue T, et al. Disease-specific analyses of unrelated cord blood transplantation compared with unrelated bone marrow transplantation in adult patients with acute leukemia. Blood 2009;113(8):1631–8.
50. Kumar P, Defor TE, Brunstein C, et al. Allogeneic hematopoietic stem cell transplantation in adult acute lymphocytic leukemia: impact of donor source on survival. Biol Blood Marrow Transplant 2008;14(12):1394–400.
51. Aversa F. Haploidentical haematopoietic stem cell transplantation for acute leukaemia in adults: experience in Europe and the United States. Bone Marrow Transplant 2008;41(5):473–81.
52. Aversa F, Tabilio A, Terenzi A, et al. Successful engraftment of T-cell-depleted haploidentical "three-loci" incompatible transplants in leukemia patients by addition of recombinant human granulocyte colony-stimulating factor-mobilized peripheral blood progenitor cells to bone marrow inoculum. Blood 1994;84(11): 3948–55.
53. Aversa F, Tabilio A, Velardi A, et al. Treatment of high-risk acute leukemia with T-cell-depleted stem cells from related donors with one fully mismatched HLA haplotype. N Engl J Med 1998;339(17):1186–93.
54. Aversa F, Terenzi A, Tabilio A, et al. Full haplotype-mismatched hematopoietic stem-cell transplantation: a phase II study in patients with acute leukemia at high risk of relapse. J Clin Oncol 2005;23(15):3447–54.
55. Ciceri F, Labopin M, Aversa F, et al. A survey of fully haploidentical hematopoietic stem cell transplantation in adults with high-risk acute leukemia: a risk factor analysis of outcomes for patients in remission at transplantation. Blood 2008; 112(9):3574–81.
56. Huang XJ, Liu DH, Liu KY, et al. Treatment of acute leukemia with unmanipulated HLA-mismatched/haploidentical blood and bone marrow transplantation. Biol Blood Marrow Transplant 2009;15(2):257–65.
57. Barrett J, Gluckman E, Handgretinger R, et al. Point-counterpoint: haploidentical family donors versus cord blood transplantation. Biol Blood Marrow Transplant 2011;17(Suppl 1):S89–93.
58. Ballen KK, Spitzer TR. The great debate: haploidentical or cord blood transplant. Bone Marrow Transplant 2011;46(3):323–9.
59. Arnold R, Massenkeil G, Bornhauser M, et al. Nonmyeloablative stem cell transplantation in adults with high-risk ALL may be effective in early but not in advanced disease. Leukemia 2002;16(12):2423–8.
60. Martino R, Giralt S, Caballero MD, et al. Allogeneic hematopoietic stem cell transplantation with reduced-intensity conditioning in acute lymphoblastic leukemia: a feasibility study. Haematologica 2003;88(5):555–60.
61. Ram R, Storb R, Sandmaier BM, et al. Non-myeloablative conditioning with allogeneic hematopoietic cell transplantation for the treatment of high-risk acute lymphoblastic leukemia. Haematologica 2011;96(8):1113–20.
62. Stein AS, Palmer JM, O'Donnell MR, et al. Reduced-intensity conditioning followed by peripheral blood stem cell transplantation for adult patients with high-risk acute lymphoblastic leukemia. Biol Blood Marrow Transplant 2009; 15(11):1407–14.
63. Marks DI, Wang T, Perez WS, et al. The outcome of full-intensity and reduced-intensity conditioning matched sibling or unrelated donor transplantation in adults with Philadelphia chromosome-negative acute lymphoblastic leukemia in first and second complete remission. Blood 2010;116(3):366–74.
64. Mohty M, Labopin M, Volin L, et al. Reduced-intensity versus conventional myeloablative conditioning allogeneic stem cell transplantation for patients with

acute lymphoblastic leukemia: a retrospective study from the European Group for Blood and Marrow Transplantation. Blood 2010;116(22):4439–43.

65. Brunstein CG, Barker JN, Weisdorf DJ, et al. Umbilical cord blood transplantation after nonmyeloablative conditioning: impact on transplantation outcomes in 110 adults with hematologic disease. Blood 2007;110(8):3064–70.

66. Bachanova V, Verneris MR, DeFor T, et al. Prolonged survival in adults with acute lymphoblastic leukemia after reduced-intensity conditioning with cord blood or sibling donor transplantation. Blood 2009;113(13):2902–5.

67. Small TN, Papadopoulos EB, Boulad F, et al. Comparison of immune reconstitution after unrelated and related T-cell-depleted bone marrow transplantation: effect of patient age and donor leukocyte infusions. Blood 1999;93(2):467–80.

68. Jakubowski AA, Small TN, Kernan NA, et al. T cell-depleted unrelated donor stem cell transplantation provides favorable disease-free survival for adults with hematologic malignancies. Biol Blood Marrow Transplant 2011;17(9): 1335–42.

69. Patel B, Kirkland KE, Szydlo R, et al. Favorable outcomes with alemtuzumab-conditioned unrelated donor stem cell transplantation in adults with high-risk Philadelphia chromosome-negative acute lymphoblastic leukemia in first complete remission. Haematologica 2009;94(10):1399–406.

70. O'Brien S, Thomas D, Ravandi F, et al. Outcome of adults with acute lymphocytic leukemia after second salvage therapy. Cancer 2008;113(11):3186–91.

71. Kolb HJ, Schattenberg A, Goldman JM, et al. Graft-versus-leukemia effect of donor lymphocyte transfusions in marrow grafted patients. European Group for Blood and Marrow Transplantation Working Party Chronic Leukemia. Blood 1995;86(5):2041–50.

72. Kolb HJ, Schmid C, Barrett AJ, et al. Graft-versus-leukemia reactions in allogeneic chimeras. Blood 2004;103(3):767–76.

73. Loren AW, Porter DL. Donor leukocyte infusions for the treatment of relapsed acute leukemia after allogeneic stem cell transplantation. Bone Marrow Transplant 2008;41(5):483–93.

74. Choi SJ, Lee JH, Lee JH, et al. Treatment of relapsed acute lymphoblastic leukemia after allogeneic bone marrow transplantation with chemotherapy followed by G-CSF-primed donor leukocyte infusion: a prospective study. Bone Marrow Transplant 2005;36(2):163–9.

75. Collins RH Jr, Goldstein S, Giralt S, et al. Donor leukocyte infusions in acute lymphocytic leukemia. Bone Marrow Transplant 2000;26(5):511–6.

76. Porter DL, Levine BL, Bunin N, et al. A phase 1 trial of donor lymphocyte infusions expanded and activated ex vivo via CD3/CD28 costimulation. Blood 2006;107(4):1325–31.

77. Oka Y, Elisseeva OA, Tsuboi A, et al. Human cytotoxic T-lymphocyte responses specific for peptides of the wild-type Wilms' tumor gene (WT1) product. Immunogenetics 2000;51(2):99–107.

78. Oka Y, Udaka K, Tsuboi A, et al. Cancer immunotherapy targeting Wilms' tumor gene WT1 product. J Immunol 2000;164(4):1873–80.

79. Rezvani K, Yong AS, Savani BN, et al. Graft-versus-leukemia effects associated with detectable Wilms tumor-1 specific T lymphocytes after allogeneic stem-cell transplantation for acute lymphoblastic leukemia. Blood 2007;110(6):1924–32.

80. Brentjens RJ. Novel Approaches to Immunotherapy for B-cell Malignancies. Curr Oncol Rep 2004;6(5):339–47.

81. Sadelain M, Brentjens R, Riviere I. The promise and potential pitfalls of chimeric antigen receptors. Curr Opin Immunol 2009;21(2):215–23.

82. Sadelain M, Riviere I, Brentjens R. Targeting tumours with genetically enhanced T lymphocytes. Nat Rev Cancer 2003;3(1):35–45.
83. Johnson LA, Morgan RA, Dudley ME, et al. Gene therapy with human and mouse T-cell receptors mediates cancer regression and targets normal tissues expressing cognate antigen. Blood 2009;114(3):535–46.
84. Morgan RA, Dudley ME, Wunderlich JR, et al. Cancer regression in patients after transfer of genetically engineered lymphocytes. Science 2006;314(5796): 126–9.
85. Dossett ML, Teague RM, Schmitt TM, et al. Adoptive immunotherapy of disseminated leukemia with TCR-transduced, CD8+ T cells expressing a known endogenous TCR. Mol Ther 2009;17(4):742–9.
86. Xue SA, Gao L, Hart D, et al. Elimination of human leukemia cells in NOD/SCID mice by WT1-TCR gene-transduced human T cells. Blood 2005;106(9):3062–7.
87. Khong HT, Restifo NP. Natural selection of tumor variants in the generation of "tumor escape" phenotypes. Nat Immunol 2002;3(11):999–1005.
88. Gottschalk S, Ng CY, Perez M, et al. An Epstein-Barr virus deletion mutant associated with fatal lymphoproliferative disease unresponsive to therapy with virus-specific CTLs. Blood 2001;97(4):835–43.
89. Park JH, Brentjens RJ. Adoptive immunotherapy for B-cell malignancies with autologous chimeric antigen receptor modified tumor targeted T cells. Discov Med 2010;9(47):277–88.
90. Hollyman D, Stefanski J, Przybylowski M, et al. Manufacturing validation of biologically functional T cells targeted to CD19 antigen for autologous adoptive cell therapy. J Immunother 2009;32(2):169–80.
91. Singh H, Figliola MJ, Dawson MJ, et al. Reprogramming CD19-specific T cells with IL-21 signaling can improve adoptive immunotherapy of B-lineage malignancies. Cancer Res 2011;71(10):3516–27.
92. Tammana S, Huang X, Wong M, et al. 4-1BB and CD28 signaling plays a synergistic role in redirecting umbilical cord blood T cells against B-cell malignancies. Hum Gene Ther 2010;21(1):75–86.
93. Kowolik CM, Topp MS, Gonzalez S, et al. CD28 costimulation provided through a CD19-specific chimeric antigen receptor enhances in vivo persistence and antitumor efficacy of adoptively transferred T cells. Cancer Res 2006;66(22): 10995–1004.
94. Hoyos V, Savoldo B, Quintarelli C, et al. Engineering CD19-specific T lymphocytes with interleukin-15 and a suicide gene to enhance their anti-lymphoma/leukemia effects and safety. Leukemia 2010;24(6):1160–70.
95. Chmielewski M, Kopecky C, Hombach AA, et al. IL-12 Release by Engineered T Cells Expressing Chimeric Antigen Receptors Can Effectively Muster an Antigen-Independent Macrophage Response on Tumor Cells That Have Shut Down Tumor Antigen Expression. Cancer Res 2011;71(17): 5697–706.
96. Brentjens RJ, Latouche JB, Santos E, et al. Eradication of systemic B-cell tumors by genetically targeted human T lymphocytes co-stimulated by CD80 and interleukin-15. Nat Med 2003;9(3):279–86.
97. Brentjens RJ, Santos E, Nikhamin Y, et al. Genetically targeted T cells eradicate systemic acute lymphoblastic leukemia xenografts. Clin Cancer Res 2007; 13(18 Pt 1):5426–35.
98. Cooper LJ, Al-Kadhimi Z, DiGiusto D, et al. Development and application of CD19-specific T cells for adoptive immunotherapy of B cell malignancies. Blood Cells Mol Dis 2004;33(1):83–9.

99. Cooper LJ, Al-Kadhimi Z, Serrano LM, et al. Enhanced antilymphoma efficacy of CD19-redirected influenza MP1-specific CTLs by cotransfer of T cells modified to present influenza MP1. Blood 2005;105(4):1622–31.

100. Cooper LJ, Topp MS, Serrano LM, et al. T-cell clones can be rendered specific for CD19: toward the selective augmentation of the graft-versus-B-lineage leukemia effect. Blood 2003;101(4):1637–44.

101. Imai C, Mihara K, Andreansky M, et al. Chimeric receptors with 4-1BB signaling capacity provoke potent cytotoxicity against acute lymphoblastic leukemia. Leukemia 2004;18(4):676–84.

102. Loskog A, Giandomenico V, Rossig C, et al. Addition of the CD28 signaling domain to chimeric T-cell receptors enhances chimeric T-cell resistance to T regulatory cells. Leukemia 2006;20(10):1819–28.

103. Rossig C, Bollard CM, Nuchtern JG, et al. Epstein-Barr virus-specific human T lymphocytes expressing antitumor chimeric T-cell receptors: potential for improved immunotherapy. Blood 2002;99(6):2009–16.

104. Topp MS, Kufer P, Gokbuget N, et al. Targeted therapy with the T-cell-engaging antibody blinatumomab of chemotherapy-refractory minimal residual disease in B-lineage acute lymphoblastic leukemia patients results in high response rate and prolonged leukemia-free survival. J Clin Oncol 2011; 29(18):2493–8.

105. Milone MC, Fish JD, Carpenito C, et al. Chimeric receptors containing CD137 signal transduction domains mediate enhanced survival of T cells and increased antileukemic efficacy in vivo. Mol Ther 2009;17(8):1453–64.

106. Kochenderfer JN, Feldman SA, Zhao Y, et al. Construction and preclinical evaluation of an anti-CD19 chimeric antigen receptor. J Immunother 2009;32(7): 689–702.

107. Wang J, Jensen M, Lin Y, et al. Optimizing adoptive polyclonal T cell immunotherapy of lymphomas, using a chimeric T cell receptor possessing CD28 and CD137 costimulatory domains. Hum Gene Ther 2007;18(8):712–25.

108. Kochenderfer JN, Wilson WH, Janik JE, et al. Eradication of B-lineage cells and regression of lymphoma in a patient treated with autologous T cells genetically engineered to recognize CD19. Blood 2010;116(20):4099–102.

109. Brentjens RJ, Riviere I, Park JH, et al. Safety and persistence of adoptively transferred autologous CD19-targeted T cells in patients with relapsed or chemotherapy refractory B-cell leukemias. Blood 2011. [Epub ahead of print].

110. Porter DL, Levine BL, Kalos M, et al. Chimeric antigen receptor-modified T cells in chronic lymphoid leukemia. N Engl J Med 2011;365(8):725–33.

111. Kalos M, Levine BL, Porter DL, et al. T cells with chimeric antigen receptors have potent antitumor effects and can establish memory in patients with advanced leukemia. Sci Transl Med 2011;3(95):95ra73.

112. Savoldo B, Micklethwaite K, Cooper L, et al. Monoculture-derived T lymphocytes providing multiple virus specificity and anti-leukemia activity for recipients of hematopoietic stem cells or umbilical cord blood transplants [abstract 3909]. Blood 2008;112(11):3909.

113. Serrano LM, Pfeiffer T, Olivares S, et al. Differentiation of naive cord-blood T cells into CD19-specific cytolytic effectors for posttransplantation adoptive immunotherapy. Blood 2006;107(7):2643–52.

114. Micklethwaite KP, Savoldo B, Hanley PJ, et al. Derivation of human T lymphocytes from cord blood and peripheral blood with antiviral and antileukemic specificity from a single culture as protection against infection and relapse after stem cell transplantation. Blood 2010;115(13):2695–703.

115. Grzywacz B, Miller JS, Verneris MR. Use of natural killer cells as immunotherapy for leukaemia. Best Pract Res Clin Haematol 2008;21(3):467–83.
116. Ruggeri L, Capanni M, Urbani E, et al. Effectiveness of donor natural killer cell alloreactivity in mismatched hematopoietic transplants. Science 2002; 295(5562):2097–100.
117. Fujisaki H, Kakuda H, Shimasaki N, et al. Expansion of highly cytotoxic human natural killer cells for cancer cell therapy. Cancer Res 2009;69(9):4010–7.
118. Imai C, Iwamoto S, Campana D. Genetic modification of primary natural killer cells overcomes inhibitory signals and induces specific killing of leukemic cells. Blood 2005;106(1):376–83.
119. Li L, Liu LN, Feller S, et al. Expression of chimeric antigen receptors in natural killer cells with a regulatory-compliant non-viral method. Cancer Gene Ther 2010;17(3):147–54.

Novel Therapeutic Approaches for Acute Lymphoblastic Leukemia

Mark R. Litzow, MD[a,b,*]

KEYWORDS

- Acute lymphoblastic leukemia • Monoclonal antibody therapy
- Chemotherapy • Kinase inhibitor therapy

The notable success of therapy for acute lymphoblastic leukemia (ALL) in children, for whom cure rates now exceed 80% to 90%, is even more remarkable when one considers that much of this success has occurred through alteration in drug dosing and schedule rather than the introduction of new agents.[1] In adults, morphologic complete remission rates are now more than 90%. Relapse is common and cure rates, up until recently, have only been in the 30% to 40% range.[2] Despite these poor results, treatment outcomes in all age groups with ALL have improved when one compares results from the early 1980s to the early 2000s.[3] The poorer outcomes in adults are multifactorial, but largely relate to a higher incidence of poor-risk cytogenetic features and lessened ability to tolerate intensive chemotherapy regimens that are often used in pediatric patients.[4]

Patients presenting to adult oncologists traditionally were treated with similarly intensive regimens regardless of whether they were adolescents, young adults, or middle-aged to older individuals. In the past 10 years, multiple retrospective comparisons of the outcomes of adolescents and young adults comparing those of similar age treated on pediatric-intensive regimens versus adult-intensive regimens have been made. Most of these studies have reported that survival outcomes are significantly better in adolescents and young adults (AYA) who receive therapy with pediatric regimens as compared with adult regimens. One of the first reports came from a review of data from the Children's Cancer Group (CCG) in comparison with data from the Cancer and Leukemia Group B (CALGB). A comparison of 197 CCG patients with

Disclosure: The author has received consulting fees from Talon Therapeutics and Micromet.

[a] Division of Hematology, Mayo Clinic, 200 First Street, South West, Rochester, MN 55905, USA
[b] Myeloid Disease-Oriented Group, Division of Hematology, Mayo Clinic, 200 First Street, South West, Rochester, MN 55905, USA
* Corresponding author. Division of Hematology, Mayo Clinic, 200 First Street, South West, Rochester, MN 55905.
E-mail address: litzow.mark@mayo.edu

124 CALGB patients showed that although the complete response (CR) rates were identical at 90% between the two groups, in the CCG study there was a 67% overall survival (OS) at 7 years compared with 46% for the CALGB cohort (P<.001). For the CCG patients, central nervous system (CNS) prophylaxis was more intensive and given earlier in the course; moreover, doses of nonmyelosuppressive drugs such as asparaginase, vincristine, and corticosteroids were much higher in the CCG regimens than in the CALGB regimens.[5] At least 6 other retrospective comparisons have largely demonstrated similar results, although the reader is cautioned that treatments in some of these studies were often quite different and incorporated blood and marrow transplantation (BMT) in different ways.[6–8] There has been much speculation as to why patients treated on pediatric regimens have improved outcomes, and whether this relates to the higher doses of nonmyelosuppressive drugs, greater adherence to treatment schedules, and/or the greater experience of pediatric hematologists and oncologists in treating this disease.[9]

These reports have led to the development of pediatric-intensive regimens for the treatment of adults. The French GRAALL (Group for Research and Adult Acute Lymphoblastic Leukemia) 2003 Trial was a phase 2 study in which a pediatric-inspired regimen was used to treat patients between the ages of 15 and 60 years. The regimen contained higher doses of prednisone, asparaginase, and vincristine in comparison with the group's previous adult protocols. With a median follow-up of 42 months, the event-free survival (EFS) and OS were 55% and 60%, respectively. However, patients older than 45 years had a treatment-related death rate of 23% in contrast to a 5% rate in patients younger than 45. EFS in the younger patients was 58% versus 46% in the older patients (P = .03).[10] Other phase 2 studies have reported similar outcomes.[11,12]

Randomized trials comparing pediatric-intensive with adult-intensive regimens in adults with ALL have not been reported, and may be logistically difficult to do. An alternative approach to addressing this question is being conducted in the United States through the Intergroup Trial led by CALGB, protocol 10403. This trial is taking patients with Philadelphia chromosome–negative (Ph-neg) up to the age of 40 years and treating them with one arm of a high-risk CCG protocol. The CALGB 10403 protocol will compare the outcomes of patients treated with this regimen with pediatric patients receiving therapy on a designated arm of the CCG protocol. End points for this study include use of traditional end points such as CR rates and survival, but will also assess whether patients and physicians are able to adhere to the scheduling and dosing requirements of the protocol.[13]

Several new approaches in the therapy for ALL, including established agents used in other diseases and new agents in development, represent hope for therapeutic advances in the treatment of ALL and are outlined in detail in this review (**Box 1**).

MONOCLONAL ANTIBODY THERAPY

Immunophenotypic analysis of ALL plays a fundamental role in the diagnosis and classification of the disease. It is assuming an increasingly prominent role in the assessment of minimal residual disease in both pediatric and adult patients.[14] A prominent antigen, CD20, is expressed on B-lineage lymphocytes in the mid-stages of development and is found on 40% to 50% of B-lineage ALL, with expression rates rising to 80% to 90% in mature B-cell or Burkitt-type leukemia and lymphoma. In pediatric ALL, expression of CD20 was found to be of conflicting prognostic significance with some studies suggesting inferior EFS, which was independent of other prognostic factors such as age and karyotype.[15] Another study from St Jude Children's Hospital

---

Box 1
Novel therapeutic approaches in ALL

- Application of pediatric ALL regimens to AYA
- Monoclonal antibodies
  - Rituximab
  - Epratuzumab
  - CAT8015
  - CAT-3888
  - Inotuzumab ozogamicin
  - DT2219 ARL
  - Alemtuzumab
  - Blinatumomab
- Chemotherapy
  - NOTCH γ-secretase inhibitors
  - Forodesine
  - Decitabine
- Emerging Therapies
  - Methotrexate analogues
    - Pemetrexed
    - Talotrexin
  - Flavopiridol
  - Proteasome inhibition
    - Bortezomib
  - Mammalian target of rapamycin inhibitors
    - Rapamycin
    - RAD001 (everolimus)
    - CCI-779 (temsirolimus)
  - MDM2 inhibitors
  - MEK/ERK inhibitors
  - PIM protein kinase inhibitors

---

suggested that expression of CD20 led to better outcomes.[16] In adults, a retrospective analysis of 253 adult patients, of whom 47% expressed CD20 at a level of 20% or more, demonstrated that although CR rates were similar, disease recurrence was higher in the CD20-positive group. These patients had less lymphadenopathy but more thrombocytopenia and a poorer performance score than the CD20-negative patients. Remission duration and OS were poorer in the CD20-positive patients, and CD20 expression remained an independent predictor of outcome in multivariate analysis.[17] The GRAALL Group has also reported that in Ph-negative B-lineage ALL in patients up to the age of 55 years, CD20 expression was associated with an increased risk of relapse (39% vs 20%, $P = .02$). Overall, it did not significantly affect EFS or OS (55% vs 59% at 42 months and CD20-positive and CD20-negative groups, respectively, $P = .65$). However, in patients with a white blood cell count of greater than 30×10^9/L, EFS was much worse in the CD20-positive cohort (70% vs 24% at 42 months, $P = .006$).[18]

Rituximab, which has dramatically changed the therapy for non-Hodgkin lymphoma, has more recently been applied to therapy in CD20-positive B-lineage ALL. In a retrospective study of 282 adolescents and adults with de novo Ph-neg B-lineage ALL received a combination of hyper-CVAD plus rituximab versus a cohort who received hyper-CVAD alone. The CR duration and OS with hyper-CVAD combined with rituximab as compared with hyper-CVAD alone were significantly better. The CR duration was 70% with hyper-CVAD plus rituximab versus 38% with hyper-CVAD alone ($P<.001$), and for OS 75% with hyper-CVAD plus rituximab versus 47% for hyper-CVAD alone ($P = .003$) **(Fig. 1)**.[19] These results were reported in patients younger than 60 years. Patients older than 60 years did not have any significant differences in outcome, whether or not they received rituximab. In a series of patients between the ages of 15 and 55 years from the German ALL Study Group, 41% of patients had CD20 expression of greater than 20%. In these patients, rituximab was added to the standard combination chemotherapy regimen. The CR rates were similar between the 181 patients who received rituximab plus chemotherapy

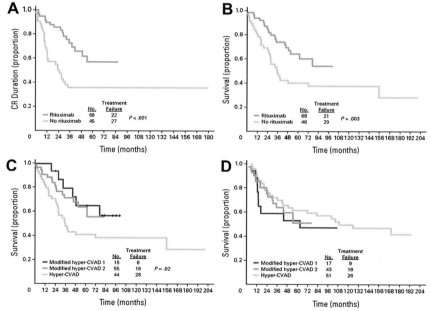

Fig. 1. Outcomes by therapy for younger patients (age younger than 60 years) with Philadelphia chromosome–negative precursor B-lineage acute lymphoblastic leukemia. In the CD20-positive subset, (A) complete remission (CR) duration and (B) survival by inclusion or exclusion of rituximab therapy, and (C) survival by hyper-CVAD (fractionated cyclophosphamide, vincristine, doxorubicin, dexamethasone) regimen (standard, modified hyper-CVAD 1 with rituximab inclusive of anthracycline intensification, or modified hyper-CVAD 2 with rituximab eliminating anthracycline intensification) are depicted. (D) Survival by regimen (without rituximab) for the CD20-negative group is also depicted. (*From* Thomas DA, O'Brien S, Faderl S, et al. Chemoimmunotherapy with a modified hyper-CVAD and rituximab regimen improves outcome in de novo Philadelphia chromosome-negative precursor B-lineage acute lymphoblastic leukemia. J Clin Oncol 2010;28:3880; with permission.)

versus the 82 patients who received chemotherapy alone. Early death rates were also similar. In standard-risk patients, achievement of minimum residual disease (MRD) negativity at day 24 was 57% with rituximab versus 24% without rituximab. Continuous CR at 5 years had a probability of 80% with rituximab versus 47% without rituximab, and overall survival was 71% with rituximab versus 57% without. For conventionally defined high-risk patients, the OS at 3 years was 55% with rituximab and 36% without rituximab. This improvement in outcome was thought to be attributable to fewer relapses in those who received rituximab.[20] Of interest, CD20 expression may actually increase following exposure to corticosteroids, as demonstrated in a group of pediatric ALL patients in whom CD20 expression was upregulated from 45% in initial samples to 81% at the end of induction therapy. This result suggests that additional patients may benefit from rituximab.[21] Rituximab is currently being studied in the therapy for newly diagnosed Ph-neg B-lineage ALL patients in phase 3 randomized trials.

Another antigen of interest in the therapy for ALL is CD22. This 135-kDa transmembrane sialoglycoprotein, a member of the immunoglobulin superfamily, is present in the cytoplasm of developing B cells. Cell surface expression occurs at a later stage of B-cell development. CD22 expression on B-cell malignancies is high, in the range of 60% to 80%.[22] A CD22 IgG$_1$ humanized monoclonal antibody known as epratuzumab has been developed. It rapidly internalizes into the cell on binding to CD22, and appears to stimulate more of an immunomodulatory effect than an antiproliferative effect with rituximab.[23] Epratuzumab has single-agent activity in aggressive B-cell non-Hodgkin lymphoma. It has been combined with rituximab and chemotherapy, demonstrating a high CR rate of 62% and a partial response (PR) rate of 33%, with EFS that appears superior to rituximab and chemotherapy alone.[24]

The Children's Oncology Group (COG) has evaluated epratuzumab in pediatric ALL patients in a pilot trial. Patients with leukemic blast expression of CD22 of greater than 25% received 4 doses of intravenous epratuzumab, 360 mg/m^2 per dose twice weekly for 4 doses and then the same dose weekly for 4 weeks in combination with chemotherapy. All patients were in marrow relapse and, of the 12 evaluable patients who received single-agent therapy, 2 patients had a minimal cytolytic response, 8 had stable disease, and 2 progressed. Nine of the 12 patients achieved a CR after combined epratuzumab and chemotherapy, for which 7 were negative by MRD.[25] The COG is conducting a phase 2 trial of 4 doses of epratuzumab in combination with chemotherapy, and other trials combining epratuzumab with chemotherapy are ongoing.

Other CD22 antibodies of interest include a combination of an antibody that is fused to a 38-kDa fragment of *Pseudomonas aeruginosa* exotoxin A. This agent is known as CAT-3888. A phase 1 trial of 23 pediatric ALL patients with heavily relapsed disease gave doses ranging from 10 to 40 μg/kg every other day for 3 to 6 doses and repeated every 21 to 28 days. Adverse events were noted to be mild and reversible; and the trial did not demonstrate a maximum tolerated dose (MTD). Objective responses were not noted, but transient clinical activity was found.[26] This immunotoxin has been modified to create higher CD22 binding affinity and is known as CAT-8015 or moxetumomab pasudotox. It has been tested in vitro and found to be highly cytotoxic to B-lineage ALL cells in preclinical studies.[27] A humanized anti-CD22 monoclonal antibody has also been conjugated to calicheamicin, and is known as inotuzumab ozogamicin (CMC544). Studies in patients with refractory non-Hodgkin lymphoma have demonstrated an objective response rate of 87% in patients with follicular lymphoma and 80% in large B-cell lymphoma.[28] In a phase 1 trial in patients with refractory and relapsed ALL of 36 evaluable patients, CD22 was expressed in more than 50% of the blasts in all patients and in more than 90% in 20 patients. Nine of 36 patients achieved a conventional CR, and an additional 11 had a marrow CR for an overall response rate of 56%. The agent was administered as an intravenous infusion over 1 hour every 3 weeks, and the median of courses administered was 2 (range 1–5). Fever and mild hypotension occurred in most patients on the first and second days of therapy. Nine patients or 25% had liver function abnormalities that were thought to be drug related, and these were severe in 4 patients. Two patients had liver biopsies showing periportal fibrosis. Twelve patients were able to proceed to allogeneic BMT, and 3 of these developed sinusoidal obstruction syndrome post transplant. Further trials using the drug in alternative schedules and in combination with other agents are planned.[29]

An interesting approach to treating B-lineage ALL is to combine antibodies in a bispecific fashion. DT22199ARL is made up of two scFv ligands recognizing CD19 and CD22, which are linked to a hybrid gene encoding the first 390 amino acids of the catalytic diphtheria toxin (DT390). This molecule has been enhanced genetically so as to improve the in vivo antileukemic activity via reverse orientation of the VH-VL domains with the addition of linkers that reduce and stabilize aggregation. In an imaging model of a bioluminescent xenograft in which progression of a human Raji-Burkitt lymphoma cell line could be tracked, it was shown that this unique molecule could prevent hindlimb paralysis by blocking metastases to the spinal cord.[30] This agent is given intravenously for 4 doses every other day for 4 hours on an inpatient basis, and is in the midst of phase 1 testing.

The anti-CD52 antibody, alemtuzumab (Campath-1H), is an unconjugated humanized monoclonal antibody. CD52 is expressed on virtually all normal and malignant T and B lymphocytes as well as monocytes and macrophages.[31]

Experience with alemtuzumab in the treatment of ALL has been relatively limited. In a phase 2 study, 6 patients with ALL and 9 patients with relapsed-refractory acute myelogenous leukemia (AML) were treated with 30 mg intravenously 3 times a week for a total of 4 to 12 weeks. All patients demonstrated myelosuppression, but 10 patients progressed while on study, and there were frequent infections.[32]

In a trial assessing the efficacy of alemtuzumab in eradicating MRD in ALL, the CALGB tested sequential cohorts of CD52-positive patients with a dose escalation of alemtuzumab to a target dose of 30 mg administered 3 times a week subcutaneously for 12 doses (4 weeks) during postremission therapy. Twenty-four patients ranging in age from 18 to 77 years were treated. The drug was generally well tolerated with mild hematologic toxicities, but grade 3 to 4 myelosuppression was evident. Two patients had transient viremia with cytomegalovirus. In 11 of 24 patients, serial assessment of MRD demonstrated a median 1-log decrease in disease burden. During subsequent postremission therapy, 8 patients developed cytomegalovirus viremia, 3 had herpes zoster reactivation, and 2 had herpes simplex infections. Further studies with a 30-mg dose are planned.[33]

Another novel approach to using monoclonal antibody therapy in the treatment of ALL is to engage the cytotoxic benefit of T cells by constructing a bispecific T-cell engaging (BiTE) antibody construct. The agent, blinatumomab, combines the variable regions of an anti-CD19 antibody directed against B cells and an anti-CD3 antibody directed against T cells. This agent physically links T cells and malignant B cells, thus triggering the T-cell receptor complex signaling cascade. Recruitment of T cells with subsequent activation occurs when the anti-CD19 antibody binds its target antigen.[34–36]

A phase 2 trial of blinatumomab at 60 $\mu g/m^2/d$ given by continuous intravenous infusion for 4 to 8 weeks demonstrated 7 PR and 4 CR for a total of 11 responses in 12 patients.[37]

In the trials with lymphoma, it was noted that in patients treated with 15 $\mu g/m^2/d$, dosing had bone marrow clearance of disease. This finding provided the rationale for using this dose by continuous infusion for 4 weeks in patients with B-lineage ALL. In a recently reported trial, patients in complete hematologic remission who had evidence of disease by MRD testing that was either persistent or recurrent were treated. Of 20 evaluable patients, 16 became MRD-negative after one 4-week cycle of therapy. Twelve of these 16 had been molecularly refractory to previous chemotherapy. The most common grade 3 or 4 toxicity was lymphopenia, with an incidence of 33%. Other adverse events included fever, chills, decrease of blood immunoglobulins, and hypokalemia. Most of these were transient. One patient had to permanently discontinue treatment because of a grade 3 seizure; this was reversible. Another patient had syncope with a convulsion.[38] Blinatumomab appears to be a promising therapy in B-lineage ALL, and further trials in patients with MRD positivity, those with morphologic relapse, and those on front-line therapy with chemotherapy are planned.

EMERGING THERAPIES

NOTCH1 is a gene encoding a transmembrane receptor that is integrally involved in normal T-cell development and regulation. Although only rare cases demonstrate a chromosomal translocation involving this gene, it was found in 2004 that more than 50% of T-cell ALL (T-ALL) cases, including different immunophenotypic subtypes, have activating mutations in the NOTCH1 receptor involving the extracellular heterodimerization domain and/or the C-terminal PEST domain of NOTCH1.[39] The NOTCH1 receptor is a ligand-activating transcription factor, which transduces extracellular signals at the cell surface into alterations in gene expression in the nucleus. The receptor has a complex structure with 4 distinct subtypes involving the Delta and Serrate family of ligands. The receptor is a class I transmembrane glycoprotein that acts as a heterodimer (**Fig. 2**).[40] NOTCH1 is active at multiple stages of T-cell development. If NOTCH1 function is ablated, there is a complete block of T-cell development. Prognostically, NOTCH1 mutations are not associated with an unfavorable prognosis, and some series have suggested that it may confer a more favorable prognosis.

Given its high frequency, NOTCH1 would appear to be the suitable target for therapeutic maneuvers. There are several steps in the activation of NOTCH1 including processing by the γ-secretase complex, an aspartyl protease that cleaves NOTCH1 at the membrane level and releases intracellular components of NOTCH1 into the cytosol.[40] By inhibiting the γ-secretase complex, it could be possible to prevent oncogenic NOTCH1 signaling in T-ALL. In Alzheimer disease, a presenilin γ-secretase complex plays an important role in disease pathogenesis. In Alzheimer disease, small-molecule γ-secretase inhibitors (GSI) block the generation of amyloidogenic Aβ peptides and may slow the progression of human dementia. Inhibitory molecules have been developed to block the processing of amyloidogenic Aβ peptides in Alzheimer disease. In vitro models showed that rapid clearance of intracellular activating NOTCH1 protein and transcriptional regulation of NOTCH1 target genes occurred with these agents.[39] MK-0752, an oral GSI, was developed for the treatment of patients with relapsed ALL. In 7 T-ALL patients treated, 4 of whom showed a mutation in NOTCH1, there were no objective clinical responses, and significant gastrointestinal (GI) toxicity and fatigue were seen. The GI toxicity was attributed to inhibition of NOTCH1 signaling in the gut.[41] It may be that the GSI tested was ineffective in this setting because these agents appear to exert a cytostatic effect as their primary mechanism and exert little or no apoptosis. Subsequent studies with GSI have shown that they can reverse glucocorticoid resistance in T-ALL, and in vitro, corticosteroids inhibit the severe secretory metaplasia that is induced by inhibition of NOTCH1

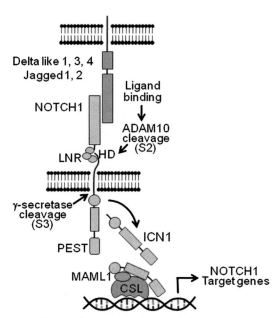

Fig. 2. The NOTCH1 signaling pathway. Interaction of the NOTCH1 receptor with Delta-like and Jagged ligands expressed on the surface of a neighbor cells triggers the proteolytic cleavage of the receptor, first by an ADAM metalloprotease (S2 cleavage) and subsequently by the γ-secretase complex (S3 cleavage), which releases the intracellular domains of NOTCH1 (ICN1) from the membrane. ICN1 translocates to the nucleus and interacts with DNA via the RBPJ/CSL DNA binding protein, and recruits the MAML1 coactivator to activate the expression of NOTCH1 target genes. (*From* Ferrando AA. The role of NOTCH1 signaling in T-ALL. Hematology 2009;353–61; with permission.)

signaling in the gut by GSI.[42] Other GSI have shown promising activity in vitro and are in early clinical trials.[43]

A genetic disorder leading to deficiency of purine nucleoside phosphorylase (PNP) results in specific T-cell immunodeficiency. This finding has suggested that inhibition of PNP could serve as a therapeutic pathway for treatment of T-ALL. The inhibition of PNP results in elevation of 2′-deoxyguanosine with accumulation of intracellular deoxyguanosine 5′-triphosphate. Accumulation of these substances induces cellular apoptosis. Bcx-1777, also known as forodesine, is a PNP inhibitor.[44] For patients with relapsed or refractory T-ALL, forodesine was infused at a dose of 40 mg/m^2 intravenously 5 days per week for a total of 6 cycles. Dose escalations to 90 mg/m^2 were permitted in patients who were not responding after the second cycle. The overall response rate in 34 patients was 32%, with 7 CR and 4 PR. A BMT was able to be performed in 2 of the patients who achieved a CR. Dose escalation to 90 mg/m^2 after cycle 2 was performed in 18 patients. Cytopenias, nausea, headache, and asthma were the adverse events noted.[45] Forodesine has also shown activity in non-Hodgkin lymphoma and chronic lymphocytic leukemia.

Hypermethylation of densely clustered cytosines (CpG islands) within the promoter region of tumor suppressor genes has been shown to induce gene silencing in ALL.[46,47] Exposure of ALL cell lines to decitabine has been shown to result in reactivation of epigenetically silenced genes and induction of apoptosis via global and gene-specific hypomethylation.[48] The pyrimidine nucleoside analogue, decitabine, is an inhibitor of DNA methyltransferase activity and can reactivate silenced genes by inhibiting methylation of cytosine residues on DNA. A phase 1 trial of decitabine in relapsed and refractory ALL initiated therapy at 10 mg/m^2 for 5 days every other week. Dose levels ranging from 10 to 120 mg/m^2 were given to 23 patients with an overall response rate of 26%. There was 1 CR with incomplete platelet recovery (CRp) and 5 complete marrow responses of blasts under 5%. Toxicities included diarrhea, fatigue, and liver function test abnormalities. Responses were noted at multiple dose levels, and global hypomethylation was seen in vitro.[49] A phase 1 trial with or without hyper-CVAD in ALL was recently reported. Patients with relapsed or refractory ALL qualified for the study without regard to the presence or absence of CNS disease, performance status, age, or level of hepatic or renal function. Patients were initially treated with single-agent decitabine, and those patients not responding or those that lost their response could be treated in the sequential phase of the trial with a combination of hyper-CVAD and decitabine. The initial dose of decitabine used was 10 mg/m^2 intravenously, daily for 5 days every 2 weeks as a single agent. When combined with hyper-CVAD, the initial dose was 5 mg/m^2 daily for 5 days on a 28-day cycle. In total, 39 patients were treated with a median age of 33 years (range 4–67 and a median white blood cell count of 5.8). Patients had received a median of 3 prior therapies (range 1–7). All patients but 9 had complex cytogenetics, with 4 of the remaining 9 having a Philadelphia chromosome. Single-agent decitabine dose levels ranged from 10 to 120 mg/m^2/d for 5 days. Seven of 30 patients (23%) treated with single-agent decitabine achieved complete marrow responses. Responses were observed at all dose levels but were transient. A dose of 60 mg/m^2 intravenously, daily for 5 days every 14 days was selected as the optimal dose because of lack of toxicity and induction of global hypomethylation. Of the 30 patients treated with decitabine alone, 16 went on to receive decitabine and hyper-CVAD in a sequential fashion. An additional 9 patients went directly to therapy with decitabine and hyper-CVAD. Doses up to 60 mg/m^2 intravenously, daily for 5 days were combined with hyper-CVAD. No significant toxicity was associated with the combination therapy. With the combination, 13 of 25 patients (52%) achieved a response including 4 CR (16%), 2 CRp (8%), and 7 complete marrow responses (28%). Median duration of response was longer than 4 months. The optimal dose of decitabine in combination with hyper-CVAD was thought to be 40 mg/m^2 intravenously, daily for 5 days. The investigators concluded that decitabine has single-agent activity and in combination with hyper-CVAD is safe.[49]

Folic acid antagonists such as the classic drug, methotrexate, were among the first agents to show activity in the treatment of ALL. A recently developed folate antagonist of interest is pemetrexed (LY-231514). Pemetrexed has been used in a phase 1 trial of patients with relapsed or refractory acute leukemia and has shown modest activity, with one patient with ALL achieving a PR at a dose level of 3.6 g/m^2. Liver dysfunction was the main nonimmunologic adverse event. The recommended phase 2 dose was 2.7 g/m^2 over 25 minutes every 3 to 4 weeks with vitamin supplementation. It was thought that the drug had limited activity as a single agent, but study of its use in combination with other agents might be considered.[50]

Another antifolate drug of interest is talotrexin, which has a higher affinity than methotrexate to dihydrofolate reductase. It achieved cell entry through a reduced folate carrier type 1 enzyme. Talotrexin has been administered as 5- to 10-minute infusion daily on days 1 to 5 over 5 to 10 minutes on a 21-day schedule, and a major response was noted in a patient with refractory ALL in an ongoing phase 1 study.[51]

Another agent of interest is the synthetic flavone derivative, flavopiridol (Alvocidib), which is derived from tree bark. It has been shown to induce apoptosis and inhibit growth against multiple human tumor cell lines, and has activity in both myeloid and lymphoid malignancies. In a phase 1 trial as a single agent, a novel bolus/infusion schedule was used whereby the initial dose is given over 30 minutes followed by a second dose infused continuously over 4 hours. The MTD in a single-agent phase 1 study in relapsed and refractory AML and ALL was found to be 40 mg/m^2 by intravenous bolus followed by 60 mg/m^2 by continuous intravenous infusion. Secretory diarrhea was the dose-limiting toxicity. As a single agent, disease activity was modest. Dramatic but transient reductions in circulating blasts that lasted 10 to 14 days were seen.[52] In a phase 1 trial in which flavopiridol was given as a daily 1-hour infusion for 3 days in combination with cytarabine and mitoxantrone to patients with refractory-relapsed AML or ALL, 40% of patients demonstrated direct leukemic cytotoxicity with a greater than 50% drop in peripheral blast counts and tumor lysis in 9 of a total of 34 patients. The overall response rate was 12.5% in the ALL patients, whereas it was 31% in 26 AML patients.[53]

Bortezomib is the first agent in a class of drugs that inhibits the proteasome. This process represents a new mechanism for inducing apoptosis in malignant cells. Bortezomib has been extensively studied in multiple myeloma and relapsed non-Hodgkin lymphoma, treatment of which by these agents is approved by the Food and Drug Administration. Preclinical data suggest bortezomib might have single-agent activity in ALL.[54] In a phase 1 trial with bortezomib in relapsed and refractory acute leukemia, the MTD was determined to be 1.25 mg/m^2 using a twice-weekly schedule for 4 out of 6 weeks. Proteasome inhibition was dose dependent and was 68% at the limiting dose of 1.5 mg/m^2. Five of 15 patients showed evidence of hematologic improvement.[55] In 12 pediatric patients (9 with ALL and 3 with AML), a phase 1 study was conducted, and the recommended phase 2 dose was suggested to be 1.3 mg/m^2 per dose given twice weekly for 2 weeks followed by 1 week of rest. Unfortunately, no objective responses were seen in this study.[56] However, bortezomib has been combined with conventional ALL agents in children including doxorubicin, pegylated asparaginase, dexamethasone, and vincristine in a phase 1 study in which the bortezomib was dose escalated on days 1, 4, 8, and 11. In this combination, 6 CR were seen among 9 evaluable patients with a dose of bortezomib of 1.3 mg/m^2.[57]

A serine and threonine kinase, the mammalian target of rapamycin (mTOR) acts through the PI3K-AKT transduction pathway and regulates antiapoptotic and proliferative signals. Examples of agents that inhibit mTOR include the first-generation drug, sirolimus (rapamycin), and second-generation analogues such as everolimus (RAD001) and temsirolimus (CCI-779). Induction of apoptosis by rapamycin has been demonstrated in B-lineage ALL cell lines in vitro, and has been shown to have in vivo activity against B-precursor leukemia/lymphoma in transgenic mice.[58]

An in vivo model of pediatric ALL has been used to demonstrate that everolimus induces autophagy in ALL cells. In this study, everolimus increased Beclin-1 expression with focal degradation of cytoplasmic areas sequestered by autophagic structures as demonstrated by electron microscopy.[59] In this study, where nonobese diabetic/severe combined immunodeficient (NOD/SCID) mice were inoculated with childhood B-cell ALL cells, everolimus increased the median survival of mice from 21 to 42 days. When combined with vincristine, they had significantly increased survival compared with either treatment alone. Everolimus induced cell cycle arrest in a $G_{0/1}$ phase, and reduced levels of cyclin-dependent kinases 4 and 6 and dephosphorylation of the retinoblastoma protein.[60]

Murine double minute (MDM2) protein has been shown to be overexpressed in pediatric ALL. It is often associated with a wild-type p53 phenotype and resistance to chemotherapy. Inhibition of the MDM2-p53 interaction by nutlin-3 can induce p53 activity and result in apoptosis, as has been shown in adult T-cell leukemia cells.[61]

R05045337 (RG-7112) is an oral formulation of nutlin-3 that is in phase 1 testing, administered either daily for 10 days or every other day for 11 of every 28 days.

Mitogen-activated protein kinase (MEK) can enhance proliferation and survival in leukemic cells when activated. MEK inhibitors might be therapeutic in ALL. BCL-2 interacting mediator of cell death (BIM), a proapoptotic protein, is inactivated by extra-cellular signal-regulated kinase (ERK)-mediated phosphorylation. In ALL cells, BIM is upregulated by dexamethasone. The use of MEK-ERK inhibitors in combination with dexamethasone may induce synergistic enhancement of apoptosis in vitro.[62] Several MEK inhibitors are in clinical trials. The serine-threonine PIM kinases are upregulated in several hematologic malignancies and play important roles in multiple signal trans-duction pathways. T-lymphoblastic leukemia/lymphoma cells have been found to be sensitive to small-molecule inhibitors of PIM protein kinases in vitro, and in vivo in immunodeficient mice inoculated with these malignant cells.[63]

SUMMARY

Therapy for ALL in adults remains a tremendous challenge for clinicians. The use of pediatric-intensive regimens in young and middle-aged adults shows promise in improving outcomes. The addition of monoclonal antibody therapy to chemotherapy appears to hold great promise in lessening relapse rates. The anti-CD20 antibody, rit-uximab, which has been of such benefit in patients with non-Hodgkin lymphoma, now seems poised to bring significant benefit to adults with ALL. Other monoclonal anti-body approaches are in earlier stages of development, but will likely be of significant benefit. The BiTE antibody, blinatumomab, represents an exciting new approach in this arena.

As new molecular abnormalities are identified in ALL, these will certainly become new targets for drug development. The increasing use of MRD testing by molecular or flow cytometric techniques will also be invaluable in further refining prognostication in ALL in helping with the selection of patients most likely to benefit from BMT.

Several new small molecules and chemotherapeutic agents will, it is hoped, also find a niche in the therapy for ALL. Early examples including *NOTCH1* inhibitors; hypo-methylating agents such as decitabine, folic acid, antagonists, flavopiridol, bortezo-mib, and mTOR inhibitors will all hopefully find a role in the therapy for this challenging disorder. Although many challenges remain, there is hope that the therapy for adults with ALL can make significant progress in the next few years, in comparison with the relative plateau that has been experienced over the last several decades.

REFERENCES

1. Pui CH, Evans WE. Treatment of acute lymphoblastic leukemia. N Engl J Med 2006;354:166.
2. Fielding A. The treatment of adults with acute lymphoblastic leukemia. Hema-tology Am Soc Hematol Educ Program 2008;381.
3. Pulte D, Gondos A, Brenner H. Improvement in survival in younger patients with acute lymphoblastic leukemia from the 1980s to the early 21st century. Blood 2009;113:1408.
4. Moorman AV, Harrison CJ, Buck GA, et al. Karyotype is an independent prog-nostic factor in adult acute lymphoblastic leukemia (ALL): analysis of cytogenetic data from patients treated on the Medical Research Council (MRC) UKALLXII/ Eastern Cooperative Oncology Group (ECOG) 2993 trial. Blood 2007;109:3189.
5. Stock W, La M, Sanford B, et al. What determines the outcomes for adolescents and young adults with acute lymphoblastic leukemia treated on cooperative

group protocols? A comparison of Children's Cancer Group and Cancer and Leukemia Group B studies. Blood 2008;112:1646.

6. Litzow MR. Evolving paradigms in the therapy of Philadelphia chromosome-negative acute lymphoblastic leukemia in adults. Hematology Am Soc Hematol Educ Program 2009;362.

7. Ramanujachar R, Richards S, Hann I, et al. Adolescents with acute lymphoblastic leukaemia: emerging from the shadow of paediatric and adult treatment protocols. Pediatr Blood Cancer 2006;47:748.

8. Ribera JM, Oriol A. Acute lymphoblastic leukemia in adolescents and young adults. Hematol Oncol Clin North Am 2009;23:1033.

9. Schiffer CA. Differences in outcome in adolescents with acute lymphoblastic leukemia: a consequence of better regimens? better doctors? both? J Clin Oncol 2003;21:760.

10. Huguet F, Leguay T, Raffoux E, et al. Pediatric-inspired therapy in adults with Philadelphia chromosome-negative acute lymphoblastic leukemia: the GRAALL-2003 Study. J Clin Oncol 2009;27:911.

11. Ribera JM, Oriol A, Sanz MA, et al. Comparison of the results of the treatment of adolescents and young adults with standard-risk acute lymphoblastic leukemia with the Programa Espanol de Tratamiento en Hematologia pediatric-based protocol ALL-96. J Clin Oncol 2008;26:1843.

12. Storring JM, Minden MD, Kao S, et al. Treatment of adults with BCR-ABL negative acute lymphoblastic leukaemia with a modified paediatric regimen. Br J Haematol 2009;146:76.

13. Phase II study of combination chemotherapy in adolescents and young adults with newly diagnosed acute lymphoblastic leukemia in. National Cancer Institute; 2011. Available at: http://clinicaltrials.gov/ct2/results. Accessed September 28, 2011.

14. Campana D. Minimal residual disease in acute lymphoblastic leukemia. Hematology Am Soc Hematol Educ Program 2010;2010:7.

15. Borowitz MJ, Shuster J, Carroll AJ, et al. Prognostic significance of fluorescence intensity of surface marker expression in childhood B-precursor acute lymphoblastic leukemia. A Pediatric Oncology Group Study. Blood 1997;89:3960.

16. Jeha S, Behm F, Pei D, et al. Prognostic significance of CD20 expression in childhood B-cell precursor acute lymphoblastic leukemia. Blood 2006;108:3302.

17. Thomas DA, O'Brien S, Jorgensen JL, et al. Prognostic significance of CD20 expression in adults with de novo precursor B-lineage acute lymphoblastic leukemia. Blood 2009;113:6330.

18. Maury S, Huguet F, Leguay T, et al. Adverse prognostic significance of CD20 expression in adults with Philadelphia chromosome-negative B-cell precursor acute lymphoblastic leukemia. Haematologica 2010;95:324.

19. Thomas DA, O'Brien S, Faderl S, et al. Chemoimmunotherapy with a modified hyper-CVAD and rituximab regimen improves outcome in de novo Philadelphia chromosome-negative precursor B-lineage acute lymphoblastic leukemia. J Clin Oncol 2010;28:3880.

20. Hoelzer D, Huettmann A, Kaul F, et al. Immunochemotherapy with rituximab improves molecular CR rate and outcome in CD20+ B-lineage standard and high-risk patients; results of 263 CD20+ patients studied prospectively in GMALL study 07/2003 [abstract: 170]. Blood 2010;116:77.

21. Dworzak MN, Schumich A, Printz D, et al. CD20 up-regulation in pediatric B-cell precursor acute lymphoblastic leukemia during induction treatment: setting the stage for anti-CD20 directed immunotherapy. Blood 2008;112:3982.

22. Coleman M, Goldenberg DM, Siegel AB, et al. Epratuzumab. Clin Cancer Res 2003;9:3991s.
23. Carnahan J, Stein R, Qu Z, et al. Epratuzumab, a CD22-targeting recombinant humanized antibody with a different mode of action from rituximab. Mol Immunol 2007;44:1331.
24. Micallef IN, Maurer MJ, Wiseman GA, et al. Epratuzumab with rituximab, cyclophosphamide, doxorubicin, vincristine, and prednisone chemotherapy (ER-CHOP) in patients with previously untreated diffuse large B-cell lymphoma. Blood 2011;118:4053.
25. Raetz EA, Cairo MS, Borowitz MJ, et al. Chemoimmunotherapy reinduction with epratuzumab in children with acute lymphoblastic leukemia in marrow relapse: a Children's Oncology Group Pilot Study. J Clin Oncol 2008;26:3756.
26. Wayne AS, Kreitman RJ, Findley HW, et al. Anti-CD22 immunotoxin RFB4(dsFv)-PE38 (BL22) for CD22-positive hematologic malignancies of childhood: preclinical studies and phase I clinical trial. Clin Cancer Res 2010;16:1894.
27. Wayne AS, Bhojwani D, Jeha S, et al. Phase I clinical trial of the anti-CD22 immunotoxin CAT-8015 (HA22) for pediatric acute lymphoblastic leukemia (ALL). Blood 2009;114:839.
28. Dang NH, Smith MR, Offner F, et al. Anti-CD22 immunoconjugate inotuzumab ozogamicin (CMC-544) + rituximab: clinical activity including survival in patients with recurrent/refractory follicular or 'aggressive' lymphoma. Blood 2009;114:584.
29. Jabbour E. Inotuzumab ozogamicin (IO; CMC544), a CD22 monoclonal antibody attached to calicheamycin, produces complete response (CR) plus complete marrow response (mCR) of greater than 50% in refractory relapse (R-R) acute lymphocytic leukemia (ALL) [abstract: 6507]. J Clin Oncol 2011;29:420s.
30. Vallera D, Hua C, Andrew RS, et al. Genetic alteration of a bispecific ligand-directed toxin targeting human CD19 and CD22 receptors resulting in improved efficacy against systemic B cell malignancy. Leuk Res 2009;33:1233.
31. Keating MJ, O'Brien S, Ferrajoli A. Alemtuzumab: a novel monoclonal antibody. Expert Opin Biol Ther 2001;1:1059.
32. Tibes R, Keating MJ, Ferrajoli A, et al. Activity of alemtuzumab in patients with CD52-positive acute leukemia. Cancer 2006;106:2645.
33. Stock W, Sanford B, Lozanski G, et al. Alemtuzumab can be incorporated into front-line therapy of adult acute lymphoblastic leukemia (ALL): final phase I results of a cancer and Leukemia Group B Study (CALGB 10102). Blood 2009;114:838.
34. Baeuerle PA, Reinhardt C. Bispecific T-cell engaging antibodies for cancer therapy. Cancer Res 2009;69:4941.
35. Bargou R, Leo E, Zugmaier G, et al. Tumor regression in cancer patients by very low doses of a T cell-engaging antibody. Science 2008;321:974.
36. Nagorsen D, Bargou R, Ruttinger D, et al. Immunotherapy of lymphoma and leukemia with T-cell engaging BiTE antibody blinatumomab. Leuk Lymphoma 2009;50:886.
37. Nagorsen D, Zugmaier G, Viardot A, et al. Confirmation of safety, efficacy and response duration in non-Hodgkin lymphoma patients treated with 60 mcg/m^2/d of BiTE(R) antibody blinatumomab. Blood 2009;114:2723.
38. Topp MS, Kufer P, Gokbuget N, et al. Targeted therapy with the T-cell-engaging antibody blinatumomab of chemotherapy-refractory minimal residual disease in B-lineage acute lymphoblastic leukemia patients results in high response rate and prolonged leukemia-free survival. J Clin Oncol 2011;29:2493.

39. Weng AP, Ferrando AA, Lee W, et al. Activating mutations of NOTCH1 in human T cell acute lymphoblastic leukemia. Science 2004;306:269.

40. Ferrando AA. The role of NOTCH1 signaling in T-ALL. Hematology 2009;353–61.

41. Deangelo DJ, Stone RM, Silverman LB, et al. A phase I clinical trial of the notch inhibitor MK-0752 in patients with T-cell acute lymphoblastic leukemia/lymphoma (T-ALL) and other leukemias. J Clin Oncol (Meeting Abstracts) 2006;24:6585.

42. Real PJ, Tosello V, Palomero T, et al. [Gamma]-secretase inhibitors reverse glucocorticoid resistance in T cell acute lymphoblastic leukemia. Nat Med 2009;15:50.

43. Wei P, Walls M, Qiu M, et al. Evaluation of selective γ-secretase inhibitor PF-03084014 for its antitumor efficacy and gastrointestinal safety to guide optimal clinical trial design. Mol Cancer Ther 2010;9:1618.

44. Furman RR, Hoelzer D. Purine nucleoside phosphorylase inhibition as a novel therapeutic approach for B-cell lymphoid malignancies. Semin Oncol 2007;34:S29.

45. Furman RR, Gore L, Ravandi F, et al. Forodesine IV (Bcx-1777) is clinically active in relapsed/refractory T-cell leukemia: results of a phase II study (interim report). Blood 2006;108:1851.

46. Bueso-Ramos C, Xu Y, McDonnell TJ, et al. Protein expression of a triad of frequently methylated genes, p73, p57Kip2, and p15, has prognostic value in adult acute lymphocytic leukemia independently of its methylation status. J Clin Oncol 2005;23:3932.

47. Zheng S, Ma X, Zhang L, et al. Hypermethylation of the 5′ CpG island of the FHIT gene is associated with hyperdiploid and translocation-negative subtypes of pediatric leukemia. Cancer Res 2004;64:2000.

48. Hui Y, Koyu H, Blanca SG, et al. Antileukemia activity of the combination of 5-aza-2′ -deoxycytidine with valproic acid. Leuk Res 2005;29:739.

49. Garcia-Manero G, Thomas DA, Ryting ME, et al. Final report of a phase I trial of decitabine with or without hyperCVAD in relapsed acute lymphocytic leukemia (ALL) [abstract: 867]. Blood 2010;116:379.

50. Abdel-Karim I, Plunkett WK Jr, O'Brien S, et al. A phase I study of pemetrexed in patients with relapsed or refractory acute leukemia. Invest New Drugs 2011;29:323.

51. Giles F, Rizzieri DA, George S, et al. A phase I study of Talvesta(R) (Talotrexin) in relapsed or refractory leukemia or myelodysplastic syndrome. Blood 2006;108:1968.

52. Blum W, Phelps MA, Klisovic RB, et al. Phase I clinical and pharmacokinetic study of a novel schedule of flavopiridol in relapsed or refractory acute leukemias. Haematologica 2010;95:1098.

53. Karp JE, Passaniti A, Gojo I, et al. Phase I and pharmacokinetic study of flavopiridol followed by 1-β -d-arabinofuranosylcytosine and mitoxantrone in relapsed and refractory adult acute leukemias. Clin Cancer Res 2005;11:8403.

54. Houghton PJ, Morton CL, Kolb EA, et al. Initial testing (stage 1) of the proteasome inhibitor bortezomib by the pediatric preclinical testing program. Pediatr Blood Cancer 2008;50:37.

55. Cortes J, Thomas D, Koller C, et al. Phase I study of bortezomib in refractory or relapsed acute leukemias. Clin Cancer Res 2004;10:3371.

56. Horton TM, Pati D, Plon SE, et al. A phase 1 study of the proteasome inhibitor bortezomib in pediatric patients with refractory leukemia: a Children's Oncology Group Study. Clin Cancer Res 2007;13:1516.

57. Messinger Y, Gaynon P, Raetz E, et al. Phase I study of bortezomib combined with chemotherapy in children with relapsed childhood acute lymphoblastic leukemia (ALL): a report from the therapeutic advances in childhood leukemia (TACL) consortium. Pediatr Blood Cancer 2010;55:254.

58. Brown VI, Fang J, Alcorn K, et al. Rapamycin is active against B-precursor leukemia in vitro and in vivo, an effect that is modulated by IL-7-mediated signaling. Proc Natl Acad Sci U S A 2003;100:15113.
59. Crazzolara R, Bradstock KF, Bendall LJ. RAD001 (everolimus) induces autophagy in acute lymphoblastic leukemia. Autophagy 2009;5:727.
60. Crazzolara R, Cisterne A, Thien M, et al. Potentiating effects of RAD001 (everolimus) on vincristine therapy in childhood acute lymphoblastic leukemia. Blood 2009;113:3297.
61. Hasegawa H, Yamada Y, Iha H, et al. Activation of p53 by Nutlin-3a, an antagonist of MDM2, induces apoptosis and cellular senescence in adult T-cell leukemia cells. Leukemia 2009;23:2090.
62. Rambal AA, Panaguiton ZL, Kramer L, et al. MEK inhibitors potentiate dexamethasone lethality in acute lymphoblastic leukemia cells through the pro-apoptotic molecule BIM. Leukemia 2009;23:1744.
63. Lin YW, Beharry ZM, Hill EG, et al. A small molecule inhibitor of PIM protein kinases blocks the growth of precursor T-cell lymphoblastic leukemia/lymphoma. Blood 2010;115:824.

Novel Transplant Strategies in Adults with Acute Leukemia

Oana Paun, MD, Hillard M. Lazarus, MD*

KEYWORDS

• Acute leukemia • Allogeneic hematopoietic cell transplantation
• Treatment-related mortality

More than 50 years have passed from the initial report from Dr E. Donnall Thomas and colleagues describing the safety (no marrow emboli) and efficacy (some donor engraftment) of bone marrow transplanted into 6 patients with a variety of malignant and nonmalignant disorders.[1,2] Worldwide, autologous and allogeneic hematopoietic cell transplantation (HCT) is regularly used as a curative treatment option for patients with various disorders, including acute leukemia. Both the chemoradiation or chemotherapy used in the preparative regimen and effects of the graft mediated via the immunologic graft-versus-leukemia (GVL) effect[3] contribute to the success of this approach. At present, acute myeloid leukemia (AML) is the most common indication for HCT; although HCT remains the preferred therapy for a distinct subset of AML patients, acute lymphoblastic leukemia (ALL) patients are also often considered for this therapy.[4] The past decade has witnessed dramatic improvements in the reduction of treatment-related mortality (TRM), in part attributable to improved supportive care but also due to better graft selection and donor-to-recipient matching regimens.[5–7] The emergence of reduced-intensity conditioning (RIC) in place of myeloablative conditioning (MAC) broadens the applicability of this modality to patients who formerly would be excluded from HCT because of advanced age or comorbid conditions. The demonstration that the graft-versus-leukemia effect eradicates disseminated cancer has fueled efforts to develop immunotherapeutic approaches to tumors.[2] Despite these advances, HCT remains plagued by the risk of relapse or failure due to graft-versus-host disease (GVHD), infectious complications, and TRM. New approaches are emerging that may improve overall patient outcome; many of these novel strategies are reviewed herein.

GRAFT SOURCES

The earliest HCT transplants used grafts obtained from histocompatible siblings and subsequently from the patients themselves if they were in complete remission

Department of Medicine, University Hospitals Case Medical Center, Case Comprehensive Cancer Center, 11100 Euclid Avenue, Cleveland, OH 44106, USA
* Corresponding author.
E-mail address: Hillard.Lazarus@case.edu

Hematol Oncol Clin N Am 25 (2011) 1319–1339
doi:10.1016/j.hoc.2011.08.001
0889-8588/11/$ – see front matter © 2011 Elsevier Inc. All rights reserved.

hemonc.theclinics.com

Table 1
Graft sources for allogeneic hematopoietic cell transplantation and percentage of all transplants

	Match Probability (%)	Percentage of All Transplants
HLA-compatible sibling	30	54
HLA-compatible unrelated donor	35–80	38
Umbilical cord blood	10–90	5
Haploidentical donor	99	<5

(autologous). The past decade has seen the emergence of a significant shift to the use of alternative donors, as shown in **Table 1**.[8]

The increase in the donor pool has contributed significantly to the sustained increase in the number of AML allogeneic transplants performed in the last decade. It is hypothesized that the source of the hematopoietic progenitor cells may play a role in exerting different donor-versus-host immune effects. **Fig. 1** summarizes the results of consecutive patients undergoing first allogeneic HCT from various graft sources for hematologic malignancy after a high-dose total body irradiation containing conditioning regimen at the Fred Hutchinson Cancer Research Center (FHCRC) and University of Minnesota between 2001 and 2008.

AUTOLOGOUS HCT

Autologous HCT is considered an alternative postremission therapy in patients with favorable-risk and intermediate-risk cytogenetics AML, whereas it cannot be recommended to patients with high-risk cytogenetics.[9–11] Outcome after autologous HCT is at least as good as after the use of postremission chemotherapy, and may offer an advantage in specific subsets of AML.[9,12] Fernandez and colleagues[13] reported recently the results of a prospective, randomized phase 3 trial evaluating the use of gemtuzumab ozogamicin (GO) in an intensive consolidation approach followed by autologous HCT. A total of 657 patients with a median age of 47 years (range 17–60 years) in first complete remission (CR1) after cytarabine and standard-dose or high-dose daunorubicin induction received 2 cycles of consolidation with high-dose cytarabine followed by peripheral blood progenitor cell collection, then were randomized to receive GO (n = 132) or not (n = 138) and proceeded to autologous HCT. The subgroups of favorable-risk and intermediate-risk AML had 4-year disease-free survival rates of 60% and 40% and overall survival rates of 80% and 49.3%, respectively, while addition of a single dose of GO in this setting did not improve outcomes. For younger AML patients in CR1, autologous HCT should be considered in patients with favorable and intermediate cytogenetic risk who do not have an allogeneic donor.

This modality does not appear to have a role in ALL.[14]

ALLOGENEIC HCT
Bone Marrow

Bone marrow as a graft source has fallen out of favor over the past 15 years; data from the Center for International Blood and Marrow Transplant Research show that in 2008 only 12% of the related donor grafts and 14% of the unrelated donor grafts were derived from bone marrow as opposed to peripheral blood. The field anxiously awaits the results of the recently completed Blood and Marrow Transplant Clinical Trials Network

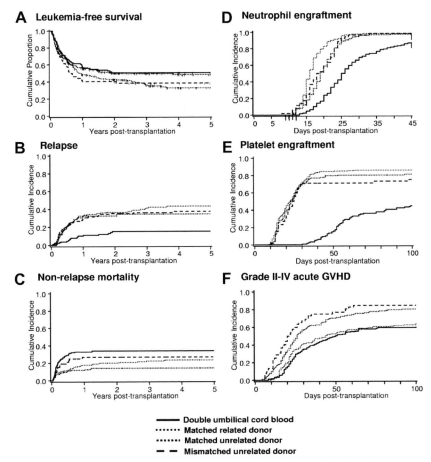

Fig. 1. Clinical outcomes. (*A*) Leukemia-free survival, (*B*) relapse, (*C*) Nonrelapse mortality, (*D*) neutrophil engraftment, (*E*) platelet engraftment, and (*F*) grade II to IV acute graft-versus-host disease (GVHD) after double umbilical cord blood, matched related donor, matched unrelated donor, and mismatched unrelated donor transplantation. (*Reproduced from* Brunstein CG, Gutman JA, Weisdorf DJ, et al. Allogeneic hematopoietic cell transplantation for hematologic malignancy: relative risks and benefits of double umbilical cord blood. Blood 2010;116(22):4695; with permission.)

(BMT CTN) prospective, randomized trial BMT CTN 0201, comparing bone marrow with mobilized peripheral blood as source of matched unrelated donor grafts.

Peripheral Blood

Dividing, nonleukemic DNA-synthesizing cells were first identified in peripheral blood in the 1950s, suggesting the existence of a small number of circulating cells of "multipotential character."[15] With the development of continuous-flow apheresis and the widespread implementation of hematopoietic growth factor mobilization treatment, blood rapidly replaced bone marrow as the graft source of choice.[16] Newer strategies include the use of plerixafor, a novel small-molecule CXCR4 chemokine antagonist that enhances mobilization of hematopoietic progenitor cells from volunteer donors,[17] with or without granulocyte colony-stimulating factor (G-CSF) (filgrastim).

Umbilical Cord Blood

This graft source first was used in 1988[18] in a Fanconi anemia patient who had a healthy HLA-identical sibling. The main practical advantages of using umbilical cord blood (UCB) as an alternative source of hematopoietic progenitor cells are many, including the relative ease of procurement, the absence of risks for mothers and donors, the reduced likelihood of transmitting infections, and rapid availability.[19] Further, for a given degree of HLA match, UCB grafts are associated with a reduced degree of GVHD when compared with a matched unrelated donor graft, yet retain the GVL effect.[20] Finally, no donor isohemagglutinins are produced in an ABO-incompatible HCT[21] when UCB is used.

One major challenge associated with the use of UCB for transplantation is the relatively low cell dose available; this impediment contributes, at least in part, to the slower engraftment and elevated risk of engraftment failure associated with UCB HCT. Several strategies have been proposed to improve the effectiveness of UCB transplants with respect to the rates and kinetics of engraftment. These approaches include the infusion of 2 UCB units and ex vivo expansion of UCB grafts using a variety of techniques including multipotent mesenchymal stromal cells (MSCs), the copper chelator tetraethylenepentamine (TEPA), and the Notch ligand (see later discussion).

Double cord blood transplant

Whereas double UCB HCT may provide significantly more rapid neutrophil engraftment[22,23] compared with use of single units, engraftment delays and failure rates remain higher when compared with bone marrow or mobilized blood sources. Furthermore, an area of continued investigation is to explain the observation of why only one unit will ultimately predominate.

In transplant recipients receiving 2 or more UCB units,[24–26] one of the UCB units predominates, usually by 4 to 6 weeks after transplant. Infusion of the UCB that does not engraft may augment engraftment via immune activation, inhibition of recipient-mediated immune rejection, or the combination.[27] On the other hand, relapse rates appear lower with 2 than with 1 unit.[28,29] To date, there have been no convincing data that infusion of 2 rather than 1 UCB unit is superior; given the significantly higher cost and other issues, the standard of care remains uncertain.

Ex vivo UCB unit expansion: MSCs

De Lima and colleagues at the MD Anderson Cancer Center[30] recently reported the early findings of a study whereby they ex vivo cocultured one of two UCB units infused in the course of a double UCB HCT. For expansion, they used either third-party haploidentical family member marrow-derived MSCs or commercially available mesenchymal progenitor cells (Angioblast Systems, Inc, New York, NY). Thirty-two patients received a MAC regimen consisting of fludarabine, melphalan, thiotepa, and antithymocyte globulin (ATG). The culture yielded a median 14-fold increase in total nucleated cells and 40-fold increase in CD34$^+$ cells. Median time to neutrophil and platelet engraftment was 15 (range 9–42) days and 40 (range 13–62) days; there were no toxicities attributable to the expanded cells. The expanded unit contributed only to early blood cell recovery; long-term engraftment was provided by the unexpanded unit.

Ex vivo UCB unit expansion: TEPA

Peled and co-workers[31] described a NOD/SCID mouse model in which the linear polyamine copper chelator TEPA augmented long-term ex vivo expansion of UCB-derived CD34$^+$ cells and increased their engraftment potential. Subsequently, the

MD Anderson Cancer Center group conducted a clinical trial in which 10 high-risk hematologic malignancy patients (n = 5 ALL; n = 2 AML) received high-dose cytotoxic therapy followed by infusion of a UCB unit that had been cryopreserved in 2 fractions.[32] The GVHD prophylaxis regimen was combination tacrolimus with "mini-methotrexate" (3 days). One of the fractions was administered unexpanded, whereas the other component was CD133-selected and expanded in vitro in media containing stem cell factor (SCF), FLT-3 ligand, interleukin (IL)-6, thrombopoietin, and TEPA. The total nucleated cell dose in the manipulated component was expanded 219-fold and the CD34$^+$ cell content increased sixfold. Despite the fact that the mean total nucleated cell content infused was low (1.8×10^7/kg), 9 of 10 patients engrafted at times comparable with those associated with infusion of unmanipulated single UCB units, for example, neutrophils at 30 days and platelets at 48 days. These data demonstrate that a graft with low cell numbers can be used successfully and justify exploring this approach in a larger patient series, in which methotrexate should be omitted from the GVHD prophylaxis regimen.

Ex vivo UCB unit expansion: Notch ligand

The Notch signaling pathway has been known to play an important role in hematopoiesis.[33] Hence, the investigators at the FHCRC initiated a phase 1 MAC UCB HCT trial in 10 high-risk acute leukemia patients who were given one nonmanipulated and one ex vivo manipulated UCB graft.[34] One UCB unit was thawed and the CD34^{+-} selected cells were expanded in serum-free media containing the Notch ligand Delta1 supplemented with SCF, thrombopoietin, FLT-3, IL-3, and IL-6. CD34$^+$ cells were expanded (mean) 164-fold, and median (range) time to attain neutrophil recovery greater than 500/μL was 16 (range 7–34) days; these numbers compare favorably with values of 26 (range 16–48) days ($P = .002$) from a concurrently treated cohort of 20 patients undergoing double UCB transplantation.

These novel UCB expansion projects are the subject of several investigations in various stages, undertaken by academic centers as well as corporate partners.

Haploidentical Bone Marrow

Given the limited numbers of matched related donors and difficulties in identifying and obtaining matched unrelated donor grafts, several investigators have pursued HCT using haploidentical relatives as donors. In this setting the donor could be a sibling, parent, or child. The initial trials were reported from the center in Perugia, Italy[35]; this group used T-cell–depleted peripheral blood progenitor cell grafts that were associated with a low rate of GVHD. This approach, however, was hampered by a high rate of graft rejection, slow immune recovery, and substantial TRM, often due to opportunistic infection. The group at Johns Hopkins uses unmodified haploidentical marrow followed by posttransplantation treatment with cyclophosphamide.[36,37] The thought is that donor alloreactive T cells will be eliminated during their proliferative phase early after infusion into the recipient. Their data show a lower rate of severe acute and chronic GVHD and TRM, but engraftment failure rates are higher.

More recently, The BMT CTN conducted two parallel, multicenter, phase 2 RIC trials for leukemia and lymphoma patients who lacked suitable related donors.[38] The graft source was either unrelated double UCB or HLA-haploidentical related donor bone marrow transplantation. For both trials, the conditioning regimen incorporated cyclophosphamide, fludarabine, and single-fraction 200 cGy total body irradiation (TBI). The 1-year probabilities of overall and progression-free survival were 54% and 46%, respectively, after double UCB transplantation (n = 50) and 62% and 48%, respectively, after haploidentical marrow transplantation (n = 50). Neutrophil recoveries were similar, and 100-day cumulative incidence of grade II to IV acute GVHD was 40% after double UCB and 32% after haploidentical marrow transplantation. Nonrelapse mortality and relapse incidence at 1 year after double UCB transplantation were 24% and 31%, respectively, with corresponding results of 7% and 45%, respectively, after haploidentical marrow transplantation.

These studies broaden the range of HCT, as almost every patient can count on an adequately matched UCB or haploidentical donor. Further work is needed to directly compare these approaches and optimize their outcome.

PARADIGMS IN CONDITIONING

The intensity of the chemoradiation or chemotherapy used for the conditioning (or preparative) regimen has been a source of continuous debate in the area of transplant efficacy. With greater understanding of patient tolerance to therapy, the approach to the patient has resulted in the recognition of 3 large categories of preparative regimens: MAC, RIC, and nonmyeloablative conditioning (NMA) regimens.[39,40] In fact, for the latter (NMA) approach, prompt hematologic recovery could be expected within 28 days without hematopoietic progenitor cell rescue, often with resulting mixed chimerism. Various NMA or RIC regimens have been used as an alternative to MAC to reduce toxicity in patients with an impaired performance status or in those subjects with visceral organ compromise. RIC and NMA HCT rely more on the allogeneic effect of the infused graft mediating a GVL effect rather than the antitumor effect of high-dose chemotherapy. RIC regimens continue to be hindered by the morbidity and mortality of GVHD.[41] The details of many of these approaches have been published elsewhere.

No one regimen has been demonstrated to be superior, and most centers rely on the conditioning with which they have generated the most experiences. So far, it has been established that survival in older patients after RIC HCT is comparable with that in younger patients, with no significant differences in nonrelapse mortality and overall survival between patients older than 55 and those younger than 55 years; as expected, the data show significantly lower 1-year infection-related mortality after RIC than after MAC.

Novel Preparative Regimens: Chemotherapeutic Agents

Taking advantage of the new developments in pharmacotherapy, several investigators have initiated newer approaches.

Clofarabine-based

Clofarabine, a new potent purine nucleoside antimetabolite that inhibits DNA polymerase and ribonucleotide reductase, is approved by the Food and Drug Administration for the treatment of relapsed or refractory childhood ALL. Biochemical and clinical studies suggest synergy with cytarabine and significant activity in acute leukemia; hence, this agent has been combined in preparative regimens. Ricci and colleagues[42] reported a combination of clofarabine, cytarabine, and TBI followed by allogeneic HCT in 12 poor-risk children, adolescents, and young adults with acute leukemia. Clofarabine was dose-escalated to the maximum tolerated dose of 52 mg/m^2/d for 5 days. TRM at 100 days was 0%; 2 patients had progressive disease while 8 patients remain alive in continuous complete remission at a median (range) of 209 (40–770) days. At the 2011 BMT tandem meeting, Agura and colleagues[43] described preliminary results of a single-institution phase 2 clofarabine and busulfan RIC regimen in 20 hematologic malignancy (n = 16 AML) patients. Eleven subjects with active malignancy attained complete remission by day 30; 7 experienced relapse and overall,

12 died but 6 remain in remission at a median (range) follow-up of 31 (13–41) months. Kirschbaum and colleagues[44] performed a phase 1 dose-escalation study of clofarabine and melphalan in 16 AML patients, median age 63 (range 30–66) years. The investigators did not identify dose-limiting toxicities; 2 patients expired early from multiorgan toxicities. Only 2 subjects relapsed and 11 remain in remission at a median (range) of 23 (4–35) months after HCT. The regimen of 5 days of clofarabine 40 $mg/m^2/d$ plus 1 day of melphalan 100 mg/m^2 appears to be an effective combination worthy of additional study. These clofarabine-containing regimens appear to be relatively well tolerated and show promising antileukemic activity.

Treosulfan-based
Treosulfan, pharmacologically similar to busulfan but more potent in vitro, is a bifunctional, alkylating agent with myeloablative as well as immunosuppressive properties.[45] Unlike busulfan, treosulfan does not appear to require dose adjustment and has an excellent toxicity profile. Furthermore, in contrast to busulfan, treosulfan is active against both primitive and committed hematopoietic progenitor cells.[46] Danylesko and colleagues[47] recently reviewed this agent in HCT. Several interesting studies reported included a prospective, multicenter RIC trial from France[48] that combined treosulfan (12 $mg/m^2/d$ for 3 days) with fludarabine (30 $mg/m^2/d$ for 5 days) and ATG (2.5 mg/kg/d for 2 days) in 56 hematologic malignancy patients. Therapy was well tolerated and median overall survival was not reached at a median follow-up of 13 months, with a 52% 3-year probability of survival.

Nemecek and colleagues[49] undertook a prospective, multicenter trial in 60 patients (n = 44 AML) at high risk for relapse or TRM. Median (range) age was 46 (5–60) years. Therapy consisted of treosulfan 12 to 14 $mg/m^2/d$ for 3 days and fludarabine 30 $mg/m^2/d$ for 5 days, followed by HCT from HLA-identical siblings (n = 30) or unrelated donors (n = 30). All patients engrafted, and the 2-year nonrelapse mortality was 8%. With a median follow-up of 22 months, 2-year relapse-free survival for all patients was 58% and 88% for patients without high-risk cytogenetics. The cumulative incidence of relapse at 2 years was 33%. Newell and colleagues[50] reported the results of a single-institution double UCB HCT protocol in 15 hematologic malignancy patients aged 4 to 63 (median 48) years including 7 AML subjects. Conditioning consisted of a regimen of treosulfan 14 $mg/m^2/d$ for 3 days, fludarabine 30 $mg/m^2/d$ for 5 days, and low-dose TBI 200 cGy. Median time to neutrophil recovery was 22.5 days and only one patient failed to engraft. Treosulfan appears to be an effective and well tolerated, interesting new addition to the HCT armamentarium, although there are no clinical HCT studies directly comparing this agent with busulfan alone or in combination.

Plerixafor and G-CSF
Plerixafor recently has been incorporated into conditioning regimens. The marrow microenvironment contributes to leukemia cell chemoresistance for those cells residing in niches. Preclinical models indicate that inhibition of the chemokine receptor CXCR4 will mobilize leukemia cells into the circulation and facilitate sensitization to cytotoxic therapy. Konopleva and colleagues[51] at the MD Anderson Cancer Center reported in preliminary fashion a phase 1/2 study in which G-CSF and plerixafor therapy were initiated in escalating dose before the start of a standard fludarabine and busulfan regimen. The investigators showed preferential mobilization of clonal leukemia cells over normal cells in this 27-patient study, without toxicities ascribed to the G-CSF/plerixafor treatment. This approach will require validation in a larger series and longer follow-up to determine efficacy.

Novel Preparative Regimens: Radiation

Selective radiation approaches

While TBI is used to prevent immunologic graft rejection and can eradicate residual malignant cells, toxic effects may be significant, and include cardiac toxicity, pulmonary fibrosis, renal failure and, especially in the pediatric population, an excess number of secondary malignancies.[52–54] Some investigators have attempted to improve on TBI using helical tomotherapy, a modality that integrates computed tomography image-guided radiotherapy and intensity-modulated radiation therapy into a single device.[55] This technique can deliver conformal targeted radiation to the marrow and lymphatic systems.[56,57] Rosenthal and colleagues[58] recently described the results of a phase 1/2 investigation using total marrow and lymph node irradiation (TMLI) to augment RIC transplantation for 33 advanced, poor-risk hematologic malignancy patients with a median age of 55 years. The addition of TMLI 1200 cGy (administered as 150 cGy/fraction in 8 fractions over 4 days) to fludarabine 25 mg/m^2/d for 5 days and melphalan 140 mg/m^2/d for 1 day, did not appear to increase toxicity of this chemotherapy preparative regimen. At 1 year after HCT, overall survival, event-free survival, and nonrelapse-related mortality rates were 75%, 65%, and 19%, respectively. The addition of TMLI to RIC is feasible and safe, and the centers equipped with this device can offer it to patients with advanced hematologic malignancies who might not otherwise be candidates for RIC.

Targeted myeloablative radioimmunotherapy

An alternative strategy for acute leukemia patients undergoing HCT is myeloablative radioimmunotherapy (RIT), a technique that targets radiotherapy to the bone marrow using radiolabeled monoclonal antibodies.[59] Candidate isotopes usually are the β-emitter radionuclides (^{131}I, ^{90}Y, ^{188}Re), which are conjugated to monoclonal antibodies including anti-CD33, anti-CD45, and anti-CD66. The cross-firing β particles create a field radiation effect, potentially killing antigen-negative resident marrow tumor cells. Most clinical studies have used ^{131}I, a long-lived β-particle emitter, whose γ emissions allow dosimetry studies to be performed easily, but require patient isolation. ^{90}Y is a pure β emitter and the absence of γ emission allows outpatient administration of high doses, but dosimetry calculations are extremely complex. ^{188}Re is another radioisotope suitable for biodistribution and dosimetry as it also has γ emission.[60,61] On the other hand, α particles are helium nuclei emitted from the decay of radioisotopes. RIT using α emitters, such as ^{213}Bi, ^{225}Ac, and ^{211}At, should result in less nonspecific toxicity to normal bystander cells and provide a more efficient single-cell killing than β-emitting constructs. Clinical experiences have been very limited.

Although the efficacy of RIT depends on a variety of factors, the most important appears to be biodistribution. Kletting and colleagues[62,63] described physiologically based pharmacokinetic models to estimate biodistribution and maximize anti-CD45 antibody and anti-CD66 RIT efficacy. These approaches have not yet penetrated clinical practice. On the other hand, Schulz and colleagues[64] recently reported an open-label, single-center pilot study of 30 pediatric and adolescent patients undergoing HCT for malignant (n = 16) and nonmalignant (n = 14) disorders using treatment with a ^{90}Y-labeled anti-CD66 monoclonal antibody. This patient population was considered at high risk for nonrelapse mortality due to advanced disease, ongoing severe infections, second HCT, and significant visceral organ damage. The therapeutic ^{90}Y activity was calculated to deliver a marrow dose of 3000 to 4000 cGy to patients in the malignant group and 1600 to 2000 cGy in the nonmalignant group. Patients also received additional conditioning with either TBI-based or intravenous busulfan, melphalan, and fludarabine-containing therapy. No excess acute organ toxicity was observed in any of the patient groups. Twenty-three patients are alive at a median (range) of 35 (19–71) months after HCT. The overall nonrelapse mortality in this extremely poor-risk group was only 13%, and supports continued exploration of this approach.

Pretargeted myeloablative radioimmunotherapy

While the use of radiolabeled antibodies has shown promise in both imaging and therapeutic applications, the clinical adoption has not fulfilled the original expectations, due either to poor image resolution and contrast in scanning, or to insufficient radiation doses delivered selectively to tumors for therapy. Pretargeting involves the separation of the localization of tumor with an anticancer antibody from the subsequent delivery of the imaging or therapeutic radionuclide.[65]

Pretargeted RIT (PRIT)[66] circumvents the issue of suboptimal therapeutic index (target-to-nontarget ratio) by separating the prolonged-circulating antibody construct ("targeting vehicle") from the therapeutic radioisotope ("effector"). Conceptually, this sequential administration allows for maximal antibody targeting to take place prior to delivery of the therapeutic radionuclide while maintaining targeting specificity. PRIT substantially reduces whole-body radiation because of radionuclide delivery via small molecules that yield rapid tumor uptake and fast renal excretion of nontumor-bound radioactivity. Synthetic chasers ("clearing agents") have been introduced as an additional refinement to PRIT.[67–69] At present, this technique has not yet been implemented in clinical practice but holds considerable promise as a means of enhancing the therapeutic index of RIT.

GVHD PREVENTION STRATEGIES

The prevention of GVHD remains an elusive goal in the quest to improve overall patient outcome after HCT. For many decades, numerous investigators have used either administration of pharmacologic agents to the patient or manipulation of the graft. A full discussion of GVHD prophylaxis is beyond the scope of this review, and the authors focus here on graft manipulation.

T-Cell Depletion of the Graft

Although T-cell depletion strategies have resulted in lower rates of acute GVHD, these techniques have unfortunately met high engraftment failure, increased post-HCT relapse rates, inability to reduce chronic GVHD rates, high cost, and the need for special expertise.

Soiffer and colleagues[70] reported on whether immune modulation with anti–T-cell antibody infusion abrogates the therapeutic benefits of transplantation in a RIC setting. The study included 1676 patients aged 21 to 69 years with ALL, AML, chronic myeloid leukemia (CML), myelodysplastic syndrome, chronic lymphocytic leukemia (CLL), non-Hodgkin lymphoma, and Hodgkin lymphoma. All patients received alkylating agent plus fludarabine; 792 received allografts from an HLA-matched sibling donor, 884 from an HLA-matched unrelated donor. Outcomes after in vivo T-cell depletion (n = 584 ATG; n = 213 alemtuzumab) were compared with T-cell–replete (n = 879) transplantation. Grade 2 to 4 acute GVHD was lower with alemtuzumab than with ATG or T-cell–replete regimens (19% vs 38% vs 40%, P<.0001), and chronic GVHD was lower with alemtuzumab and ATG regimens in comparison with T-cell–replete approaches (24% vs 40% vs 52%, P<.0001). However, relapse was more frequent with alemtuzumab and ATG than with T-cell–replete regimens (49%, 51%, and 38%, respectively, P<.001). Disease-free survival was lower with alemtuzumab and ATG than with T-cell–replete regimens (30%, 25%, and 39%, respectively, $P<.001$). Corresponding probabilities of overall survival were 50%, 38%, and 46% ($P = .008$). These data suggest adopting a cautious approach to routine use of in vivo T-cell depletion with RIC regimens.

Recently, Devine and colleagues[71] within BMT CTN performed a phase 2 single-arm multicenter study in 44 AML CR1 (n = 37) and CR2 (n = 7) patients with a median (range) age of 48.5 (21–59) years. These investigators administered MAC chemotherapy, fractionated TBI (1375 cGy), and immune-magnetically selected CD34-enriched, T-cell–depleted allografts from HLA-identical siblings. No pharmacologic GVHD prophylaxis was given. All patients engrafted; the incidence of grade II to IV acute GVHD was 22.7%, and the incidence of extensive chronic GVHD at 24 months was 6.8% with a 17% relapse rate at 36 months for CR1 patients. Disease-free survival for CR1 patients was 72.8% at 12 months and 58% at 36 months. The BMT CTN investigators demonstrated that a MAC HCT can be performed in a multi-center setting using a uniform method of T-cell depletion that results in a low risk of extensive chronic GVHD and relapse for AML patients in CR1. Such a strategy should be studied in a comparative fashion.

Treg Therapy for GVHD Prevention

Forty years ago Gershon and Kondo[72] discovered the so-called suppressor T cells, a subpopulation of T cells that dampen the immune response. The field was reignited in 1995 when Sakaguchi and colleagues,[73] using a murine model, identified CD4$^+$ T cells coexpressing CD25 (the IL-2 receptor α chain) as a thymus-derived population of peripheral T cells capable of inhibiting autoimmunity otherwise resulting from neonatal thymectomy. Secondary transfer of murine T cells depleted of the CD4$^+$ CD25$^+$ subpopulation resulted in systemic autoimmunity, including a "graft-versus-host like wasting disease." Further models suggested that donor regulatory T cells (Tregs) can reliably suppress GVHD,[74,75] possibly sparing leukemia-specific immune responses.[76] In the milieu of preclinical promise, Brunstein and colleagues[77] reported the "first-in-human" clinical trial of ex vivo expansion of CD4$^+$CD25$^+$FoxP3$^+$ T regulatory cell enrichment from cryopreserved UCB. Twenty-three patients with a median (range) age of 52 (24–68) years were given intravenous cyclophosphamide 50 mg/kg, intravenous fludarabine 40 mg/m^2/d for 5 days, single-fraction TBI 200 cGy, and double UCB HCT followed by the expanded cell population. No infusional toxicities were observed and UCB Tregs were detected for up to 14 days. When compared with 108 identically treated historical controls who did not receive Treg infusions, the incidence of grade II to IV acute GVHD was reduced from 61% to 43% ($P = .05$). This maneuver was not associated with deleterious effects on risks of infection, relapse, or early mortality, and merits further consideration.

Di Ianni and the Perugia group[78] evaluated the impact of early infusion of Tregs, followed by conventional T cells (Tcons), on GVHD prevention and immunologic reconstitution in 28 high-risk hematologic malignancy patients (n = 22 AML) who underwent HLA-haploidentical HCT after single-fraction TBI 800 cGy, thiotepa 4 mg/kg/d for 2 days, cyclophosphamide 35 mg/kg/d for 2 days, and fludarabine 40 mg/m^2/d for 5 days. These investigators showed for the first time in humans that adoptive transfer of Tregs prevented GVHD in the absence of posttransplantation immunosuppression, as only 2 patients developed grade II or greater acute GVHD and no patient developed chronic GVHD. Although 13 subjects died of infection or visceral organ injury, at a median follow-up of 12 months, 12 patients remain alive at a median (range) of 12 (9–21) months after haploidentical HCT. This approach clearly is associated with the need for considerable expertise and is hampered by high rates of opportunistic infection.

POSTTRANSPLANT MANEUVERS
Immune Reconstitution with Exogenous Cytokines

The investigations examining the use of IL-2 in the HCT setting have yielded mixed results. The best evidence for IL-2 enhancement of donor T-cell function after alloge-neic HCT comes from reports of patients who failed to respond to donor lymphocyte infusion (DLI) for relapsed disease but achieved complete remission after treatment with IL-2.[79,80] More recently, Zorn and colleagues[81] examined the effect of low-dose IL-2 infusions on Treg populations after HCT in patients who also received infusions of donor CD4[+] lymphocytes. This study suggested that administration of low-dose IL-2 combined with adoptive CD4[+] cellular therapy may provide a mecha-nism to preferentially expand Treg cells in vivo, thus decreasing GVHD.

At present, there are several recently completed and ongoing allogeneic HCT clinical trials that hope to define the use of IL-2 (NCT00003962, "IL-2 following BMT in treating patients with hematologic cancer," NCT00539695, "Low dose IL-2 for GVHD as GVHD prophylaxis after stem cell transplantation," NCT00941928, "Haploi-dentical NK cells with epratuzumab [IL-2] for relapsed ALL").

Donor Lymphocyte Infusion

DLI can be effective in inducing remission in patients with residual or relapsed disease after allogeneic HCT[82,83] and can be useful in converting the recipient to full-donor chimerism.[84,85] Preemptive DLI administration in patients at high risk for relapse also has been investigated as a result of the data showing a GVL effect in CML and other hematologic malignancies relapsing after allogeneic HCT.[86] Lutz and colleagues[87] reported the impact of prophylactic DLI in 26 of 85 ALL allograft recipi-ents. Twelve of 13 patients who had mixed chimerism converted to complete donor chimerism; 18 of 26 patients developed GVHD and are alive at a median follow-up of 42 (range 14–72) months after HCT. Although some of these analyses report the effectiveness of DLI when given in the prophylactic setting, the majority of patients are ineligible for this strategy because of the onset of GVHD or disease progression before the planned infusion after HCT. Further, although DLI provides "proof of prin-ciple" for a direct and curative effect of allogeneic cellular therapy in the treatment of relapsed CML, this positive result has failed to translate to other hematologic malig-nancies.[88] Although data support the antitumor effects of DLI in AML, ALL, myeloma, and lymphoma in some recipients, the overall long-term outcomes have been disap-pointing, in part owing to complications of GVHD as well as lack of durable disease control. Current research focuses on modifying DLI to enhance its antileukemic effect, but the fact remains that adequate data regarding the specific target antigens neces-sary for GVL induction are lacking in the majority of clinical scenarios. Other interven-tions may be more attractive alternatives than DLI (see later discussion).

Chimeric Antigen Receptor–Redirected T Lymphocytes

Both T-cell depletion of the graft and posttransplant immune suppression may be effective in abating GVHD incidence and severity, but are associated with a reduction in the GVL effect. To broaden the clinical application of adoptive immunotherapy, investigators have generated T cells by introducing chimeric antigen receptors (CARs) to redirect specificity. CARs combine antigen specificity and T-cell–activating properties in a single fusion molecule. First-generation CARs included as their signaling domain the cytoplasmic region of the CD3ζ or Fc receptor γ chain, effectively redirecting T-cell cytotoxicity, but failed to enable T-cell proliferation and survival on repeated antigen exposure. Receptors encompassing both CD28 and CD3ζ are the prototypes for second-generation CARs, which now are rapidly expanding to a diverse array of receptors with different functional properties.[89] The concept of the genetic redirection of T cells by means of a chimeric receptor linking the antigen-binding moiety of a mouse monoclonal antibody (mAb) in the form of a single-chain fragment variable (scFv) region to the signal transduction machinery of T cells is actively translated into clinical trials.[90] The current research focuses on 4 areas: (1) reprogramming the T cells themselves or insertion of transgenes for improved safety, replicative potential, homing, effector function, and in vivo persistence, especially within the tumor microenvironment; (2) manipulating the recipient to improve target tumor-associated antigens expression and survival of infused T cells; and (3) adapting the gene therapy platform to deliver CARs capable of initiating an antigen-dependent, fully competent activation signal. A few highly committed and experienced centers are incorporating these approaches into the HCT posttransplant therapy in select patients at high-risk for relapse.

Porter and colleagues[91] at the University of Pennsylvania recently reported the successful infusion of a lentiviral vector CD19-specific autologous T-cell modified CAR (coupled with CD137 and CD3ζ) in a refractory CLL patient. The cells were expanded more than 1000-fold; apart from tumor lysis syndrome, the only other grade III to IV toxic effects were lymphopenia and hypogammaglobulinemia. The engineered cells persisted in vivo at high concentration in the blood and bone marrow for 6 months and continued to express the CAR. A specific immune response was detected in the bone marrow, accompanied by loss of normal B cells and leukemia cells that expressed CD19. Complete remission was ongoing 10 months after treatment.

ANCILLARY APPROACHES
Multipotent Mesenchymal Stromal Cells

In addition to hematopoietic progenitor and stem cells, the bone marrow contains a population of primitive cells known as MSCs. These cells secrete hematopoietic colony-stimulating factors and cytokines both constitutively and after stimulation into the marrow microenvironment, and also exhibit immunosuppressive properties. Expanding from studies using preclinical animal models and from clinical autologous HCT, Lazarus and colleagues[92] hypothesized that cotransplantation of marrow-derived, culture-expanded MSCs and hematopoietic progenitor cells (HPCs) obtained from HLA-identical sibling donors after myeloablative therapy could facilitate engraftment and prevent or reduce GVHD. In this open-label, multicenter trial, 46 acute leukemia patients (median age 44.5 years) underwent MAC followed by intravenous infusion of culture-expanded MSCs and allogeneic HPCs. The MSC infusion was not associated with toxicity, and hematopoietic engraftment was brisk. The incidence of both acute and chronic GVHD appeared to be reduced. Subsequently, several allogeneic HCT trials have examined the use of MSCs as prophylaxis as well as therapy for GVHD. Given the technical and logistic constraints of using sibling donors as the source for MSCs, several protocols have used cotransplantation of third-party donor MSCs. Studies have demonstrated short-term safety of the procedure and reduced nonrelapse mortality.[92,93] In a landmark case report, Le Blanc and colleagues[94] described successful therapy for a 9-year-old boy who had treatment-resistant grade IV acute GVHD in the course of an HLA-matched unrelated donor transplant. Using third-party MSCs obtained from his haploidentical mother, the severe GVHD of the gastrointestinal tract and liver were eradicated. In a follow-up study, 6 of 8 additional patients with steroid-refractory GVHD experienced a favorable clinical response to MSC infusions.[95] A European Blood and Marrow Transplant Group (EBMT)-sponsored multicenter phase 2 trial used single or multiple MSC infusions collected from a variety of sources (HLA-identical allograft donors, haploidentical family donors, and unrelated HLA-mismatched donors) as therapy for 55 patients experiencing steroid-resistant, severe acute GVHD.[96] Again, MSC infusions took place without side effects and a complete response was documented in 30 (55%) subjects. Follow-up investigations, however, including a phase 3 study sponsored by Osiris Therapeutics (Baltimore, MD, USA) using third-party, non-HLA–matched MSCs, have shown mixed results in the treatment of acute GVHD.[97] The use of MSCs is an area of intense investigation and cannot be recommended as part of routine clinical care. Unresolved issues include the source of the MSCs, the culture expansion conditions, timing and dosing of infusions, and route of administration. Several ongoing programs are exploring multipotent adult progenitor cells (MAPCs), cells similar to MSCs but expanded under different conditions and possessing greater proliferative and regenerative properties. A recent report in which both the cell dose and the number of MAP cells (Athersys, Inc, Cleveland, OH, USA) infusions were escalated infused shortly after a MAC-matched unrelated donor HCT was promising; this investigation likely will be followed by a phase 2 study.[98]

The major advantages of using cellular therapies such as MSCs and MAPCs for GVHD prophylaxis or therapy are that these cells not only can stimulate hematopoiesis, but their immunosuppressive properties appear to be selective and may not lead to an increase in opportunistic infections.[99,100]

Intra–Bone Marrow Injection of Cord Blood Cells

As previously stated, the significant limitations of UCB transplant are the low number of nucleated cells contained in a unit and the fact that engraftment is significantly slower when compared with other graft sources.[23,101,102] Animal models have suggested that injection of HPCs directly into the marrow space may improve homing and engraftment after transplantation.[103–106]

In this context Frassoni and colleagues[107] performed a phase 1/2 MAC HCT study in 32 leukemia patients who received a single UCB unit injected directly in the iliac crest. No complications occurred during the infusion, and neutrophil and platelet engraftment appeared to be accelerated. A follow-up study[108] by the same group noted that 72 of 75 consecutive hematologic malignancy patients (median age 45 years) engrafted at a median (range) of 23 (14–44) days for neutrophils and 35 (16–70) days for platelets, despite the use of a lower total nucleated cell dose infused. Brunstein and colleagues[109] at the University of Minnesota explored intraosseous administration of UCB grafts in 10 MAC double UCB HCT patients (median age 35 years). One unit was designated randomly for intra–bone marrow delivery, whereas the second unit was administered intravenously. The median infused graft total nucleated cell dose was 3.7×10^7/kg with no difference between intravenous and intraosseous units; median times to neutrophil engraftment and platelet recovery were 21 and 69 days, respectively, with no advantage over conventional double UCB unit transplantation. This finding may reflect that above an infused cell threshold, route of administration may not provide additional benefit, and the intraosseous route of administration remains investigational.

Enhancing Homing and Engraftment Capabilities of Hematopoietic Cells

Engraftment of hematopoietic progenitor and stem cells encompasses at least 2 separate but interrelated events, including homing of cells to the bone marrow, and then nurturing them for survival, proliferation, self-renewal, and differentiation, within the marrow microenvironment. A ligand-receptor interaction strongly implicated in homing and engraftment of hematopoietic stem and progenitor cells is stromal cell–derived factor-1 (SDF-1/CXCL12) and CXCR4.[110,111] SDF-1/CXCL12 not only acts as a chemotactic (directed cell migration) agent but also enhances survival of early hematopoietic cells. Christopherson and colleagues[112] reported that CD26/DPPIV was active in truncating SDF-1/CXCL12 into a molecule that had no chemotactic activity, and used a preclinical model to demonstrate enhanced ability of cells to better and more efficiently home to marrow of lethally irradiated mice, resulting in greatly enhanced engrafting capacity.[113] These observations have provided the impetus to undertake a human clinical trial model for testing the feasibility of CD26/DPPIV inhibition to enhance engrafting capability of limited numbers of human UCB cells present in single cord blood collections, in patients with malignant disorders. Candidate agents are being studied.

EXPERT OPINION

The standard of care in HCT for hematologic malignancies has been established based on therapies undertaken on a relatively uncommon population of young patients with minimal comorbidities who are able to withstand the difficulties of using a MAC modality. The majority of the population, however, is elderly and likely has multiple comorbidities. RIC and NMA clearly have been demonstrated to be successfully performed in some subjects in the latter category. Unfortunately, the same problems that affect recipients of MAC HCT can hamper success in the RIC and NMA HCT, that is, TRM, relapse, and GVHD. Newer approaches are being developed to overcome these persistent limitations, as discussed in this review. The authors expect that in the next few years, investigators will further define the immunologic landscape of grafting and the postgrafting dynamics. Goals include harnessing GVL and developing strategies for further abatement of GVHD. The field clearly has an emphasis on pursuing a rational, targeted approach, as proven feasible by options such as radioimmunotherapy, CARs, Treg enhancement, and MSCs. Finding the optimal individualized strategy for patients, however, depends on the development of well-designed, randomized, multicenter, prospective trials. Enrollment of patients into clinical trials cannot be overemphasized.

REFERENCES

1. Thomas ED, Lochte HL Jr, Lu WC, et al. Intravenous infusion of bone marrow in patients receiving radiation and chemotherapy. N Engl J Med 1957;257(11): 491–6.
2. Appelbaum FR. Hematopoietic-cell transplantation at 50. N Engl J Med 2007; 357(15):1472–5.
3. Horowitz MM, Gale RP, Sondel PM, et al. Graft-versus-leukemia reactions after bone marrow transplantation. Blood 1990;75(3):555–62.
4. Koreth J, Schlenk R, Kopecky KJ, et al. Allogeneic stem cell transplantation for acute myeloid leukemia in first complete remission: systematic review and meta-analysis of prospective clinical trials. JAMA 2009;301(22):2349–61.
5. Gooley TA, Chien JW, Pergam SA, et al. Reduced mortality after allogeneic hematopoietic-cell transplantation. N Engl J Med 2010;363(22):2091–101.
6. Horan JT, Logan BR, Agovi-Johnson MA, et al. Reducing the risk for transplantation-related mortality after allogeneic hematopoietic cell transplantation: how much progress has been made? J Clin Oncol 2011;29(7):805–13.

7. Lee SJ, Klein J, Haagenson M, et al. High-resolution donor-recipient HLA matching contributes to the success of unrelated donor marrow transplantation. Blood 2007;110(13):4576–83.
8. Ferrara JL, Anasetti C, Stadtmauer E, et al. Blood and marrow transplant clinical trials network state of the science symposium 2007. Biol Blood Marrow Transplant 2007;13(11):1268–85.
9. Whitman SP, Ruppert AS, Marcucci G, et al. Long-term disease-free survivors with cytogenetically normal acute myeloid leukemia and MLL partial tandem duplication: a Cancer and Leukemia Group B study. Blood 2007;109(12): 5164–7.
10. Schlenk RF, Benner A, Hartmann F, et al. Risk-adapted postremission therapy in acute myeloid leukemia: results of the German multicenter AML HD93 treatment trial. Leukemia 2003;17(8):1521–8.
11. Breems DA, Lowenberg B. Acute myeloid leukemia and the position of autologous stem cell transplantation. Semin Hematol 2007;44(4):259–66.
12. Dohner H, Estey EH, Amadori S, et al. Diagnosis and management of acute myeloid leukemia in adults: recommendations from an international expert panel, on behalf of the European LeukemiaNet. Blood 2010;115(3): 453–74.
13. Fernandez HF, Sun Z, Litzow MR, et al. Autologous transplantation gives encouraging results for young adults with favorable-risk acute myeloid leukemia, but is not improved with gemtuzumab ozogamicin. Blood 2011; 117(20):5306–13.
14. Goldstone AH, Richards SM, Lazarus HM, et al. In adults with standard-risk acute lymphoblastic leukemia, the greatest benefit is achieved from a matched sibling allogeneic transplantation in first complete remission, and an autologous transplantation is less effective than conventional consolidation/maintenance chemotherapy in all patients: final results of the International ALL Trial (MRC UKALL XII/ECOG E2993). Blood 2008;111(4):1827–33.
15. Bond VP, Cronkite EP, Fliedner TM, et al. Deoxyribonucleic acid synthesizing cells in peripheral blood of normal human beings. Science 1958;128(3317): 202–3.
16. Korbling M, Freireich EJ. Twenty-five years of peripheral blood stem cell transplantation. Blood 2011;117(24):6411–6.
17. Cashen AF, Lazarus HM, Devine SM. Mobilizing stem cells from normal donors: is it possible to improve upon G-CSF? Bone Marrow Transplant 2007;39(10): 577–88.
18. Gluckman E, Broxmeyer HA, Auerbach AD, et al. Hematopoietic reconstitution in a patient with Fanconi's anemia by means of umbilical-cord blood from an HLA-identical sibling. N Engl J Med 1989;321(17):1174–8.
19. Gluckman E. History of cord blood transplantation. Bone Marrow Transplant 2009;44(10):621–6.
20. Eapen M, Rubinstein P, Zhang MJ, et al. Outcomes of transplantation of unrelated donor umbilical cord blood and bone marrow in children with acute leukaemia: a comparison study. Lancet 2007;369(9577):1947–54.
21. Snell M, Chau C, Hendrix D, et al. Lack of isohemagglutinin production following minor ABO incompatible unrelated HLA mismatched umbilical cord blood transplantation. Bone Marrow Transplant 2006;38(2):135–40.
22. Barker JN, Weisdorf DJ, Wagner JE. Creation of a double chimera after the transplantation of umbilical-cord blood from two partially matched unrelated donors. N Engl J Med 2001;344(24):1870–1.

23. Barker JN, Weisdorf DJ, DeFor TE, et al. Transplantation of 2 partially HLA-matched umbilical cord blood units to enhance engraftment in adults with hematologic malignancy. Blood 2005;105(3):1343–7.

24. Brunstein CG, Fuchs EJ, Carter SL, et al. Alternative donor transplantation after reduced intensity conditioning: results of parallel phase 2 trials using partially HLA-mismatched related bone marrow or unrelated double umbilical cord blood grafts. Blood 2011;118(2):282–8.

25. Avery S, Shi W, Lubin M, et al. Influence of infused cell dose and HLA match on engraftment after double-unit cord blood allografts. Blood 2011;117(12): 3277–85 [quiz: 3478].

26. Fanning LR, Hegerfeldt Y, Tary-Lehmann M, et al. Allogeneic transplantation of multiple umbilical cord blood units in adults: role of pretransplant-mixed lymphocyte reaction to predict host-vs-graft rejection. Leukemia 2008;22(9):1786–90.

27. Gutman JA, Turtle CJ, Manley TJ, et al. Single-unit dominance after double-unit umbilical cord blood transplantation coincides with a specific CD8+ T-cell response against the nonengrafted unit. Blood 2010;115(4):757–65.

28. Verneris MR, Brunstein CG, Barker J, et al. Relapse risk after umbilical cord blood transplantation: enhanced graft-versus-leukemia effect in recipients of 2 units. Blood 2009;114(19):4293–9.

29. Kindwall-Keller TL, Hegerfeldt Y, Meyerson HJ, et al. Prospective study of single vs. two unit umbilical cord blood transplantation following reduced intensity conditioning in adults with hematologic malignancies. Bone Marrow Transplant 2011, in press.

30. de Lima M, Robinson S, McMannis J, et al. Mesenchymal stem cell (MSC) based cord blood (CB) expansion (Exp) leads to rapid engraftment of platelets and neutrophils [abstract: #362]. Blood 2010;116.

31. Peled T, Landua E, Mandel J, et al. Linear polyamine copper chelator tetraethylenepentamine augments long-term ex vivo expansion of cord blood-derived CD34+ cells and increases their engraftment potential in NOD/SCID mice. Exp Hematol 2004;32(6):547–55.

32. de Lima M, McMannis J, Gee A, et al. Transplantation of ex vivo expanded cord blood cells using the copper chelator tetraethylenepentamine: a phase I/II clinical trial. Bone Marrow Transplant 2008;41(9):771–8.

33. Tanavde VM, Malehorn MT, Lumkul R, et al. Human stem-progenitor cells from neonatal cord blood have greater hematopoietic expansion capacity than those from mobilized adult blood. Exp Hematol 2002;30(7):816–23.

34. Delaney C, Ratajczak MZ, Laughlin MJ. Strategies to enhance umbilical cord blood stem cell engraftment in adult patients. Expert Rev Hematol 2010;3(3): 273–83.

35. Aversa F, Tabilio A, Velardi A, et al. Treatment of high-risk acute leukemia with T-cell-depleted stem cells from related donors with one fully mismatched HLA haplotype. N Engl J Med 1998;339(17):1186–93.

36. Luznik L, O'Donnell PV, Symons HJ, et al. HLA-haploidentical bone marrow transplantation for hematologic malignancies using nonmyeloablative conditioning and high-dose, posttransplantation cyclophosphamide. Biol Blood Marrow Transplant 2008;14(6):641–50.

37. Fuchs EJ, Huang XJ, Miller JS. HLA-haploidentical stem cell transplantation for hematologic malignancies. Biol Blood Marrow Transplant 2010; 16(1 Suppl):S57–63.

38. Brunstein CG, Fuchs EJ, Carter SL, et al. Alternative donor transplantation after reduced intensity conditioning: results of parallel phase 2 trials using partially

HLA-mismatched related bone marrow or unrelated double umbilical cord blood grafts. Blood 2011;118(2):282–8.

39. Giralt S, Ballen K, Rizzo D, et al. Reduced-intensity conditioning regimen workshop: defining the dose spectrum. Report of a workshop convened by the center for international blood and marrow transplant research. Biol Blood Marrow Transplant 2009;15(3):367–9.

40. Bacigalupo A, Ballen K, Rizzo D, et al. Defining the intensity of conditioning regimens: working definitions. Biol Blood Marrow Transplant 2009;15(12): 1628–33.

41. Ringden O, Labopin M, Ehninger G, et al. Reduced intensity conditioning compared with myeloablative conditioning using unrelated donor transplants in patients with acute myeloid leukemia. J Clin Oncol 2009;27(27):4570–7.

42. Ricci AM, Geyer LA, Harrison D, et al. Preliminary results of phase I/II study of clofarabine (CLO) in combination with cytarabine and total body irradiation (TBI) followed by allogeneic stem cell transplantation (AlloSCT) in children, adolescents and young adults (CAYA) with poor-risk acute leukemia. Biol Blood Marrow Transplant 2011;17(2):S186.

43. Agura E, Berryman RB, Pineiro L, et al. Preliminary results of phase II trial of clofarabine with parenteral busulfan (CLO/BU) followed by allogeneic related or unrelated donor transplantation for the treatment of hematologic malignancies [abstract: #399]. Biol Blood Marrow Transplant 2011;17:S298–9.

44. Kirschbaum MH, Stein AS, Popplewell L, et al. A phase I study in adults of clofarabine combined with high-dose melphalan as reduced intensity conditioning for allogeneic transplantation. Biol Blood Marrow Transplant 2011. [Epub ahead of print].

45. Sjoo F, Hassan Z, Abedi-Valugerdi M, et al. Myeloablative and immunosuppressive properties of treosulfan in mice. Exp Hematol 2006;34(1):115–21.

46. Westerhof GR, Ploemacher RE, Boudewijn A, et al. Comparison of different busulfan analogues for depletion of hematopoietic stem cells and promotion of donor-type chimerism in murine bone marrow transplant recipients. Cancer Res 2000;60(19):5470–8.

47. Danylesko I, Shimoni A, Nagler A. Treosulfan-based conditioning before hematopoietic SCT: more than a BU look-alike. Bone Marrow Transplant 2011. [Epub ahead of print].

48. Michallet M, Sobh M, Morisset S, et al. Phase II prospective multicenter study of treosulfan based reduced intensity conditioning in allogeneic hematopoietic stem cell transplantation for hematological malignancies from 10/10 HLA identical unrelated donor. Blood 2010;116 [abstract: #2353].

49. Nemecek ER, Guthrie KA, Sorror ML, et al. Conditioning with treosulfan and fludarabine followed by allogeneic hematopoietic cell transplantation for high-risk hematologic malignancies. Biol Blood Marrow Transplant 2011;17(3):341–50.

50. Newell L, Milano F, Gutman J, et al. Treosulfan-based conditioning is sufficient to promote engraftment in cord blood transplantation. Biol Blood Marrow Transplant 2011;17(Suppl):S227–8.

51. Konopleva M, Zihihong Z, Wang R-Y, et al. A phase I/II trial of plerixafor/G-CSF combined with IV Bu/Flu conditioning regimen in AML/MDS patients undergoing allogeneic stem cell transplantation. Blood 2010;116 [abstract: #2358].

52. Curtis RE, Rowlings PA, Deeg HJ, et al. Solid cancers after bone marrow transplantation. N Engl J Med 1997;336(13):897–904.

53. Lowsky R, Lipton J, Fyles G, et al. Secondary malignancies after bone marrow transplantation in adults. J Clin Oncol 1994;12(10):2187–92.

54. Socie G, Curtis RE, Deeg HJ, et al. New malignant diseases after allogeneic marrow transplantation for childhood acute leukemia. J Clin Oncol 2000;18(2):348–57.
55. Mackie TR, Balog J, Ruchala K, et al. Tomotherapy. Semin Radiat Oncol 1999; 9(1):108–17.
56. Wong JY, Rosenthal J, Liu A, et al. Image-guided total-marrow irradiation using helical tomotherapy in patients with multiple myeloma and acute leukemia undergoing hematopoietic cell transplantation. Int J Radiat Oncol Biol Phys 2009;73(1):273–9.
57. Wong JY, Liu A, Schultheiss T, et al. Targeted total marrow irradiation using three-dimensional image-guided tomographic intensity-modulated radiation therapy: an alternative to standard total body irradiation. Biol Blood Marrow Transplant 2006;12(3):306–15.
58. Rosenthal J, Wong J, Stein A, et al. Phase 1/2 trial of total marrow and lymph node irradiation to augment reduced-intensity transplantation for advanced hematologic malignancies. Blood 2011;117(1):309–15.
59. Buchmann I, Meyer RG, Mier W, et al. Myeloablative radioimmunotherapy in conditioning prior to haematological stem cell transplantation: closing the gap between benefit and toxicity? Eur J Nucl Med Mol Imaging 2009;36(3): 484–98.
60. Griffiths GL, Goldenberg DM, Knapp FF Jr, et al. Direct radiolabeling of mono-clonal antibodies with generator-produced rhenium-188 for radioimmunother-apy: labeling and animal biodistribution studies. Cancer Res 1991;51(17): 4594–602.
61. Kotzerke J, Glatting G, Seitz U, et al. Radioimmunotherapy for the intensification of conditioning before stem cell transplantation: differences in dosimetry and biokinetics of 188Re- and 99mTc-labeled anti-NCA-95 MAbs. J Nucl Med 2000;41(3):531–7.
62. Kletting P, Bunjes D, Reske SN, et al. Improving anti-CD45 antibody radioimmu-notherapy using a physiologically based pharmacokinetic model. J Nucl Med 2009;50(2):296–302.
63. Kletting P, Kull T, Bunjes D, et al. Radioimmunotherapy with anti-CD66 antibody: improving the biodistribution using a physiologically based pharmacokinetic model. J Nucl Med 2010;51(3):484–91.
64. Schulz AS, Glatting G, Hoenig M, et al. Radioimmunotherapy-based condi-tioning for hematopoietic cell transplantation in children with malignant and nonmalignant diseases. Blood 2011;117(17):4642–50.
65. Goldenberg DM, Chatal JF, Barbet J, et al. Cancer imaging and therapy with bispecific antibody pretargeting. Update Cancer Ther 2007;2(1):19–31.
66. Walter RB, Press OW, Pagel JM. Pretargeted radioimmunotherapy for hemato-logic and other malignancies. Cancer Biother Radiopharm 2010;25(2):125–42.
67. Goodwin DA, Meares CF. Pretargeting: general principles; October 10–12, 1996. Cancer 1997;80(Suppl 12):2675–80.
68. Press OW, Corcoran M, Subbiah K, et al. A comparative evaluation of conven-tional and pretargeted radioimmunotherapy of CD20-expressing lymphoma xenografts. Blood 2001;98(8):2535–43.
69. Pagel JM, Hedin N, Subbiah K, et al. Comparison of anti-CD20 and anti-CD45 antibodies for conventional and pretargeted radioimmunotherapy of B-cell lymphomas. Blood 2003;101(6):2340–8.
70. Soiffer RJ, Lerademacher J, Ho V, et al. Impact of immune modulation with anti-T-cell antibodies on the outcome of reduced-intensity allogeneic hematopoietic stem cell transplantation for hematologic malignancies. Blood 2011;117(25):6963–70.

71. Devine SM, Carter S, Soiffer RJ, et al. Low risk of chronic graft-versus-host disease and relapse associated with T cell-depleted peripheral blood stem cell transplantation for acute myelogenous leukemia in first remission: results of the blood and marrow transplant clinical trials network protocol 0303. Biol Blood Marrow Transplant 2011;17(9):1343–51.

72. Gershon RK, Kondo K. Cell interactions in the induction of tolerance: the role of thymic lymphocytes. Immunology 1970;18(5):723–37.

73. Sakaguchi S, Sakaguchi N, Asano M, et al. Immunologic self-tolerance maintained by activated T cells expressing IL-2 receptor alpha-chains (CD25). Breakdown of a single mechanism of self-tolerance causes various autoimmune diseases. J Immunol 1995;155(3):1151–64.

74. Hoffmann P, Ermann J, Edinger M, et al. Donor-type CD4(+)CD25(+) regulatory T cells suppress lethal acute graft-versus-host disease after allogeneic bone marrow transplantation. J Exp Med 2002;196(3):389–99.

75. Taylor PA, Lees CJ, Blazar BR. The infusion of ex vivo activated and expanded CD4(+)CD25(+) immune regulatory cells inhibits graft-versus-host disease lethality. Blood 2002;99(10):3493–9.

76. Edinger M, Hoffmann P, Ermann J, et al. CD4+CD25+ regulatory T cells preserve graft-versus-tumor activity while inhibiting graft-versus-host disease after bone marrow transplantation. Nat Med 2003;9(9):1144–50.

77. Brunstein CG, Miller JS, Cao Q, et al. Infusion of ex vivo expanded T regulatory cells in adults transplanted with umbilical cord blood: safety profile and detection kinetics. Blood 2011;117(3):1061–70.

78. Di Ianni M, Falzetti F, Carotti A, et al. Tregs prevent GVHD and promote immune reconstitution in HLA-haploidentical transplantation. Blood 2011;117(14):3921–8.

79. Slavin S, Naparstek E, Nagler A, et al. Allogeneic cell therapy with donor peripheral blood cells and recombinant human interleukin-2 to treat leukemia relapse after allogeneic bone marrow transplantation. Blood 1996;87(6): 2195–204.

80. Nadal E, Fowler A, Kanfer E, et al. Adjuvant interleukin-2 therapy for patients refractory to donor lymphocyte infusions. Exp Hematol 2004;32(2):218–23.

81. Zorn E, Mohseni M, Kim H, et al. Combined CD4+ donor lymphocyte infusion and low-dose recombinant IL-2 expand FOXP3+ regulatory T cells following allogeneic hematopoietic stem cell transplantation. Biol Blood Marrow Transplant 2009;15(3):382–8.

82. Morris E, Thomson K, Craddock C, et al. Outcomes after alemtuzumab-containing reduced-intensity allogeneic transplantation regimen for relapsed and refractory non-Hodgkin lymphoma. Blood 2004;104(13):3865–71.

83. Bethge WA, Hegenbart U, Stuart MJ, et al. Adoptive immunotherapy with donor lymphocyte infusions after allogeneic hematopoietic cell transplantation following nonmyeloablative conditioning. Blood 2004;103(3):790–5.

84. Marks DI, Lush R, Cavenagh J, et al. The toxicity and efficacy of donor lymphocyte infusions given after reduced-intensity conditioning allogeneic stem cell transplantation. Blood 2002;100(9):3108–14.

85. Rondelli D, Barosi G, Bacigalupo A, et al. Allogeneic hematopoietic stem-cell transplantation with reduced-intensity conditioning in intermediate- or high-risk patients with myelofibrosis with myeloid metaplasia. Blood 2005;105(10): 4115–9.

86. Goldstein SC, Porter DL. Allogeneic immunotherapy to optimize the graft-versus-tumor effect: concepts and controversies. Expert Rev Hematol 2010; 3(3):301–14.

87. Lutz C, Massenkeli G, Nagy M, et al. A pilot study of prophylatic donor lympho-cyte infusions to prevent relapse in adult acute lymphoblastic leukemias after allogenic hemefoprietic stem cell transplantation. Bone Marrow Transplant 2008;41(9):805–12.

88. Tomblyn M, Lazarus HM. Donor lymphocyte infusions: the long and wind-ing road: how should it be traveled? Bone Marrow Transplant 2008;42(9): 569–79.

89. Sadelain M, Brentjens R, Riviere I. The promise and potential pitfalls of chimeric antigen receptors. Curr Opin Immunol 2009;21(2):215–23.

90. Jena B, Dotti G, Cooper LJ. Redirecting T-cell specificity by introducing a tumor-specific chimeric antigen receptor. Blood 2010;116(7):1035–44.

91. Porter DL, Levine BL, Kalos M, et al. Chimeric antigen receptor-modified T cells in chronic lymphoid leukemia. N Engl J Med 2011;365(8):725–33.

92. Lazarus HM, Koc ON, Devine SM, et al. Cotransplantation of HLA-identical sibling culture-expanded mesenchymal stem cells and hematopoietic stem cells in hematologic malignancy patients. Biol Blood Marrow Transplant 2005;11(5): 389–98.

93. Baron F, Lechanteur C, Willems E, et al. Cotransplantation of mesenchymal stem cells might prevent death from graft-versus-host disease (GVHD) without abrogating graft-versus-tumor effects after HLA-mismatched allogeneic transplantation following nonmyeloablative conditioning. Biol Blood Marrow Transplant 2010;16(6):838–47.

94. Le Blanc K, Rasmusson I, Sundberg B, et al. Treatment of severe acute graft-versus-host disease with third party haploidentical mesenchymal stem cells. Lancet 2004;363(9419):1439–41.

95. Ringden O, Uzunel M, Rasmusson I, et al. Mesenchymal stem cells for treatment of therapy-resistant graft-versus-host disease. Transplantation 2006;81(10): 1390–7.

96. Le Blanc K, Frassoni F, Ball L, et al. Mesenchymal stem cells for treatment of steroid-resistant, severe, acute graft-versus-host disease: a phase II study. Lancet 2008;371(9624):1579–86.

97. Caimi PF, Reese J, Lee Z, et al. Emerging therapeutic approaches for multipo-tent mesenchymal stromal cells. Curr Opin Hematol 2010;17(6):505–13.

98. Maziarz R, Bachier C, Goldstein S, et al. Stromal cell therapy for prophylaxis of acute GVHD: preliminary results from a phase 1 trial. Biol Blood Marrow Trans-plant 2011;17(Suppl):222–3 [abstract: #189].

99. Karlsson H, Samarasinghe S, Ball LM, et al. Mesenchymal stem cells exert differential effects on alloantigen and virus-specific T-cell responses. Blood 2008;112(3):532–41.

100. Potian JA, Aviv H, Ponzio NM, et al. Veto-like activity of mesenchymal stem cells: functional discrimination between cellular responses to alloantigens and recall antigens. J Immunol 2003;171(7):3426–34.

101. Laughlin MJ, Eapen M, Rubinstein P, et al. Outcomes after transplantation of cord blood or bone marrow from unrelated donors in adults with leukemia. N Engl J Med 2004;351(22):2265–75.

102. Rocha V, Labopin M, Sanz G, et al. Transplants of umbilical-cord blood or bone marrow from unrelated donors in adults with acute leukemia. N Engl J Med 2004;351(22):2276–85.

103. Zhong JF, Zhan Y, Anderson WF, et al. Murine hematopoietic stem cell distribu-tion and proliferation in ablated and nonablated bone marrow transplantation. Blood 2002;100(10):3521–6.

104. Wang J, Kimura T, Asada R, et al. SCID-repopulating cell activity of human cord blood-derived CD34- cells assured by intra-bone marrow injection. Blood 2003; 101(8):2924–31.
105. Kushida T, Inaba M, Hisha H, et al. Intra-bone marrow injection of allogeneic bone marrow cells: a powerful new strategy for treatment of intractable autoimmune diseases in MRL/lpr mice. Blood 2001;97(10):3292–9.
106. Mazurier F, Doedens M, Gan OI, et al. Rapid myeloerythroid repopulation after intrafemoral transplantation of NOD-SCID mice reveals a new class of human stem cells. Nat Med 2003;9(7):959–63.
107. Frassoni F, Gualandi F, Podesta M, et al. Direct intrabone transplant of unrelated cord-blood cells in acute leukaemia: a phase I/II study. Lancet Oncol 2008;9(9): 831–9.
108. Frassoni F, Varaldo R, Gualandi F, et al. The intra-bone marrow injection of cord blood cells extends the possibility of transplantation to the majority of patients with malignant hematopoietic diseases. Best Pract Res Clin Haematol 2010; 23(2):237–44.
109. Brunstein CG, Barker JN, Weisdorf DJ, et al. Intra-BM injection to enhance engraftment after myeloablative umbilical cord blood transplantation with two partially HLA-matched units. Bone Marrow Transplant 2009;43(12):935–40.
110. Dar A, Kollet O, Lapidot T. Mutual, reciprocal SDF-1/CXCR4 interactions between hematopoietic and bone marrow stromal cells regulate human stem cell migration and development in NOD/SCID chimeric mice. Exp Hematol 2006;34(8):967–75.
111. Spiegel A, Kalinkovich A, Shivtiel S, et al. Stem cell regulation via dynamic interactions of the nervous and immune systems with the microenvironment. Cell Stem Cell 2008;3(5):484–92.
112. Christopherson KW 2nd, Hangoc G, Broxmeyer HE. Cell surface peptidase CD26/dipeptidylpeptidase IV regulates CXCL12/stromal cell-derived factor-1 alpha-mediated chemotaxis of human cord blood CD34+ progenitor cells. J Immunol 2002;169(12):7000–8.
113. Christopherson KW 2nd, Hangoc G, Mantel CR, et al. Modulation of hematopoietic stem cell homing and engraftment by CD26. Science 2004;305(5686): 1000–3.

Index

Note: Page numbers of article titles are in **boldface** type.

A

AC220, investigational therapy for AML with, 1202
Acute lymphoblastic leukemia (ALL), 1119–1339
  cellular therapies in, **1281–1301**
    hematopoietic stem cell transplantation, 1281–1287
      allogeneic for relapsed and refractory, 1287
      alternative-donor allogeneic, 1284–1286
      HLA-matched donor allogeneic as first remission therapy, 1282–1284
      reduced-intensity conditioning allogeneic, 1286
      T-cell depletion to lower risk of GvHD, 1286–1287
      unrelated allogeneic, 1284
    novel adoptive, 1287–1293
      clinical trials, 1289–1293
      donor lymphocyte infusion, 1287–1288
      genetically modified T cells, 1289
      genetically modified tumor-targeted T cells, 1288–1289
  current therapeutic strategies in, **1255–1279**
  current therapeutic strategies in adults, **1255–1279**
    diagnosis, 1256–1257
    induction treatment, 1258–1260
      L-asparaginase and coagulation problems during, 1259–1260
      steroid prephase, 1258–1259
      supportive care, 1258
    long-term consequences of, 1269
    overview, 1255
    postremission treatment, 1260–1264
      allogeneic hematopoietic stem cell transplant, 1262–1263
      choice of myeloablative conditioning regimen, 1263
      CNS-directed prophylaxis, 1260–1261
      consolidation and maintenance, 1261
      nonmyeloablative reduced-intensity conditioning, 1264
    prognostic factors, 1257–1258
      minimal residual disease, 1257–1258
    relapsed disease, 1268–1269
    specific scenarios in, 1264–1268
      CNS involvement, 1264–1265
      in older adults, 1266–1267
      in younger adults, 1265–1266
      Philadelphia-positive, 1267–1268
  novel therapeutic approaches, **1303–1317**
    emerging therapies, 1304–1309
    monoclonal antibody therapy, 1304–1309

Hematol Oncol Clin N Am 25 (2011) 1341–1350
doi:10.1016/S0889-8588(11)00150-X
0889-8588/11/$ – see front matter © 2011 Elsevier Inc. All rights reserved.

hemonc.theclinics.com

Acute (*continued*)
    prognostic factors in, 1174–1177
        at presentation, 1174–1176
        pharmacogenetics, 1176–1177
        response-based, 1176–1177
Acute myeloid leukemia (AML), 1119–1161, 1189–1213
    cytogenetics in, **1135–1161**
        as a prognostic factor, 1140–1145
            in children, 1144–1145
            in older adults, 1145
            in younger adults, 1142–1144
        entities recognized in WHO classification, 1136–1139
        future perspective, 1147–1150
        influence of patient age on, 1139–1140
        limitations for risk stratification, 1145–1147
    induction and postremission strategies in, **1189–1213**
        in older adults, 1196–1201
            intensive chemotherapy, 1198–1199
            reduced-intensity therapies, 1199–1201
        in younger adults, 1190–1196
            allogeneic hematopoietic stem cell transplantation, 1193–1195
            autologous hematopoietic stem cell transplantation, 1195–1196
            induction, 1190–1192
            intensive chemotherapy, 1193
            maintenance, 1196
        investigational agents, 1201–1204
            chemosensitization strategies, 1203
            FLT3 and other molecular targets, 1201–1203
            novel chemotherapeutic agents, 1203–1204
    novel mutations in epigenetic modifiers in, *DNMT3$_A$*, 1126–1128
        IDH1 and *IDH2,* 1123–1126
        in pediatric AML, 1128
        potential use for minimal residual disease detection, 1128–1129
        TET2, 1120–1123
    prognostic factors in, 1163–1174
        disease-related, 1164–1169
        molecular markers, 1169–1172
        patient-related, 1163–1164
        response-related, 1172–1173
        scores, 1173–1174
        secondary AML, 1172
Acute promyelocytic leukemia (APL), curing all patients with, **1215–1233**
    consolidation therapy, 1219–1220
    in search of chemotherapy-free cure for, 1224–1225
    increasing cure rates with early death reduction, 1223–1224
    induction therapy, 1216–1219
    maintenance (postconsolidation) therapy, 1220–1221
    minimal residual disease monitoring, 1221–1223
    role of arsenic trioxide, 1225–1227
Age, patient, influence on cytogenetic profile in AML, 1139–1140
    prognostic factor in AML, 1163

Alemtuzumab, for ALL therapy, 1308
All-trans retinoic acid, in therapy of APL, **1215–1233**
ALL. *See* Acute lymphoblastic leukemia.
Allogeneic hematopoietic cell transplant, for adults with acute leukemia, 1320–1324
     bone marrow, 1320–1321
     haploidentical bone marrow, 1323–1324
     in ALL, 1262–1263
     in older adults, 1199
     peripheral blood, 1321
     postremission in younger adults, 1193–1195
     umbilical cord blood, 1322–1323
Ambiguous lineage, acute leukemias of mixed phenotype and, **1235–1253**
AML. *See* Acute myeloid leukemia.
Anthracyclines, in therapy of APL, 1217–1219
APL. *See* Acute promyelocytic leukemia.
Arsenic trioxide, role of, in therapy of APL, 1225–1227
Asparaginase, L-, and coagulation problems during induction therapy for ALL, 1259–1260
Autologous hematopoietic cell transplant, for adults with acute leukemia, 1320
     postremission AML in younger adults, 1195–1196

B

Biphenotypic leukemias, **1235–1253**
Blinatumomab, for ALL therapy, 1308–1309
Bone marrow, for allogeneic hematopoietic cell transplant in adults with acute leukemia, 1320–1321
     haploidentical, 1323–1324
Bortezomin, for ALL therapy, 1312

C

CAT-3888, for ALL therapy, 1307–1308
CAT-8015, for ALL therapy, 1307–1308
Central nervous system (CNS), involvement of, in ALL, 1264–1265
Chemosensitization strategies, investigational therapy for AML with, 1203
Chemotherapeutic agents, conditioning for hematopoietic cell transplant in adults acute leukemia, 1324–1325
     clofarabine-based, 1324–1325
     plerixafor and G-CSF, 1325
     treosulfan-based, 1325
Chemotherapy, for ALL, novel approaches to, 1309–1311
     decitabine, 1310–1311
     forodesine, 1310
     NOTCH-1, 1309–1310
    for AML induction therapy, in older adults, 1196–1201
     in younger adults, 1190–1192
    for APL, anthracyclines in, 1217–1219
    intensive, for AML in older adults, 1198–1199
    intensive, for postremission AML in younger adults, 1193
    novel investigational agents for AML, 1203
    reduced-intensity, for AML in older adults, 1199–1201
Children. *See* Pediatrics.

Chimeric antigen receptors, post-transplant, in adult acute leukemia, 1329–1330
Classification, of acute leukemias of mixed phenotype and ambiguous origin, **1235–1253**
    historical development and diagnostic criteria, 1239–1244
        before 1991, 1239–1240
        European Group for Immunologic Characterization of Leukemias Criteria,
            1240–1242
        limitations of current criteria, 1244
        WHO criteria, 1242–1244
    of AML, cytogenetic entities recognized by WHO, 1136–1139
Clofarabine, conditioning for hematopoietic cell transplant with, 1324–1325
Coagulation problems, L-asparaginase and, during induction therapy for ALL, 1259–1260
Comorbidities, prognostic factor in AML, 1164
Conditioning, for hematopoietic cell transplant in adults acute leukemia, 1324–1327
Consolidation therapy, for ALL, 1261
    for APL, 1219–1220
Cord blood cells, intra-bone marrow injection of, in adult acute leukemia treatment, 1331
Core binding factor, prognostic factor in AML, 1169
CPX-351, investigational therapy for AML with, 1202
Cyogenetics, in acute leukemias of mixed phenotype and ambiguous origin, 1245–1247
Cytarabine (Ara-C), in therapy of APL, 1216–1219
Cytogenetics, in AML, **1135–1161**
      as a prognostic factor, 1140–1145, 1165–1169
        in children, 1144–1145
        in older adults, 1145
        in younger adults, 1142–1144
      entities recognized in WHO classification, 1136–1139
      future perspective, 1147–1150
      influence of patient age on, 1139–1140
      limitations for risk stratification, 1145–1147
    prognostic factor in AML, 1165–1169
Cytokines, post-transplant immune reconstitution with exogenous in adult acute
    leukemia, 1329

D

Decitabine, for ALL chemotherapy, 1310–1311
DNMT3A, novel mutations in AML, 1126–1128
    potential use for minimal residual disease detection, 1128–1129
Donor lymphocyte infusion, in ALL, 1287–1288
    post-transplant in acute leukemias, 1329
DT22199ARL, for ALL therapy, 1308

E

Elacytarabine, investigational therapy for AML with, 1202
Engraftment, enhancing capabilities of, in adult acute leukemia treatment, 1331–1332
Epigenetic modifiers, novel mutations in AML, **1119–1133**
      $DNMT3_A$, 1126–1128
      IDH1 and *IDH2,* 1123–1126
      in pediatric AML, 1128
      potential use for minimal residual disease detection, 1128–1129
      TET2, 1120–1123

Epratuzumab, for ALL therapy, 1307
European Group for Immunologic Characterization of Leukemias Criteria, 1240–1242
Everolimus, for ALL therapy, 1312
Extracellular signal-regulated kinase (ERK), in ALL therapy, 1314

F

Flavopiridol, for ALL therapy, 1311–1312
Forodesine, for ALL chemotherapy, 1310
FTL3-selective tyrosine kinase inhibitors, investigational therapy for AML with, 1201–1203

G

Gender, patient, prognostic factor in AML, 1164
Graft sources, for hematopoietic cell transplantation for acute leukemia in adults,
    1319–1320
Graft-*versus*-host disease (GvHD), prevention strategies, for hematopoietic cell transplant,
    1327–1329
        T regulation therapy, 1328–1329
        T-cell depletion of graft, 1327–1328

H

Hematopoietic stem cell transplantation. *See* Transplant strategies.

I

IDH1 and *IDH2,* novel mutations in AML, 1123–1126
        potential use for minimal residual disease detection, 1123–1126
Immune reconstitution, post-transplant, in adult acute leukemia, 1329
Immunophenotype, leukemias of mixed phenotype and lineage, **1235–1253**
    prognostic factor in AML, 1165
Induction therapy, for ALL, 1258–1260
        dealing with problems and delays during, 1259–1260
        steroid prephase, 1258–1259
        supportive care, 1258
    for AML, in older adults, 1196–1201
        in younger adults, 1190–1192
    for APL, 1216–1219
Inotuzumab, for ALL therapy, 1307–1308

L

L-Asparaginase, and coagulation problems during induction therapy for ALL, 1259–1260
Leukemia, 1119–1339
    acute lymphoblastic (ALL), adult, 1255–1317
        cellular therapies in, **1281–1301**
            hematopoietic stem cell transplantation, 1281–1287
            novel adoptive cellular therapies, 1287–1293
        current therapeutic strategies in, **1255–1279**
            diagnosis, 1256–1257

Leukemia (*continued*)
        induction treatment, 1258–1260
        long-term consequences of, 1269
        overview, 1255
        postremission treatment, 1260–1264
        prognostic factors, 1257–1258
        relapsed disease, 1268–1269
        specific scenarios in, 1264–1268
     novel therapeutic approaches, **1303–1317**
        emerging therapies, 1304–1309
        monoclonal antibody therapy, 1304–1309
  acute myeloid (AML), 1119–1161, 1189–1213
     cytogenetics in, **1135–1161**
        as a prognostic factor, 1140–1145
        entities recognized in WHO classification, 1136–1139
        future perspective, 1147–1150
        influence of patient age on, 1139–1140
        limitations for risk stratification, 1145–1147
     induction and postremission strategies in, **1189–1213**
        for older adults, 1196–1201
        for younger adults, 1190–1196
        investigational agents, 1201–1204
     novel mutations in epigenetic modifiers in, *DNMT3$_A$*, 1126–1128
        IDH1 and *IDH2,* 1123–1126
        in pediatric AML, 1128
        potential use for minimal residual disease detection, 1128–1129
        TET2, 1120–1123
  acute promyelocytic (APL), curing all patients with, **1215–1233**
     consolidation therapy, 1219–1220
     in search of chemotherapy-free cure for, 1224–1225
     increasing cure rates with early death reduction, 1223–1224
     induction therapy, 1216–1219
     maintenance (postconsolidation) therapy, 1220–1221
     minimal residual disease monitoring, 1221–1223
     role of arsenic trioxide, 1225–1227
  novel transplant strategies in adult acute, **1319–1339**
     allogeneic hematopoietic cell transplant, 1320–1324
        bone marrow, 1320–1321
        haploidentical bone marrow, 1323–1324
        peripheral blood, 1321
        umbilical cord blood, 1322–1323
     ancillary approaches, 1330–1332
        enhancing homing and engraftment capabilities of hematopoietic cells,
          1331–1332
        intra-bone marrow injection of cord blood cells, 1331
        multipotent mesenchymal stem cells, 1330–1331
     autologous hematopoietic cell transplant, 1320
     expert opinion, 1332
     graft sources, 1319–1320
     GvHD prevention strategies, 1327–1329
        T-cell depletion of graft, 1327–1328

T-regulation therapy, 1328–1329
    paradigms in conditioning, 1324–1327
        chemotherapeutic agents, 1324–1325
        radiation, 1325–1327
    post-transplant maneuvers, 1329–1330
        chimeric antigen receptor-redirected T lymphocytes, 1329–1330
        donor lymphocyte infusion, 1329
        immune reconstitution with exogenous cytokines, 1329
of mixed phenotype and ambiguous origin, **1235–1253**
    historical development and diagnostic criteria, 1239–1244
        before 1991, 1239–1240
        European Group for Immunologic Characterization of Leukemias Criteria,
            1240–1242
        limitations of current criteria, 1244
        WHO criteria, 1242–1244
    molecular and cytogenetic findings, 1245–1247
    prevalence and prognosis, 1244–1245
    treatment, 1247–1248
prognostic factors in adult acute, ALL, 1174–1177
    AML, 1163–1174
Liver function abnormalities, L-asparaginase and, during induction therapy for ALL, 1260
Lymphoblastic leukemia. See Acute lymphoblastic leukemia (ALL).

M

Maintenance therapy, for ALL, 1261
    for APL, 1220–1221
    postremission, for AML in younger adults, 1196
Mammalian target of rapamycin (mTOR) inhibitors, for ALL therapy, 1312
Mesenchymal stem cells, multipotent, in adult acute leukemia treatment, 1330–1331
Methotrexate analogues, for ALL therapy, 1311
Midostaurin, investigational therapy for AML with, 1202
Minimal residual disease, and prognosis in ALL, 1257–1258
    detection of, with epigenetic gene mutations, 1128–1129
    monitoring for, for APL, 1221–1223
Mitogen-activated protein kinase, in ALL therapy, 1314
Mixed-phenotype acute leukemias, **1235–1253**
Molecular markers, prognostic factor in AML, 1169–1172
Molecular studies, in acute leukemias of mixed phenotype and ambiguous origin,
    1245–1247
Monoclonal antibody therapy, for acute lymphoblastic leukemia, 1304–1309
        alemtuzumab, 1308
        blinatumomab, 1308–1309
        CAT-8015, 1307–1308
        CAT3888, 1307–1308
        DT2219ARL, 1308
        epratuzumab, 1307
        inotuzumab, 1307–1308
        rituximab, 1306–1307
Murine double minute (MDM2) protein, for ALL therapy, 1312–1313
Mutations, in epigenetic modifiers mutations in AML, **1119–1133**
        $DNMT3_A$, 1126–1128

Mutations (*continued*)
    IDH1 and *IDH2,* 1123–1126
    in pediatric AML, 1128
    potential use for minimal residual disease detection, 1128–1129
    TET2, 1120–1123
Myeloid leukemia. *See* Acute myeloid leukemia (AML).

N

Natural killer (NK) cells, genetically modified CD-19 targeted, clinical trials in ALL,
    1293–1294
NOTCH-1, for ALL chemotherapy, 1309–1310

P

Pancreatitis, L-asparaginase and, during induction therapy for ALL, 1260
Pediatrics., prognostic significance of cytogenetics in AML, 1144–1145
Pemetrexed, for ALL therapy, 1311
Peripheral blood, for allogeneic hematopoietic cell transplant in adults with acute leukemia,
    1321
Pharmacogenetics, prognosis in ALL, 1177
Philadelphia chromosome, positive for, in ALL 1267–1268
Plerixafor, conditioning for hematopoietic cell transplant with, 1325
Postremission strategies, for AML in younger adults, 1190–1196
        allogeneic hematopoietic stem cell transplantation, 1193–1195
        autologous hematopoietic stem cell transplantation, 1195–1196
        intensive chemotherapy, 1193
        maintenance, 1196
Prognostic factors, in acute leukemias of mixed phenotype and ambiguous origin,
    1244–1245
    in ALL, 1174–1177, 1257–1258
        at presentation, 1174–1176
        pharmacogenetics, 1176–1177
        response-based, 1176–1177
    in AML, 1163–1174
        cytogenetics, 1140–1145
          in children, 1144–1145
          in older adults, 1145
          in younger adults, 1142–1144
        disease-related, 1164–1169
        molecular markers, 1169–1172
        patient-related, 1163–1164
        response-related, 1172–1173
        scores, 1173–1174
        secondary AML, 1172
Promyelocytic leukemia. *See* Acute promyelocytic leukemia (APL).

R

Race, patient, prognostic factor in AML, 1164
Radiation, conditioning for hematopoietic cell transplant in adults acute leukemia,
    1325–1327

    selective approaches, 1326
    targeted myeloablative radioimmunotherapy, 1326–1327
Radioimmunotherapy, targeted myeloablative, conditioning for hematopoietic cell
    transplant with, 1326–1327
Rapamycin, for ALL therapy, 1312
Reduced-intensity therapies, for AML in older adults, 1199–1201
Relapse, of ALL, treatment for, 1268–1269
Response, to therapy, as prognostic factor in ALL, 1176–1177
    as prognostic factor in AML, 1172–1173
Retinoic acid, all-trans, in therapy of APL, **1215–1233**
Risk stratification, of AML, limits of cytogenetics for, 1145–1147
Rituximab, for ALL therapy, 1306

S

Sapacitabine, investigational therapy for AML with, 1202
Secondary AML, prognostic factors in, 1172
Socioeconomic status, prognostic factor in AML, 1164

T

T cells, genetically modified, in novel therapies for ALL, 1288–1292
        clinical trials with CD19-targeted, 1289–1292
        tumor-targeted, 1288–1289
Talotrexin, for ALL therapy, 1311
Temsirolimus, for ALL therapy, 1312
TET2, novel mutations in AML, 1120–1123
        potential use for minimal residual disease detection, 1128–1129
Tipifarnib, investigational therapy for AML with, 1202
Transplant strategies, for ALL, 1262–1263, 1281–1287
        hematopoietic stem cell transplantation in, 1281–1287
            allogeneic for relapsed and refractory, 1287
            alternative-donor allogeneic, 1284–1286
            HLA-matched donor allogeneic as first remission therapy, 1282–1284
            reduced-intensity conditioning allogeneic, 1286
            T-cell depletion to lower risk of GvHD, 1286–1287
            unrelated allogeneic, 1284
        myeloablative conditioning regimens, 1263
        nonmyeloablative reduced-intensity conditioning, 1263
    for older adults with AML, 1199
        allogeneic hematopoietic stem cell, 1193–1195
        autologous hematopoietic stem cell, 1195–1196
    novel, for adults with acute leukemia, **1319–1339**
        allogeneic hematopoietic cell transplant, 1320–1324
            bone marrow, 1320–1321
            haploidentical bone marrow, 1323–1324
            peripheral blood, 1321
            umbilical cord blood, 1322–1323
        ancillary approaches, 1330–1332
            enhancing homing and engraftment capabilities of hematopoietic cells,
                1331–1332
            intra-bone marrow injection of cord blood cells, 1331

Transplant (*continued*)
>   multipotent mesenchymal stem cells, 1330–1331
>   autologous hematopoietic cell transplant, 1320
>   expert opinion, 1332
>   graft sources, 1319–1320
>   GvHD prevention strategies, 1327–1329
>   T-cell depletion of graft, 1327–1328
>   T-regulation therapy, 1328–1329
>   paradigms in conditioning, 1324–1327
>   chemotherapeutic agents, 1324–1325
>   radiation, 1325–1327
>   post-transplant maneuvers, 1329–1330
>   chimeric antigen receptor-redirected T lymphocytes, 1329–1330
>   donor lymphocyte infusion, 1329
>   immune reconstitution with exogenous cytokines, 1329

Treosulfan, conditioning for hematopoietic cell transplant with, 1325

U

Umbilical cord blood, for allogeneic hematopoietic cell transplant in adults with acute
>   leukemia, 1322–1323

Undifferentiated acute leukemias, **1235–1253**

V

Vosaroxin, investigational therapy for AML with, 1202

W

White blood cell count, prognostic factor in AML, 1164–1165

World Health Organization (WHO) classification, of acute leukemias of ambiguous lineage,
>   1235–1239
>   criteria, third and fourth editions, 1242–1244
>   limitations of, 1244
>   of AML, cytogenetic entities recognized in, 1136–1139

Moving?

Make sure your subscription moves with you!

To notify us of your new address, find your **Clinics Account Number** (located on your mailing label above your name), and contact customer service at:

Email: journalscustomerservice-usa@elsevier.com

800-654-2452 (subscribers in the U.S. & Canada)
314-447-8871 (subscribers outside of the U.S. & Canada)

Fax number: 314-447-8029

Elsevier Health Sciences Division
Subscription Customer Service
3251 Riverport Lane
Maryland Heights, MO 63043

*To ensure uninterrupted delivery of your subscription, please notify us at least 4 weeks in advance of move.